PANCE®:
POWER PRACTICE

PANCE®:
POWER PRACTICE

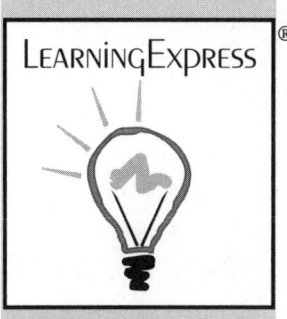

LEARNINGEXPRESS®

NEW YORK

Library of Congress Cataloging-in-Publication Data:
PANCE : power practice.—1st ed.

     p.   cm.

  Physician Assistant National Certifying Examination

  ISBN-13: 978-1-57685-897-4

  ISBN-10: 1-57685-897-9

  I. LearningExpress (Organization)   II. Title: Physician Assistant National Certifying Examination.

  [DNLM: 1. Physician Assistants—United States—Examination Questions.   2. Certification—United States—Examination Questions.   3. Test Taking Skills—United States. W 18.2]

  610.7372069076—dc23

2011040877

Printed in the United States of America

9 8 7 6 5 4 3 2 1

First Edition

ISBN: 978-1-57685-897-4

For more information or to place an order, contact LearningExpress at:

  2 Rector Street

  26th Floor

  New York, NY 10006

Or visit us at:

  www.learningexpressllc.com

CONTENTS

CONTRIBUTORS ▶

Mehdi Amri is currently a medical student at University of Sydney in Australia. He earned his undergraduate degree from the University of Toronto with a specialization in biochemistry. He has experience as a tutor for various standardized medical and dental exams.

Ann Cohen is a freelance writer/editor based in New York City. A graduate of the University of Pennsylvania, she has spent 20 years in the nonprofit sector, 10 of them as director of development and communications for a medical research institute. Ms. Cohen is a co-author of *The Complete Idiot's Guide to Dangerous Diseases and Epidemics* and served as editorial consultant on *Timebomb*, a book about multi-drug-resistant tuberculosis in Russia. She has also contributed to a number of test preparation books, including those for PCAT, NCLEX-RN, Advanced Placement Study in English Language, English Composition, U.S. Government and Politics, U.S. History and World History, and the MAT.

Diana Dou is a certified Physician Assistant, with an emphasis on gastroenterology and hepatalogy. She is a graduate of the Surgical Physician Assistant program at Weill Cornell Medical College, and has a B.S. in Nutritional Sciences from Cornell University.

Kate Lieberman is a certified Physician Assistant, with clinical experience in a pediatric emergency department, internal medicine, women's health, and travel medicine. She is a graduate of the Touro College School of Health Sciences and the University of Massachusetts–Amherst.

Joe Knight has over 20 years' experience as a family practice Physician Assistant. He has been a peer reviewer for the *Journal of the American Academy of Physician Assistants* (*JAAPA*), reviewing and critiquing manuscripts submitted to JAAPA for publication. He is currently a medical, science, and history writer for various professional journals and consumer magazines. Joe is also a retired Air Force Captain, and presently lives in California.

Robert Shifko received his Bachelor of Science degree in Nuclear Medicine from Edinboro University of Pennsylvania. He continued his education receiving graduate level certification in Epidemiology and Biostatistics from Drexel University Graduate School of Public Health. With 18 years' experience in a healthcare setting he has certifications in Nuclear Medicine, Epidemiology, Biostatistics, and Radiation Health Physics. He currently performs research for the University of Pittsburgh's Department of Pharmacology and assists in the creation of standardized tests for medical professionals, including PANCE.

Shan Siddiqi is a freelance writer and current medical student at the University of Sydney in Australia. He earned his undergraduate degree from the University of Missouri with a major in chemistry (medicinal) and minors in medical physics, radio environmental sciences, and biology. His research background centers around projects in medicinal chemistry and clinical pharmacology, often in combination with molecular biology and microbiology. Combined with his background in writing preparation materials for a variety of medical examinations, his background in clinical research and his graduate medical training help to create a solid foundation for producing PANCE preparation materials.

1 ▶ INTRODUCTION TO THE PANCE

Congratulations! If you are reading this book, it means that you have graduated or are about to graduate from an accredited physician assistant program and are interested in preparing for the Physician Assistant National Certifying Examination (PANCE), which will enable you to designate yourself as a certified physician assistant (PA-C).

One of the most important ways to begin preparing for the PANCE is to become familiar with the format of the exam, the process of registering for the exam, the subjects the exam covers, what to expect on test day, and so on. This chapter will help you get started. Note: The information in this chapter is current as of the date of publication. For the most recent information, refer to the official National Commission on Certification of Physician Assistants (NCCPA) PANCE website, www.nccpa.net/Pance.aspx.

Overview of the PANCE

The PANCE is a computer-based 300-question multiple-choice exam that tests your basic medical and surgical knowledge. The questions are written as clinical vignettes; each question has five answer choices. Some questions may contain graphics, such as EKGs, rhythm strips, dermatological photos, and radiographs. Other questions contain lab data; if you are given lab data in a question, you can click on the data and a screen with normal values will pop up for reference. Generic names of drugs are always provided, and trade names are provided in parentheses after the generic name only if deemed necessary by the NCCPA.

On the PANCE, the questions are separated into five sections of 60 questions each; you will have 60 minutes to complete each section. You can answer questions within a section in any order, mark questions for review, and change answers within the section during the time allotted for that section. However, once you have exited a section, or time has expired, you cannot go back to it.

You will have a total of 45 minutes of scheduled break time between sections. You are responsible for managing this time. If you take an unscheduled break while you are working on a section, the time will be deducted from the 60 minutes that you have to complete that section.

Your computer screen will show the amount of break time you have left.

Registering for the Exam

To be eligible to take the PANCE, you must graduate from a physician assistant program accredited by the Accreditation Review Commission on Education for the Physician Assistant (ARC-PA). You can register for the exam on the NCCPA website up to 90 days before your expected graduation date.

The cost to take the exam is $475, which must be paid in advance. Once you have paid, an online personal record will be created for you, and you will be emailed instructions for scheduling your exam. The earliest date you'll be able to take the exam is seven days after you graduate, and the latest is 180 days (six months) from the beginning of your exam time frame.

If you don't pass the exam on your first try, you must wait 90 days before taking it again. You can only take the PANCE once in any 90-day period, and a maximum of three times in any one calendar year. You have up to six attempts within a six-year period to pass the PANCE. If you don't pass within that time frame, you lose your eligibility to take the PANCE and must complete another ARC-PA accredited physician assistant program before attempting the exam again. If you need any special testing accommodations, you must so indicate when you apply for the exam, and submit appropriate documentation for approval by the NCCPA.

What to Expect at the Test Center

The PANCE is administered by Pearson Vue at a secure testing center. Plan to arrive at least 30 minutes before your test is scheduled to begin. Make sure to bring two forms of valid and current (i.e., not expired) identification: a primary ID and a secondary ID, or two primary IDs. Your primary ID must contain your preprinted name, a photograph of you, and your signature. Acceptable primary IDs typically include your driver's license, passport, or other government-issued identification card. Your second form of identification must contain your printed name and signature, but does not have to have a photograph. Acceptable secondary IDs typically include credit cards, social security cards, student IDs, and employee IDs. The first and last name on the ID must match the name on your records in the NCCPA's and

Pearson Vue's databases. Check the NCCPA website for further guidance on what name difference will and will not be accepted. A digital fingerprint or palm scan and photograph of you will be taken at the test center. You will not be allowed to bring any personal belongings into the testing room, but you can store them in a locker that will be assigned to you. Make sure to bring a drink and healthy snacks to store in your locker. You can access these belongings during a scheduled break, but not during an unscheduled break.

During the Test

As noted previously, the PANCE is a computer-based exam. You will be instructed on the use of the computer equipment, and have the opportunity to complete a short tutorial before your test begins. You won't have access to paper or pen/pencils, but if you want, you will be given a whiteboard and erasable marker to use during the exam. As noted previously, you will have a total of 45 minutes for scheduled breaks between sections of the test, and any unscheduled breaks taken during a section are deducted from the time allowed for that section. A digital fingerprint or palm scan is required each time you re-enter the test room. The test room is also audio- and video-monitored by test center staff, and you may be audio- or videotaped while you are taking the exam.

What Skills Are Tested?

On the PANCE, you will be tested on various organ systems and the diseases, disorders, and medical assessments you will encounter with respect to those systems. You will also be tested on the various skills and knowledge (practice task areas) needed to deal with those diseases, disorders, and assessments. Each question will address both a task area *and* an organ system.

The various organ systems and topics covered, and the percentage of questions you can expect with respect to each system, are as follows (listed from highest percentage to lowest):

- **Cardiovascular: 16%**
  Topics covered include cardiomyopathy, conduction disorders, congenital heart disease, hypertension, hypotension, coronary heart disease, vascular disease, valvular disease, and other forms of heart disease.
- **Pulmonary: 12%**
  Topics covered include infectious disorders, neoplastic disease, obstructive pulmonary disease, pleural diseases, pulmonary circulation, restrictive pulmonary disease, and other pulmonary diseases.
- **Gastrointestinal/Nutritional: 10%**
  Topics covered include the esophagus, stomach, gallbladder, liver, pancreas, small intestine/colon and rectum, hernia, infectious and noninfectious diarrhea, vitamin and nutritional deficiencies, and metabolic disorders.
- **Musculoskeletal: 10%**
  Topics covered include disorders of the shoulder, forearm/wrist/hand, back/spine, hip, knee, and ankle/foot, infectious and neoplastic diseases, osteoarthritis, osteoporosis, compartment syndrome, and rheumatologic conditions.
- **EENT (Eyes, Ear, Nose, and Throat): 9%**
  Topics covered include eye, ear, nose/sinus, and mouth/throat disorders, and benign and malignant neoplasms.
- **Reproductive: 8%**
  Topics covered include the breast, uterus, ovary, cervix, and vagina/vulva, menstrual disorders, menopause, pelvic inflammatory disease, contraceptive methods, infertility, uncomplicated pregnancy, and complicated pregnancy.
- **Endocrine: 6%**
  Topics covered include diseases of the thyroid, adrenal, and pituitary glands, diabetes mellitus, and lipid disorders.

- **Genitourinary: 6%**
  Topics covered include GU tract conditions, infectious/inflammatory conditions, neoplastic disorders, renal diseases, fluid and electrolyte disorders, and acid/base disorders.

- **Dermatologic: 5%**
  Topics covered include eczematous eruptions, papulosquamous diseases, desquamation, vesicular bullae, acneiform lesions, verrucous lesions, insects/parasites, neoplasms, hair and nails, viral diseases, bacterial infections, fungal infections, and other issues such as burns, vitiligo, melasma, and so forth.

- **Neurologic: 6%**
  Topics covered include diseases of the peripheral nerve, headaches, and infectious, movement, vascular, and other neurologic disorders.

- **Psychiatry/Behavioral Science: 6%**
  Topics covered include psychoses, and anxiety, attention-deficit/hyperactivity, autistic, eating, mood, personality, somatoform, substance use, and other behavioral/emotional disorders.

- **Hematologic: 3%**
  Topics covered include anemias, coagulation disorders, and malignancies.

- **Infectious Diseases: 3%**
  Topics covered include fungal, bacterial, mycobacterial, parasitic, spirochetal, and viral diseases.

There are seven basic task areas. The percentage of questions on each task area is as follows, again listed from highest percentage to lowest:

- **Formulating Most Likely Diagnosis: 18%**
  Questions in this category assess your ability to correlate normal and abnormal diagnostic data, formulate differential diagnoses, and select the most likely diagnosis in light of the data provided in the question, and your understanding of the significance of history, physical findings, and diagnostic and laboratory studies as they relate to diagnosis.

- **Pharmaceutical Therapeutics: 18%**
  Questions in this category assess your ability to select appropriate pharmacologic therapy for various medical conditions, monitor and adjust pharmacologic regimens, and evaluate and report adverse drug reactions, and your understanding of mechanism of action, indications for use, contraindications, side effects, adverse reactions, followup and monitoring of pharmacologic regimens, risks for drug interactions, clinical presentation of drug interactions, treatment of drug interactions, drug toxicity, methods to reduce medication errors, cross-reactivity of similar medications, and recognition and treatment of allergic reactions.

- **History Taking and Performing Physical Examinations: 16%**
  Questions in this category assess your ability to conduct interviews, identify pertinent historical information, perform physical exams, associate current complaint with presented history and identify pertinent physical examination information, and your understanding of pertinent historical information associated with selected medical conditions, risk factors for development of selected medical conditions, signs and symptoms of selected medical conditions, physical examination techniques, physical examination findings associated with selected medical conditions, appropriate physical examination directed to selected medical conditions, and differential diagnosis associated with presenting symptoms or physical findings.

- **Using Laboratory and Diagnostic Studies: 14%**
  Questions in this category assess your ability to use diagnostic equipment safely and appropriately, select appropriate diagnostic or laboratory studies, collect diagnostic or laboratory specimens, and interpret diagnostic or laboratory studies results, and your understanding of the indications for initial or subsequent diagnostic or laboratory studies, cost-effectiveness of

diagnostic studies or procedures, relevance of common screening tests for selected medical conditions, normal and abnormal diagnostic ranges, risks associated with diagnostic studies or procedures, and appropriate patient education related to laboratory or diagnostic studies.

- **Clinical Intervention: 14%**
  Questions in this category assess your ability to formulate and implement treatment plans, recognize and initiate treatment for life-threatening emergencies, demonstrate technical expertise related to performing specific procedures, communicate effectively, use counseling techniques, facilitate patient adherence and active participation in treatment, and interact effectively in multidisciplinary teams, and your understanding of the management and treatment of selected medical conditions, indications, contraindications, complications, risks, benefits and techniques of selected procedures, standard precautions and special isolation conditions, sterile technique, follow-up and monitoring of therapeutic regimens, conditions that constitute medical emergencies, indications for admission or discharge from hospitals or other facilities, discharge planning, available and appropriate community resources, appropriate patient education, roles of other health professionals, end-of-life issues, and risks and benefits of alternative medicine.

- **Health Maintenance: 10%**
  Questions in this category assess your ability to use counseling and patient education techniques, communicate effectively with patients to enhance health maintenance, adapt health maintenance to the patient's context, and use information databases, and your understanding of epidemiology of selected medical conditions, early detection and prevention of selected medical conditions, relative value of common screening tests, appropriate patient education regarding preventable conditions or lifestyle modifications, healthy lifestyles, prevention of communicable diseases,

immunization schedules and recommendations for infants, children, adults, and foreign travelers, risks and benefits of immunization, human growth and development, human sexuality, occupational and environmental exposure, impact of stress on health, psychological manifestations of illness and injury, effects of aging and changing family roles on health maintenance and disease prevention, signs of abuse and neglect, and barriers to care.

- **Applying Basic Science Concepts: 10%**
  Questions in this category assess your ability to recognize normal and abnormal anatomy and physiology, relate pathophysiologic principles to specific disease processes, correlate abnormal physical examination findings to a given disease process, and correlate abnormal results of diagnostic tests to a given disease process, and your understanding of human anatomy and physiology, underlying pathophysiology, microbiology, and biochemistry.

Refer to the NCCPA content blueprint for further detail on the various topics and knowledge and cognitive skills included within the above. Again, each question will address both an organ system *and* a task area. In addition, up to 20% of the questions on the exam may be related to surgery and up to 2% may cover legal or ethical issues.

Scoring

You will receive one point for each correct answer on the PANCE. *There is no penalty for guessing or for wrong answers, so make sure you answer every question.* Your raw score will then be converted to a scaled score between 200 and 800 using an algorithm developed by the NCCPA. The NCCPA no longer publishes the percent of correct answers necessary to pass the PANCE, but the minimum passing score is 350. The NCCPA will notify you by e-mail as soon as your exam results have been posted to your personal record, which is typically about two weeks after your test date.

Once You Are Certified/PANRE

After you have passed the PANCE, there is a six-year certification maintenance cycle. During every two-year period, you must take a minimum of 100 hours of continuing medical education, and by the end of the sixth year, you must have passed the Physician Assistant National Recertifying Exam (PANRE). The PANRE is very similar to the PANCE, and utilizes the same content blueprint. It contains 240 multiple-choice questions administered in four sections of 60 question each, with 60 minutes to complete each section. Unlike the PANCE, the PANRE offers a practice-focused component. You can choose to have 40% of the questions focus on adult medicine, surgery, or primary care. The remaining 60% always covers generalist content. This option gives PAs who specialize in one of these areas the ability to focus their exam more closely on their areas of practice. In general, the questions on the PANRE tend to address broader clinical issues than the PANCE, which tends to have more specific questions. According to the NCCPA, this difference is most apparent in the questions related to applying basic science concepts. If you do not pass the PANRE on your first try, you can take it three more times for a total of four attempts—twice in the fifth year after your initial certification, and twice in the sixth year. As with the PANCE, there is a 90-day waiting period between exams.

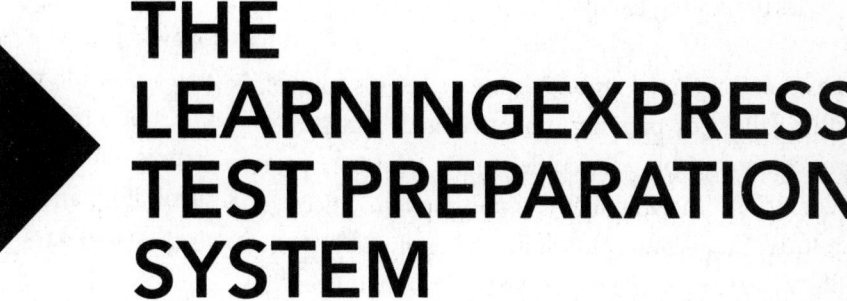

2 ▶ THE LEARNINGEXPRESS TEST PREPARATION SYSTEM

I t takes significant preparation to score well on any exam, and the PANCE is no exception. The LearningExpress Test Preparation System, developed by experts exclusively for LearningExpress, offers a number of strategies designed to facilitate the development of the skills, disciplines, and attitudes necessary for success.

Preparing for and attaining a passing score on the PANCE exam requires surmounting an assortment of obstacles. While some may prove more troublesome than others, all of them carry the potential to hinder your performance, and negatively affect your scores. Here are some examples:

- lack of familiarity with the exam format
- paralyzing test anxiety
- leaving preparation to the last minute
- not preparing
- failure to develop vital test-taking skills, such as
  - how to effectively pace through an exam
  - how to use the process of elimination to answer questions accurately
  - when and how to guess

- mental and/or physical fatigue
- test day blunders, such as
  - arriving late at the testing facility
  - taking the exam on an empty stomach
  - not accounting for fluctuations in temperature at the testing facility

The common thread among these obstacles is control. While a host of pressing, unanticipated, and sometimes unavoidable difficulties may frustrate your preparation, there remain some proven, effective strategies for placing yourself in the best possible position on exam day. These strategies can significantly improve your level of comfort with the exam, offering you not only the confidence you'll need, but also—and perhaps most importantly—a higher test score.

The LearningExpress Test Preparation System helps to put you in greater control. Here's how it works: Separated into nine steps, the system heightens your confidence level by helping you understand both the exam and your own particular set of test-taking strengths and weaknesses. It will help you structure a study plan, practice a number of effective test-taking skills, and avoid mental and physical fatigue on exam day. Each step is accompanied by an activity.

While the following list suggests an approximate time for the completion of each step, these are only guidelines for your initial introduction. The regular practice of a number of them may require a more substantial time commitment. It may also be necessary and helpful to return to one or more of them throughout the course of your preparation.

Step 1. Get Information	1 hour
Step 2. Conquer Test Anxiety	20 minutes
Step 3. Make a Plan	20 minutes
Step 4. Learn to Manage Your Time	10 minutes
Step 5. Learn to Use the Process of Elimination	20 minutes
Step 6. Guessing on the PANCE	20 minutes
Step 7. Reach Your Peak Performance Zone	10 minutes
Step 8. Make Final Preparations	10 minutes
Step 9. Make Your Preparations Count	10 minutes
Total	3 hours

We estimate that working through the entire system will take you approximately three hours. It's perfectly okay if you work at a faster or slower pace. It's up to you to decide whether you should set aside a whole afternoon or evening to work through the LearningExpress Test Preparation System in one sitting, or break it up and do just one or two steps a day for the next several days.

Step 1: Get Information

Time to complete: 1 hour
Activity: Read the Introduction to this book (Chapter 1)

Knowing more about an exam can often make it appear less daunting. The first step in the LearningExpress Test Preparation System is to determine everything you can about the type of information you will be expected to know on the PANCE, as well as how your knowledge will be assessed.

What You Should Find Out

Knowing the details will help you study efficiently and help you feel a sense of control. Here's a list of things you might want to find out:

- What skills are tested?
- How many sections are on the exam?
- How many questions are in each section?
- How much time is allotted for each section?
- How is the exam scored, and is there a penalty for guessing or for wrong answers?
- Is the test a computerized test or will you have an exam booklet?
- Will you be given scratch paper to write on?

You will find answers to these questions in Chapter 1 of this book and on the NCCPA PANCE website.

Step 2: Conquer Test Anxiety

Time to complete: 20 minutes
Activity: Take the Test Anxiety Quiz

Now that you know what's on the test, the next step is to address one of the biggest obstacles to success: *test anxiety*. Test anxiety may not only impair your performance on the exam itself, but it can also keep you from preparing properly. In Step 2, you will learn stress management techniques that will help you succeed on your exam. Practicing these techniques as you work through the activities in this book will help them become second nature to you by exam day.

Combating Test Anxiety

A little test anxiety is a good thing. Everyone gets nervous before a big exam—and if that nervousness motivates you to prepare thoroughly, so much the better. Many athletes report pre-game jitters, which they are able to harness to help them perform at their peak. Stop here and answer the questions on the Test Anxiety Quiz below to determine your level of test anxiety.

TEST ANXIETY QUIZ

You need to worry about test anxiety only if it is extreme enough to impair your performance. The following questionnaire will provide a diagnosis of your level of test anxiety. In the blank before each statement, write the number that most accurately describes your experience.

0 = Never   1 = Once or twice   2 = Sometimes   3 = Often

___I have gotten so nervous before an exam that I simply put down the books and didn't study for it.

___I have experienced disabling physical symptoms such as vomiting and severe headaches because I was nervous about an exam.

___I have simply not showed up for an exam because I was scared to take it.

___I have experienced dizziness and disorientation while taking an exam.

___I have had trouble filling in the little circles because my hands were shaking too hard.

___I have failed an exam because I was too nervous to complete it.

___**Total: Add up the numbers in the blanks above.**

Your Test Stress Score

Here are the steps you should take, depending on your score. If you scored:

- **Below 3,** your level of test anxiety is nothing to worry about; it's probably just enough to give you that little extra edge.

- **Between 3 and 6,** your test anxiety may be enough to impair your performance, and you should practice the stress management techniques in this section to try to bring your test anxiety down to manageable levels.

- **Above 6,** your level of test anxiety is a serious concern. In addition to practicing the stress management techniques listed in this section, you may want to seek additional, personal help. Call your local high school or community college and ask for the academic counselor. Tell the counselor that you have a level of test anxiety that sometimes keeps you from being able to take the exam. The counselor may be willing to help you or may suggest someone else you should talk to.

Stress Management before the Exam

If you feel your level of anxiety is getting the best of you in the weeks before the exam, here are things you can do to bring the level down:

- **Prepare.** There's nothing like knowing what to expect to put you in control of test anxiety. That's why you're reading this book. Use it faithfully, and you will be ready on test day.
- **Practice self-confidence.** A positive attitude is a great way to combat test anxiety. Stand in front of the mirror and say to your reflection, "I'm prepared. I'm confident. I'm going to ace this exam. I know I can do it." As soon as negative thoughts creep in, drown them out with these positive affirmations. If you hear them often enough, and you use the LearningExpress method to study for the PANCE, they will be true.
- **Fight negative messages.** Every time someone talks to you about how hard the exam is or how difficult it is to pass, think about your self-confidence messages. If the "someone" with the negative messages is you—telling yourself you don't do well on exams, that you just can't do this—don't listen. Turn on your recorder and listen to your self-confidence messages.
- **Visualize.** Visualizing success can help make it happen—and it reminds you of why you're doing all this work in preparing for the exam. Imagine yourself on your first day of classes or beginning the first day of your dream job.
- **Exercise.** Physical activity helps calm your body and focus your mind. Besides, being in good physical shape can actually help you do well on the exam. Go for a run, lift weights, go swimming—and exercise regularly.

Stress Management on Test Day

There are several ways you can bring down your level of test stress and anxiety on test day. They'll work best if you practice them in the weeks before the exam, so you know which ones work best for you.

- **Breathe deeply.** Take a deep breath in while you count to five. Hold it for a count of one, and then let it out on a count of five. Repeat several times.
- **Move your body.** Try rolling your head in a circle. Rotate your shoulders. Shake your hands from the wrist.
- **Visualize again.** Think of the place where you are most relaxed: lying on the beach in the sun, walking through the park, or wherever relaxes you. Now, close your eyes and imagine you're actually there. If you practice in advance, you will find that you need only a few seconds of this exercise to experience a significant increase in your sense of relaxation and well-being.

When anxiety threatens to overwhelm you *during* the test, there are still things you can do to manage your stress level:

- **Repeat your self-confidence messages.** You should have them memorized by now. Say them quietly to yourself, and believe them!
- **Visualize one more time.** This time, visualize yourself moving smoothly and quickly through the exam, answering every question correctly, and finishing just before time is up. Like most visualization techniques, this one works best if you've practiced it ahead of time.
- **Find an easy question.** Skim over the questions until you find an easy question, and then answer it. Getting even one question answered correctly gets you into the test-taking groove.

- **Take a mental break.** Everyone loses concentration once in a while during a long exam. It's normal, so you shouldn't worry about it. Instead, accept what has happened. Say to yourself, "Hey, I lost it there for a minute. My brain is taking a break." Close your eyes, and do some deep breathing for a few seconds. Then go back to work.

Try these techniques ahead of time and see if they work for you!

Step 3: Make a Plan

Time to complete: 20 minutes
Activity: Construct a study plan

There is no substitute for careful preparation and practice over time. So the most important thing you can do to better prepare yourself for your exam is to create a study plan or schedule and then follow it. This will help you avoid cramming at the last minute, which is an ineffective study technique that will only add to your anxiety.

Once you make your plan, make a commitment to follow it. Set aside at least 30 minutes every day for studying and practice. This will do more good than two hours crammed into a Saturday. If you have months before the test, you're lucky. Don't put off your studying until the week before. Start now. Even 10 minutes each weekday, with half an hour or more on weekends, can make a big difference in your score.

Step 4: Learn to Manage Your Time

Time to complete: 10 minutes to read; many hours of practice!
Activity: Practice these strategies as you take the sample exams

Steps 4, 5, and 6 of the LearningExpress Test Preparation System put you in charge of your PANCE experience by showing you test-taking strategies that work. Practice these strategies as you take the practice exams in this book and online. Then, you will be ready to use them on test day.

First, you will take control of your time on the PANCE. Start by understanding the format of the test. Each of the five blocks of 60 questions on the PANCE is timed separately. You will have 60 minutes for each and a total combined 45 minutes of break time, which you are responsible for managing on your own.

You will want to practice using your time wisely on the practice tests, while trying to avoid making mistakes at the same time as working quickly.

- **Listen carefully to directions.** By the time you get to the test, you should know how it works. But listen carefully in case something has changed.
- **Pace yourself.** Glance at your watch every few minutes and compare the time to how far you've gotten in the section. Leave some extra time for review, so that when one-quarter of the time has elapsed, you should be more than a quarter of the way through the section, and so on. If you're falling behind, pick up the pace.

- **Keep moving.** Don't spend too much time on one question. If you don't know the answer, skip the question and move on. Mark the question for review and come back to it later.
- **Don't rush.** You should keep moving; but rushing won't help. Try to keep calm and work methodically and quickly.

Step 5: Learn to Use the Process of Elimination

Time to complete: 20 minutes
Activity: Complete the worksheet on Using the Process of Elimination

After time management, the next most important tool for taking control of your test is using the process of elimination wisely. It's standard test-taking wisdom that you should always read all the answer choices before choosing your answer. This helps you find the right answer by eliminating wrong answer choices. Consider the following question. Although it is not the type of question you will see on the PANCE, the mental process that you use will be the same.

9. Sentence 6: I would like to be considered for the assistant manager position in your company my previous work experience is a good match for the job requirements posted. Which correction should be made to sentence 6?
 a. Insert *Although* before *I*.
 b. Insert a question mark after *company*.
 c. Insert a semicolon and *However* before *my*.
 d. Insert a period after *company* and capitalize *my*.
 e. No corrections are necessary.

If you happen to know that sentence 6 is a run-on sentence, and you know how to correct it, you don't need to use the process of elimination. But let's assume that, like some people, you don't. So, you look at the answer choices. *Although* sure doesn't sound like a good choice, because it would change the meaning of the sentence. So, you eliminate choice **a**; now you only have four answer choices to deal with. Write **a** on your whiteboard with an X through or beside it. Move on to the other answer choices.

If you know that the first part of the sentence does not ask a question, you can eliminate choice **b** as a possible answer. Write **b** on your whiteboard with an X through or beside it. Choice **c**, inserting a semicolon, could create a pause in an otherwise long sentence, but inserting the word *However* might not be correct. If you're not sure whether or not this answer is correct, write **c** on your whiteboard with a question mark beside it, meaning "well, maybe."

Answer choice **d** would separate a very long sentence into two shorter sentences, and it would not change the meaning. It could work, so write **d** on your whiteboard with a check mark beside it, meaning "good answer." Answer choice **e** means that the sentence is fine as it is and doesn't need any changes. The sentence could make sense as it is, but it is definitely long. Is this the best way to write the sentence? If you're not sure, write **e** on your whiteboard with a question mark beside it.

Now your whiteboard looks like this:
 a. X
 b. X
 c. ?
 d. ✔
 e. ?

You have just one check mark, for a good answer, **d**. If you're pressed for time, you should simply select choice **d**. If you have the time to be extra careful, you could compare your check mark answer to your question mark answers to make sure that it's better. (It is: Sentence 6 is a run-on, and should be separated into two shorter, complete sentences.)

It's good to have a system for marking good, bad, and maybe answers. We recommend using this one:

X = bad
✔ = good
? = maybe

If you don't like these marks, devise your own system. Just make sure you do it long before exam day—while you're working through the practice tests in this book and online—so you won't have to worry about it during the exam.

Even when you think you're absolutely clueless about a question, you can use the process of elimination to get rid of one answer choice. By doing so, you're better prepared to make an educated guess, as you will see in Step 6. More often, the process of elimination allows you to get down to only two possible right answers. Then you're in a strong position to guess, which you should do, since guessing is not penalized on the PANCE. And sometimes, even though you don't know the right answer, you find it simply by getting rid of the wrong ones, as you did in the example above.

Try using the process of elimination on the following questions. The answer explanations show one possible way you might use the process to arrive at the right answer.

USING THE PROCESS OF ELIMINATION

Use the process of elimination to answer the following questions.

1. Ilsa is as old as Meghan will be in five years. The difference between Ed's age and Meghan's age is twice the difference between Ilsa's age and Meghan's age. Ed is 29. How old is Ilsa?
   a. 4
   b. 10
   c. 19
   d. 24

2. "All drivers of commercial vehicles must carry a valid commercial driver's license whenever operating a commercial vehicle."
   According to this sentence, which of the following people need NOT carry a commercial driver's license?
   a. a truck driver idling his engine while waiting to be directed to a loading dock
   b. a bus operator backing her bus out of the way of another bus in the bus lot
   c. a taxi driver driving his personal car to the grocery store
   d. a limousine driver taking the limousine to her home after dropping off her last passenger of the evening

3. Smoking tobacco has been linked to
   a. increased risk of stroke and heart attack.
   b. all forms of respiratory disease.
   c. increasing mortality rates over the past ten years.
   d. juvenile delinquency.

4. Which of the following words is spelled correctly?
   a. incorrigible
   b. outragous
   c. domestickated
   d. understandible

Answers

Here are the answers, as well as some suggestions as to how you might have used the process of elimination to find them.

1. **d.** You should have eliminated choice **a** right off the bat. Ilsa can't be four years old if Meghan is going to be Ilsa's age in five years. The best way to eliminate other answer choices is to try plugging them in to the information given in the problem. For instance, for choice **b**, if Ilsa is 10, then Meghan must be 5. The difference between their ages is 5. The difference between Ed's age, 29, and Meghan's age, 5, is 24. Is 24 two times 5? No. Then choice **b** is wrong. You could eliminate choice **c** in the same way and be left with choice **d**.

2. **c.** Note the word *not* in the question, and go through the answers one by one. Is the truck driver in choice **a** "operating a commercial vehicle"? Yes, idling counts as "operating," so he needs to have a commercial driver's license. Likewise, the bus operator in choice **b** is operating a commercial vehicle; the question doesn't say the operator has to be on the street. The limo driver in choice **d** is operating a commercial vehicle, even if it doesn't have a passenger in it. However, the driver in choice **c** is *not* operating a commercial vehicle, but his own private car.

3. a. You could eliminate choice **b** simply because of the presence of the word *all*. Such absolutes hardly ever appear in correct answer choices. Choice **c** looks attractive until you think a little about what you know—aren't fewer people smoking these days, rather than more? So how could smoking be responsible for a higher mortality rate? (If you didn't know that mortality rate means the rate at which people die, you might keep this choice as a possibility, but you would still be able to eliminate two answers and have only two to choose from.) And choice **d** is plain silly, so you could eliminate that one, too. You are left with the correct choice, **a**.

4. a. How you used the process of elimination here depends on which words you recognized as being spelled incorrectly. If you knew that the correct spellings were *outrageous*, *domesticated*, and *understandable*, then you were home free. Surely you knew that at least one of those words was wrong!

Step 6: Guessing on the PANCE

Time to complete: 20 minutes
Activity: Complete the worksheet on Your Guessing Ability

Armed with the process of elimination, you're ready to make educated guesses. *Since there is no guessing penalty, you should be sure to answer every question on the test.*

YOUR GUESSING ABILITY

The following are ten really hard questions. You're not supposed to know the answers. Rather, this is an assessment of your ability to guess when you don't have a clue. Read each question carefully, just as if you did expect to answer it. If you have any knowledge at all of the subject of the question, use that knowledge to help you eliminate wrong answer choices. Use this answer grid to fill in your answers to the questions.

ANSWER GRID

1. ⓐ ⓑ ⓒ ⓓ
2. ⓐ ⓑ ⓒ ⓓ
3. ⓐ ⓑ ⓒ ⓓ
4. ⓐ ⓑ ⓒ ⓓ

5. ⓐ ⓑ ⓒ ⓓ
6. ⓐ ⓑ ⓒ ⓓ
7. ⓐ ⓑ ⓒ ⓓ
8. ⓐ ⓑ ⓒ ⓓ

9. ⓐ ⓑ ⓒ ⓓ
10. ⓐ ⓑ ⓒ ⓓ

1. September 7 is Independence Day in
   a. India.
   b. Costa Rica.
   c. Brazil.
   d. Australia.

2. Which of the following is the formula for determining the momentum of an object?
   a. $p = MV$
   b. $F = ma$
   c. $P = IV$
   d. $E = mc^2$

3. Because of the expansion of the universe, the stars and other celestial bodies are all moving away from each other. This phenomenon is known as
   a. Newton's first law.
   b. the big bang.
   c. gravitational collapse.
   d. Hubble flow.

4. American author Gertrude Stein was born in
   a. 1713.
   b. 1830.
   c. 1874.
   d. 1901.

5. Which of the following is NOT one of the Five Classics attributed to Confucius?
   a. *I Ching*
   b. *Book of Holiness*
   c. *Spring and Autumn Annals*
   d. *Book of History*

6. The religious and philosophical doctrine that holds that the universe is constantly in a struggle between good and evil is known as
   a. Pelagianism.
   b. Manichaeanism.
   c. neo-Hegelianism.
   d. Epicureanism.

7. The third Chief Justice of the U.S. Supreme Court was
   a. John Blair.
   b. William Cushing.
   c. James Wilson.
   d. John Jay.

8. Which of the following is the poisonous portion of a daffodil?
   a. the bulb
   b. the leaves
   c. the stem
   d. the flowers

9. The winner of the Masters golf tournament in 1953 was
  a. Sam Snead.
  b. Cary Middlecoff.
  c. Arnold Palmer.
  d. Ben Hogan.

10. The state with the highest per capita personal income in 1980 was
  a. Alaska.
  b. Connecticut.
  c. New York.
  d. Texas.

Answers

Check your answers against the following correct answers.

  1. c.
  2. a.
  3. d.
  4. c.
  5. b.
  6. b.
  7. b.
  8. a.
  9. d.
  10. a.

How Did You Do?

You may have simply gotten lucky and actually known the answer to one or two questions. In addition, your guessing was probably more successful if you were able to use the process of elimination on any of the questions. Maybe you didn't know who the third Chief Justice was (question 7), but you knew that John Jay was the first. In that case, you would have eliminated choice **d** and, therefore, improved your odds of guessing right from one in four to one in three.

According to probability, you should get two-and-a-half answers correct, so getting either two or three right would be average. If you got four or more right, you may be a really terrific guesser. If you got one or none right, you may be a really bad guesser.

Keep in mind, though, that this is only a small sample. You should continue to keep track of your guessing ability as you work through the sample questions in this book. Circle the numbers of questions you guess on as you make your guess; or, if you don't have time while you take the practice tests, go back afterward and try to remember which questions you guessed at. Remember, on a test with four answer choices, your chance of guessing correctly is one in four. So keep a separate "guessing" score for each exam. How many questions did you guess on? How many did you get right? If the number you got right is at least one-fourth of the number of questions you guessed on, you are at least an average guesser—maybe better—and you should always go ahead and guess on the real exam. If the number you got right is significantly lower than one-fourth of the number you guessed on, you would be safe in guessing anyway, but maybe you would feel more comfortable if you guessed only selectively, when you can eliminate a wrong answer or at least have a good feeling about one of the answer choices.

Step 7: Reach Your Peak Performance Zone

Time to complete: 10 minutes to read; weeks to complete!
Activity: Complete the Physical Preparation Checklist.

Physical and mental fatigue can significantly hinder your ability to perform, both as you prepare and also on the day of the exam. Poor diet choices can, as well. While drastic changes to your existing daily routine may cause a disruption too great to be helpful, modest, calculated alterations in your level of physical activity, the quality of your diet, and the amount and regularity of your rest can enhance your studies and your performance on the exam.

Exercise

If you are already engaged in a regular program of physical activity, resist allowing the pressure of the approaching exam to alter this routine. If you are not, and have not been engaged in regular physical activity, it may be helpful to begin during your preparations. Speak with someone knowledgeable about such matters to design a regime suited to your particular circumstances and needs. Whatever its form, try to keep it a regular part of your preparation as the exam approaches.

Diet

A balanced diet will help you achieve peak performance. Limit your caffeine and junk food intake as you continue on your preparation journey. Eat plenty of fruits and vegetables, along with lean proteins and complex carbohydrates. Foods that are high in lecithin (an amino acid), such as fish and beans, are especially good brain foods.

Your diet is also a matter that is particular to you, so any major alterations to it should be discussed with a person with expert knowledge of nutrition.

Rest

For your brain and body to function at optimal levels, they must have an adequate amount of rest. It will be important to determine what an adequate amount of rest is for you. Determine how much rest you need to feel at your sharpest and most alert, and make an effort to get that amount regularly as the exam approaches and particularly on the night before the exam.

It may help to record your efforts. What follows is a "Physical Preparation Checklist" for the week prior to the exam; you may find its use helpful for staying on track.

Physical Preparation Checklist

In the week leading up to the test, you may be so involved with studying (and, unfortunately, stress) that you neglect to treat your body kindly. The worksheet that follows will help you stay on track.

For each day of the week before the test, write down what physical exercise you engaged in and for how long, and what you ate for each meal. Remember, you're trying for at least half an hour of exercise every other day (preferably every day) and a balanced diet that is light on junk food. These practices are key to having your body and brain working at their peak.

PHYSICAL PREPARATION CHECKLIST

For the week before the test, write down what physical exercise you engaged in and for how long and what you ate for each meal. Remember, you're trying for at least half an hour of exercise every other day (preferably every day) and a balanced diet that's light on junk food.

Exam minus 7 days

Exercise: _____ for _____ minutes

Breakfast: _____

Lunch: _____

Dinner: _____

Snacks: _____

Exam minus 6 days

Exercise: _____ for _____ minutes

Breakfast: _____

Lunch: _____

Dinner: _____

Snacks: _____

Exam minus 5 days

Exercise: _____ for _____ minutes

Breakfast: _____

Lunch: _____

Dinner: _____

Snacks: _____

Exam minus 4 days

Exercise: _____ for _____ minutes

Breakfast: _____

Lunch: _____

Dinner: _____

Snacks: _____

Exam minus 3 days

Exercise: _____ for _____ minutes

Breakfast: _____

Lunch: _____

Dinner: _____

Snacks: _____

Exam minus 2 days

Exercise: _____ for _____ minutes

Breakfast: _____

Lunch: _____

Dinner: _____

Snacks: _____

Exam minus 1 day

Exercise: _____ for _____ minutes

Breakfast: _____

Lunch: _____

Dinner: _____

Snacks: _____

Step 8: Make Final Preparations

Time to complete: 10 minutes to read; time to complete will vary
Activity: Complete Final Preparations worksheet.

You're in control of your mind and body; you're in charge of test anxiety, your preparation, and your test-taking strategies. Now, it's time to take charge of external factors, like the testing site and the materials you need to take the test.

Find Out Where the Exam Is and Make a Trial Run

Make sure you know exactly when and where your test is being held. Do you know how to get to the exam site? Do you know how long it will take to get there? If not, make a trial run, preferably on the same day of the week at the same time of day. On the Final Preparations worksheet, make note of the amount of time it will take you to get to the test site. Plan on arriving at least 30 to 45 minutes early so you can get the lay of the land, use the bathroom, and calm down. Then figure out how early you will have to get up that morning, and make sure you get up that early every day for a week before the test.

Gather Your Materials

Make sure you have all the materials that will be required at the testing facility. Whether it's an admission ticket, an I.D., a second form of I.D., pencils, pens, calculators, a watch, or any other item that may be necessary, make sure you have put it aside. It's preferable to put them all aside together.

Arrange your clothes the evening before the exam. Dress in layers so that you can adjust readily to the temperature of the exam room.

Fuel Appropriately

Decide on a meal to eat in the time before your exam. Taking the exam on an empty stomach is something to avoid, particularly if it is an exam that spans several hours. Eating poorly and feeling lethargic are also to be avoided. Decide on a meal that will sate your hunger without adverse effect.

Step 9: Make Your Preparations Count

Time to complete: 10 minutes, plus test-taking time
Activity: Ace the PANCE!

Fast-forward to test day. You're ready. You made a study plan and followed through. You practiced your test-taking strategies while working through this book. You're in control of your physical, mental, and emotional state. You know when and where to show up and what to bring with you. In other words, you're well prepared!

When you're done with the test, you will have earned a reward. Plan a celebration. Call up your friends and plan a party, have a nice dinner with your family, or pick out a movie to see—whatever your heart desires.

And then do it. Go into the test, full of confidence, armed with test-taking strategies you've practiced until they're second nature. You're in control of yourself, your environment, and your performance on the exam. You're ready to succeed. So do it. And look forward to your future as someone who has passed the PANCE!

Getting to the Exam Site

Location of exam site: _____

Date: _____

Departure time: _____

Do I know how to get to the exam site?   Yes ___   No ___   (If no, make a trial run.)

Time it will take to get to the exam site: _____

Things to Lay Out the Night Before

Clothes I will wear   _____

Sweater/jacket   _____

Watch   _____

Photo ID   _____

Four #2 pencils and
blue or black ink pens
(if taking the paper-
based test)   _____

Other Things to Bring/Remember

_____   _____

_____   _____

_____   _____

_____   _____

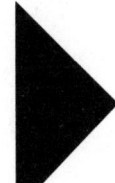

3 ▶ PRACTICE TEST 1

This is the first of two practice tests included with *PANCE: Power Practice*. Each practice test consists of questions that mirror those you will find on the official PANCE. The 300-question test, separated into 60-question sections, was developed by test experts.

Remember, on test day, you will have 60 minutes to complete each 60-question section. After you finish a section and start the next, you are not allowed to go back to answer questions in a previous section. Try to adhere to test day rules when you take these practice tests so that you have the most authentic practice experience possible.

These tests will show you how much you know and what kinds of problems you still need to study. In the answer explanations that follow the test, you will find which organ system and task area each question covers. Take note of which question types you tend to get wrong; this will help you focus your study until you take the actual exam.

Mastering these practice tests will allow you to reach your highest potential on the real PANCE. Good luck!

Practice Test 1 Answer Sheet

Section 1

1.	ⓐ ⓑ ⓒ ⓓ ⓔ		21.	ⓐ ⓑ ⓒ ⓓ ⓔ		41.	ⓐ ⓑ ⓒ ⓓ ⓔ
2.	ⓐ ⓑ ⓒ ⓓ ⓔ		22.	ⓐ ⓑ ⓒ ⓓ ⓔ		42.	ⓐ ⓑ ⓒ ⓓ ⓔ
3.	ⓐ ⓑ ⓒ ⓓ ⓔ		23.	ⓐ ⓑ ⓒ ⓓ ⓔ		43.	ⓐ ⓑ ⓒ ⓓ ⓔ
4.	ⓐ ⓑ ⓒ ⓓ ⓔ		24.	ⓐ ⓑ ⓒ ⓓ ⓔ		44.	ⓐ ⓑ ⓒ ⓓ ⓔ
5.	ⓐ ⓑ ⓒ ⓓ ⓔ		25.	ⓐ ⓑ ⓒ ⓓ ⓔ		45.	ⓐ ⓑ ⓒ ⓓ ⓔ
6.	ⓐ ⓑ ⓒ ⓓ ⓔ		26.	ⓐ ⓑ ⓒ ⓓ ⓔ		46.	ⓐ ⓑ ⓒ ⓓ ⓔ
7.	ⓐ ⓑ ⓒ ⓓ ⓔ		27.	ⓐ ⓑ ⓒ ⓓ ⓔ		47.	ⓐ ⓑ ⓒ ⓓ ⓔ
8.	ⓐ ⓑ ⓒ ⓓ ⓔ		28.	ⓐ ⓑ ⓒ ⓓ ⓔ		48.	ⓐ ⓑ ⓒ ⓓ ⓔ
9.	ⓐ ⓑ ⓒ ⓓ ⓔ		29.	ⓐ ⓑ ⓒ ⓓ ⓔ		49.	ⓐ ⓑ ⓒ ⓓ ⓔ
10.	ⓐ ⓑ ⓒ ⓓ ⓔ		30.	ⓐ ⓑ ⓒ ⓓ ⓔ		50.	ⓐ ⓑ ⓒ ⓓ ⓔ
11.	ⓐ ⓑ ⓒ ⓓ ⓔ		31.	ⓐ ⓑ ⓒ ⓓ ⓔ		51.	ⓐ ⓑ ⓒ ⓓ ⓔ
12.	ⓐ ⓑ ⓒ ⓓ ⓔ		32.	ⓐ ⓑ ⓒ ⓓ ⓔ		52.	ⓐ ⓑ ⓒ ⓓ ⓔ
13.	ⓐ ⓑ ⓒ ⓓ ⓔ		33.	ⓐ ⓑ ⓒ ⓓ ⓔ		53.	ⓐ ⓑ ⓒ ⓓ ⓔ
14.	ⓐ ⓑ ⓒ ⓓ ⓔ		34.	ⓐ ⓑ ⓒ ⓓ ⓔ		54.	ⓐ ⓑ ⓒ ⓓ ⓔ
15.	ⓐ ⓑ ⓒ ⓓ ⓔ		35.	ⓐ ⓑ ⓒ ⓓ ⓔ		55.	ⓐ ⓑ ⓒ ⓓ ⓔ
16.	ⓐ ⓑ ⓒ ⓓ ⓔ		36.	ⓐ ⓑ ⓒ ⓓ ⓔ		56.	ⓐ ⓑ ⓒ ⓓ ⓔ
17.	ⓐ ⓑ ⓒ ⓓ ⓔ		37.	ⓐ ⓑ ⓒ ⓓ ⓔ		57.	ⓐ ⓑ ⓒ ⓓ ⓔ
18.	ⓐ ⓑ ⓒ ⓓ ⓔ		38.	ⓐ ⓑ ⓒ ⓓ ⓔ		58.	ⓐ ⓑ ⓒ ⓓ ⓔ
19.	ⓐ ⓑ ⓒ ⓓ ⓔ		39.	ⓐ ⓑ ⓒ ⓓ ⓔ		59.	ⓐ ⓑ ⓒ ⓓ ⓔ
20.	ⓐ ⓑ ⓒ ⓓ ⓔ		40.	ⓐ ⓑ ⓒ ⓓ ⓔ		60.	ⓐ ⓑ ⓒ ⓓ ⓔ

Section 2

61.	ⓐ	ⓑ	ⓒ	ⓓ	ⓔ	**81.**	ⓐ	ⓑ	ⓒ	ⓓ	ⓔ	**101.**	ⓐ	ⓑ	ⓒ	ⓓ	ⓔ
62.	ⓐ	ⓑ	ⓒ	ⓓ	ⓔ	**82.**	ⓐ	ⓑ	ⓒ	ⓓ	ⓔ	**102.**	ⓐ	ⓑ	ⓒ	ⓓ	ⓔ
63.	ⓐ	ⓑ	ⓒ	ⓓ	ⓔ	**83.**	ⓐ	ⓑ	ⓒ	ⓓ	ⓔ	**103.**	ⓐ	ⓑ	ⓒ	ⓓ	ⓔ
64.	ⓐ	ⓑ	ⓒ	ⓓ	ⓔ	**84.**	ⓐ	ⓑ	ⓒ	ⓓ	ⓔ	**104.**	ⓐ	ⓑ	ⓒ	ⓓ	ⓔ
65.	ⓐ	ⓑ	ⓒ	ⓓ	ⓔ	**85.**	ⓐ	ⓑ	ⓒ	ⓓ	ⓔ	**105.**	ⓐ	ⓑ	ⓒ	ⓓ	ⓔ
66.	ⓐ	ⓑ	ⓒ	ⓓ	ⓔ	**86.**	ⓐ	ⓑ	ⓒ	ⓓ	ⓔ	**106.**	ⓐ	ⓑ	ⓒ	ⓓ	ⓔ
67.	ⓐ	ⓑ	ⓒ	ⓓ	ⓔ	**87.**	ⓐ	ⓑ	ⓒ	ⓓ	ⓔ	**107.**	ⓐ	ⓑ	ⓒ	ⓓ	ⓔ
68.	ⓐ	ⓑ	ⓒ	ⓓ	ⓔ	**88.**	ⓐ	ⓑ	ⓒ	ⓓ	ⓔ	**108.**	ⓐ	ⓑ	ⓒ	ⓓ	ⓔ
69.	ⓐ	ⓑ	ⓒ	ⓓ	ⓔ	**89.**	ⓐ	ⓑ	ⓒ	ⓓ	ⓔ	**109.**	ⓐ	ⓑ	ⓒ	ⓓ	ⓔ
70.	ⓐ	ⓑ	ⓒ	ⓓ	ⓔ	**90.**	ⓐ	ⓑ	ⓒ	ⓓ	ⓔ	**110.**	ⓐ	ⓑ	ⓒ	ⓓ	ⓔ
71.	ⓐ	ⓑ	ⓒ	ⓓ	ⓔ	**91.**	ⓐ	ⓑ	ⓒ	ⓓ	ⓔ	**111.**	ⓐ	ⓑ	ⓒ	ⓓ	ⓔ
72.	ⓐ	ⓑ	ⓒ	ⓓ	ⓔ	**92.**	ⓐ	ⓑ	ⓒ	ⓓ	ⓔ	**112.**	ⓐ	ⓑ	ⓒ	ⓓ	ⓔ
73.	ⓐ	ⓑ	ⓒ	ⓓ	ⓔ	**93.**	ⓐ	ⓑ	ⓒ	ⓓ	ⓔ	**113.**	ⓐ	ⓑ	ⓒ	ⓓ	ⓔ
74.	ⓐ	ⓑ	ⓒ	ⓓ	ⓔ	**94.**	ⓐ	ⓑ	ⓒ	ⓓ	ⓔ	**114.**	ⓐ	ⓑ	ⓒ	ⓓ	ⓔ
75.	ⓐ	ⓑ	ⓒ	ⓓ	ⓔ	**95.**	ⓐ	ⓑ	ⓒ	ⓓ	ⓔ	**115.**	ⓐ	ⓑ	ⓒ	ⓓ	ⓔ
76.	ⓐ	ⓑ	ⓒ	ⓓ	ⓔ	**96.**	ⓐ	ⓑ	ⓒ	ⓓ	ⓔ	**116.**	ⓐ	ⓑ	ⓒ	ⓓ	ⓔ
77.	ⓐ	ⓑ	ⓒ	ⓓ	ⓔ	**97.**	ⓐ	ⓑ	ⓒ	ⓓ	ⓔ	**117.**	ⓐ	ⓑ	ⓒ	ⓓ	ⓔ
78.	ⓐ	ⓑ	ⓒ	ⓓ	ⓔ	**98.**	ⓐ	ⓑ	ⓒ	ⓓ	ⓔ	**118.**	ⓐ	ⓑ	ⓒ	ⓓ	ⓔ
79.	ⓐ	ⓑ	ⓒ	ⓓ	ⓔ	**99.**	ⓐ	ⓑ	ⓒ	ⓓ	ⓔ	**119.**	ⓐ	ⓑ	ⓒ	ⓓ	ⓔ
80.	ⓐ	ⓑ	ⓒ	ⓓ	ⓔ	**100.**	ⓐ	ⓑ	ⓒ	ⓓ	ⓔ	**120.**	ⓐ	ⓑ	ⓒ	ⓓ	ⓔ

Section 3

121.	ⓐ	ⓑ	ⓒ	ⓓ	ⓔ	**141.**	ⓐ	ⓑ	ⓒ	ⓓ	ⓔ	**161.**	ⓐ	ⓑ	ⓒ	ⓓ	ⓔ
122.	ⓐ	ⓑ	ⓒ	ⓓ	ⓔ	**142.**	ⓐ	ⓑ	ⓒ	ⓓ	ⓔ	**162.**	ⓐ	ⓑ	ⓒ	ⓓ	ⓔ
123.	ⓐ	ⓑ	ⓒ	ⓓ	ⓔ	**143.**	ⓐ	ⓑ	ⓒ	ⓓ	ⓔ	**163.**	ⓐ	ⓑ	ⓒ	ⓓ	ⓔ
124.	ⓐ	ⓑ	ⓒ	ⓓ	ⓔ	**144.**	ⓐ	ⓑ	ⓒ	ⓓ	ⓔ	**164.**	ⓐ	ⓑ	ⓒ	ⓓ	ⓔ
125.	ⓐ	ⓑ	ⓒ	ⓓ	ⓔ	**145.**	ⓐ	ⓑ	ⓒ	ⓓ	ⓔ	**165.**	ⓐ	ⓑ	ⓒ	ⓓ	ⓔ
126.	ⓐ	ⓑ	ⓒ	ⓓ	ⓔ	**146.**	ⓐ	ⓑ	ⓒ	ⓓ	ⓔ	**166.**	ⓐ	ⓑ	ⓒ	ⓓ	ⓔ
127.	ⓐ	ⓑ	ⓒ	ⓓ	ⓔ	**147.**	ⓐ	ⓑ	ⓒ	ⓓ	ⓔ	**167.**	ⓐ	ⓑ	ⓒ	ⓓ	ⓔ
128.	ⓐ	ⓑ	ⓒ	ⓓ	ⓔ	**148.**	ⓐ	ⓑ	ⓒ	ⓓ	ⓔ	**168.**	ⓐ	ⓑ	ⓒ	ⓓ	ⓔ
129.	ⓐ	ⓑ	ⓒ	ⓓ	ⓔ	**149.**	ⓐ	ⓑ	ⓒ	ⓓ	ⓔ	**169.**	ⓐ	ⓑ	ⓒ	ⓓ	ⓔ
130.	ⓐ	ⓑ	ⓒ	ⓓ	ⓔ	**150.**	ⓐ	ⓑ	ⓒ	ⓓ	ⓔ	**170.**	ⓐ	ⓑ	ⓒ	ⓓ	ⓔ
131.	ⓐ	ⓑ	ⓒ	ⓓ	ⓔ	**151.**	ⓐ	ⓑ	ⓒ	ⓓ	ⓔ	**171.**	ⓐ	ⓑ	ⓒ	ⓓ	ⓔ
132.	ⓐ	ⓑ	ⓒ	ⓓ	ⓔ	**152.**	ⓐ	ⓑ	ⓒ	ⓓ	ⓔ	**172.**	ⓐ	ⓑ	ⓒ	ⓓ	ⓔ
133.	ⓐ	ⓑ	ⓒ	ⓓ	ⓔ	**153.**	ⓐ	ⓑ	ⓒ	ⓓ	ⓔ	**173.**	ⓐ	ⓑ	ⓒ	ⓓ	ⓔ
134.	ⓐ	ⓑ	ⓒ	ⓓ	ⓔ	**154.**	ⓐ	ⓑ	ⓒ	ⓓ	ⓔ	**174.**	ⓐ	ⓑ	ⓒ	ⓓ	ⓔ
135.	ⓐ	ⓑ	ⓒ	ⓓ	ⓔ	**155.**	ⓐ	ⓑ	ⓒ	ⓓ	ⓔ	**175.**	ⓐ	ⓑ	ⓒ	ⓓ	ⓔ
136.	ⓐ	ⓑ	ⓒ	ⓓ	ⓔ	**156.**	ⓐ	ⓑ	ⓒ	ⓓ	ⓔ	**176.**	ⓐ	ⓑ	ⓒ	ⓓ	ⓔ
137.	ⓐ	ⓑ	ⓒ	ⓓ	ⓔ	**157.**	ⓐ	ⓑ	ⓒ	ⓓ	ⓔ	**177.**	ⓐ	ⓑ	ⓒ	ⓓ	ⓔ
138.	ⓐ	ⓑ	ⓒ	ⓓ	ⓔ	**158.**	ⓐ	ⓑ	ⓒ	ⓓ	ⓔ	**178.**	ⓐ	ⓑ	ⓒ	ⓓ	ⓔ
139.	ⓐ	ⓑ	ⓒ	ⓓ	ⓔ	**159.**	ⓐ	ⓑ	ⓒ	ⓓ	ⓔ	**179.**	ⓐ	ⓑ	ⓒ	ⓓ	ⓔ
140.	ⓐ	ⓑ	ⓒ	ⓓ	ⓔ	**160.**	ⓐ	ⓑ	ⓒ	ⓓ	ⓔ	**180.**	ⓐ	ⓑ	ⓒ	ⓓ	ⓔ

Section 4

181.	ⓐ	ⓑ	ⓒ	ⓓ	ⓔ	201.	ⓐ	ⓑ	ⓒ	ⓓ	ⓔ	221.	ⓐ	ⓑ	ⓒ	ⓓ	ⓔ
182.	ⓐ	ⓑ	ⓒ	ⓓ	ⓔ	202.	ⓐ	ⓑ	ⓒ	ⓓ	ⓔ	222.	ⓐ	ⓑ	ⓒ	ⓓ	ⓔ
183.	ⓐ	ⓑ	ⓒ	ⓓ	ⓔ	203.	ⓐ	ⓑ	ⓒ	ⓓ	ⓔ	223.	ⓐ	ⓑ	ⓒ	ⓓ	ⓔ
184.	ⓐ	ⓑ	ⓒ	ⓓ	ⓔ	204.	ⓐ	ⓑ	ⓒ	ⓓ	ⓔ	224.	ⓐ	ⓑ	ⓒ	ⓓ	ⓔ
185.	ⓐ	ⓑ	ⓒ	ⓓ	ⓔ	205.	ⓐ	ⓑ	ⓒ	ⓓ	ⓔ	225.	ⓐ	ⓑ	ⓒ	ⓓ	ⓔ
186.	ⓐ	ⓑ	ⓒ	ⓓ	ⓔ	206.	ⓐ	ⓑ	ⓒ	ⓓ	ⓔ	226.	ⓐ	ⓑ	ⓒ	ⓓ	ⓔ
187.	ⓐ	ⓑ	ⓒ	ⓓ	ⓔ	207.	ⓐ	ⓑ	ⓒ	ⓓ	ⓔ	227.	ⓐ	ⓑ	ⓒ	ⓓ	ⓔ
188.	ⓐ	ⓑ	ⓒ	ⓓ	ⓔ	208.	ⓐ	ⓑ	ⓒ	ⓓ	ⓔ	228.	ⓐ	ⓑ	ⓒ	ⓓ	ⓔ
189.	ⓐ	ⓑ	ⓒ	ⓓ	ⓔ	209.	ⓐ	ⓑ	ⓒ	ⓓ	ⓔ	229.	ⓐ	ⓑ	ⓒ	ⓓ	ⓔ
190.	ⓐ	ⓑ	ⓒ	ⓓ	ⓔ	210.	ⓐ	ⓑ	ⓒ	ⓓ	ⓔ	230.	ⓐ	ⓑ	ⓒ	ⓓ	ⓔ
191.	ⓐ	ⓑ	ⓒ	ⓓ	ⓔ	211.	ⓐ	ⓑ	ⓒ	ⓓ	ⓔ	231.	ⓐ	ⓑ	ⓒ	ⓓ	ⓔ
192.	ⓐ	ⓑ	ⓒ	ⓓ	ⓔ	212.	ⓐ	ⓑ	ⓒ	ⓓ	ⓔ	232.	ⓐ	ⓑ	ⓒ	ⓓ	ⓔ
193.	ⓐ	ⓑ	ⓒ	ⓓ	ⓔ	213.	ⓐ	ⓑ	ⓒ	ⓓ	ⓔ	233.	ⓐ	ⓑ	ⓒ	ⓓ	ⓔ
194.	ⓐ	ⓑ	ⓒ	ⓓ	ⓔ	214.	ⓐ	ⓑ	ⓒ	ⓓ	ⓔ	234.	ⓐ	ⓑ	ⓒ	ⓓ	ⓔ
195.	ⓐ	ⓑ	ⓒ	ⓓ	ⓔ	215.	ⓐ	ⓑ	ⓒ	ⓓ	ⓔ	235.	ⓐ	ⓑ	ⓒ	ⓓ	ⓔ
196.	ⓐ	ⓑ	ⓒ	ⓓ	ⓔ	216.	ⓐ	ⓑ	ⓒ	ⓓ	ⓔ	236.	ⓐ	ⓑ	ⓒ	ⓓ	ⓔ
197.	ⓐ	ⓑ	ⓒ	ⓓ	ⓔ	217.	ⓐ	ⓑ	ⓒ	ⓓ	ⓔ	237.	ⓐ	ⓑ	ⓒ	ⓓ	ⓔ
198.	ⓐ	ⓑ	ⓒ	ⓓ	ⓔ	218.	ⓐ	ⓑ	ⓒ	ⓓ	ⓔ	238.	ⓐ	ⓑ	ⓒ	ⓓ	ⓔ
199.	ⓐ	ⓑ	ⓒ	ⓓ	ⓔ	219.	ⓐ	ⓑ	ⓒ	ⓓ	ⓔ	239.	ⓐ	ⓑ	ⓒ	ⓓ	ⓔ
200.	ⓐ	ⓑ	ⓒ	ⓓ	ⓔ	220.	ⓐ	ⓑ	ⓒ	ⓓ	ⓔ	240.	ⓐ	ⓑ	ⓒ	ⓓ	ⓔ

Section 5

241. (a) (b) (c) (d) (e)	261. (a) (b) (c) (d) (e)	281. (a) (b) (c) (d) (e)
242. (a) (b) (c) (d) (e)	262. (a) (b) (c) (d) (e)	282. (a) (b) (c) (d) (e)
243. (a) (b) (c) (d) (e)	263. (a) (b) (c) (d) (e)	283. (a) (b) (c) (d) (e)
244. (a) (b) (c) (d) (e)	264. (a) (b) (c) (d) (e)	284. (a) (b) (c) (d) (e)
245. (a) (b) (c) (d) (e)	265. (a) (b) (c) (d) (e)	285. (a) (b) (c) (d) (e)
246. (a) (b) (c) (d) (e)	266. (a) (b) (c) (d) (e)	286. (a) (b) (c) (d) (e)
247. (a) (b) (c) (d) (e)	267. (a) (b) (c) (d) (e)	287. (a) (b) (c) (d) (e)
248. (a) (b) (c) (d) (e)	268. (a) (b) (c) (d) (e)	288. (a) (b) (c) (d) (e)
249. (a) (b) (c) (d) (e)	269. (a) (b) (c) (d) (e)	289. (a) (b) (c) (d) (e)
250. (a) (b) (c) (d) (e)	270. (a) (b) (c) (d) (e)	290. (a) (b) (c) (d) (e)
251. (a) (b) (c) (d) (e)	271. (a) (b) (c) (d) (e)	291. (a) (b) (c) (d) (e)
252. (a) (b) (c) (d) (e)	272. (a) (b) (c) (d) (e)	292. (a) (b) (c) (d) (e)
253. (a) (b) (c) (d) (e)	273. (a) (b) (c) (d) (e)	293. (a) (b) (c) (d) (e)
254. (a) (b) (c) (d) (e)	274. (a) (b) (c) (d) (e)	294. (a) (b) (c) (d) (e)
255. (a) (b) (c) (d) (e)	275. (a) (b) (c) (d) (e)	295. (a) (b) (c) (d) (e)
256. (a) (b) (c) (d) (e)	276. (a) (b) (c) (d) (e)	296. (a) (b) (c) (d) (e)
257. (a) (b) (c) (d) (e)	277. (a) (b) (c) (d) (e)	297. (a) (b) (c) (d) (e)
258. (a) (b) (c) (d) (e)	278. (a) (b) (c) (d) (e)	298. (a) (b) (c) (d) (e)
259. (a) (b) (c) (d) (e)	279. (a) (b) (c) (d) (e)	299. (a) (b) (c) (d) (e)
260. (a) (b) (c) (d) (e)	280. (a) (b) (c) (d) (e)	300. (a) (b) (c) (d) (e)

Questions

Section 1
Time: 60 minutes

1. A parrot beak appearance on a barium swallow procedure is a classic finding for which of the following disorders?
   a. esophageal varices
   b. esophageal neoplasm
   c. infectious esophagitis
   d. esophageal dysmotility
   e. reflux esophagitis

2. A 21-year-old man presents with paranoid delusions and visual hallucinations. Which of the following signs or symptoms would rule out a diagnosis of schizophrenia?
   a. disorganized speech
   b. disorganized thought
   c. agraphesthesia
   d. Kayser-Fleischer rings
   e. flat affect

3. A 64-year-old female patient presents to her primary care clinic for review four months after a surgical bowel resection. The wound is healing well, but there is a small palpable lump in the region of the incision. The lump appears to become larger when she stands upright. Which of the following interventions is most appropriate for this patient?
   a. abdominal strength training
   b. regular review
   c. surgical repair
   d. antibiotic therapy
   e. drainage of the lesion

4. A 62-year-old man with a history of hypertension and hyperlipidemia complains of worsening of fatigue and shortness of breath for the past six months. He denies tobacco use or fever. A physical exam is significant for a pansystolic murmur at the apex, radiating into the axilla with associated S3 heart sound. Which of the following is the most likely diagnosis?
   a. aortic stenosis
   b. mitral stenosis
   c. chronic obstructive pulmonary disease (COPD)
   d. mitral regurgitation
   e. first-degree heart block

5. An 11-year-old Caucasian male is brought in by his mother and is complaining of chronic productive cough, dyspnea, and wheezing. He shows airflow obstruction on spirometry, and his sweat chloride concentration is 100 mEq/L on two occasions (normal value: < 60mEq/L). Which of the following is the most likely diagnosis?
   a. acute asthma exacerbation
   b. pneumonia
   c. pulmonary tuberculosis
   d. cystic fibrosis
   e. chronic obstructive pulmonary disease (COPD)

6. A 64-year-old patient presents to his primary care clinic with concerns about a six-month history of persisting muscle pain in the large muscles of his arms, legs, and trunk. His past history is significant for hypertension (managed effectively with furosemide) and hypercholesterolemia (managed effectively with atorvastatin). Physical examination reveals weakness in the muscles affected by the pain. Blood tests show an elevation in creatine kinase, while all electrolyte levels are normal. Which of the following is the most likely cause of his symptoms?
   a. polymyalgia rheumatica
   b. fibromyalgia
   c. trauma
   d. atorvastatin therapy
   e. furosemide therapy

7. A 29-year-old female presents with excessive hair growth, truncal obesity, acne, and irregular menstruation. Physical examination reveals skin discoloration. Ultrasound examination reveals a "string of pearls" appearance within the ovaries. Which of the following is the most likely diagnosis?
   a. ovarian cysts
   b. ovarian cancer
   c. polycystic ovarian syndrome
   d. endometrial cancer
   e. endometriosis

8. A 60-year-old man with a history of daily alcohol use presents with a tender, red, and warm swelling on the first metatarsal phalangeal joint of his left foot. A joint aspiration shows negatively birefringent, needle-shaped crystals. Which of the following is the most likely diagnosis?
   a. septic joint
   b. pseudogout
   c. acute gout
   d. osteoarthritis of the foot
   e. fracture of the first toe

9. The combination of sulfamethoxazole and trimethoprim is commonly known as which of the following antibiotic medications?
   a. Zithromax
   b. Bactrim
   c. Cipro
   d. penicillin
   e. erythromycin

10. A 19-year-old sexual assault victim presents for a gynecological exam. Which of the following should be included in caring for this patient?
    a. establish a sense of safety and security
    b. take complete history and give physical exam
    c. prophylactic antibiotic treatment
    d. contact patient after 24 to 48 hours for post-treatment evaluation
    e. all of the above

11. A 19-year-old male patient with cystic fibrosis presents to his primary care physician complaining of a bout of fever and green sputum production with his usual cough. Which of the following organisms is most likely to be found in a sputum culture?
    a. *Mycoplasma pneumoniae*
    b. *Streptococcus pneumoniae*
    c. *Klebsiella pneumoniae*
    d. *Haemophilus influenzae*
    e. *Pseudomonas aeruginosa*

12. A 50-year-old Hispanic man with a history of diabetes mellitus and depression presents to your clinic for a general check-up. He appears to have a rounded face and truncal obesity. His blood pressure is 145/89. His subsequent lab work is significant for an increased cortisol excretion from a 24-hour urine cortisol test. His thyroid function tests and all other lab results are within normal limits. Which of the following is the most likely diagnosis?
  a. hyperthyroidism
  b. hypothyroidism
  c. Cushing's syndrome
  d. Paget's disease
  e. obesity

13. A 23-year-old woman presents with chronic abdominal pain, is found to have anti-tTG antibodies, and is suspected to have celiac disease. Which component of her history is most specific for this condition?
  a. colicky abdominal pain
  b. foul-smelling stool
  c. perianal bleeding
  d. worsening symptoms with ingestion of gluten
  e. nosebleeds

14. A 25-year-old female presents with a left-sided and pulsating headache (HA). The headache is followed by light-sensitivity and usually lasts for a few hours. She denies nausea or vomiting. She reports increased frequency of her left-sided HA when she is under stress or during her menstrual periods. A CAT scan of the brain is negative for any lesions. Which of the following is an appropriate treatment for her condition?
  a. acetaminophen
  b. nonsteroidal anti-inflammatory drugs (NSAIDs)
  c. ergotamine with caffeine
  d. triptans
  e. all of the above

15. A 66-year-old man, post-operative day five, is found to have acute renal failure. His urinalysis shows hematuria, proteinuria, and red cell casts with some white cells. Which of the following is the most likely diagnosis based on the lab findings?
  a. acute tubular necrosis
  b. acute interstitial nephritis
  c. prerenal azotemia
  d. acute glomerulonephritis
  e. postrenal azotemia

16. A 59-year-old male presents with foul-smelling, purulent sputum, hemoptysis, and chronic cough. He has a history of recurrent pneumonia. Auscultation of the chest reveals localized chest crackles and clubbing of the fingernails. A high resolution CT scan reveals dilated, tortuous airways. Which of the following is the most likely diagnosis?
  a. pneumonia
  b. asthma
  c. bronchiectasis
  d. chronic obstructive pulmonary disease (COPD)
  e. cystic fibrosis

17. Selective serotonin reuptake inhibitors (SSRIs) regulate which of the following mechanisms, making them an effective treatment for fibromyalgia?
  a. menstrual cycles
  b. eating habits
  c. bowel habits
  d. circadian rhythms
  e. sleep patterns

18. A 15-year-old male presents with complaints of pain, excessive tearing, and light sensitivity of the left eye. Examination of the eyes is unable to confirm the presence of a foreign body within the left eye. Which of the following is the most likely diagnosis?
   a. orbital cellulitis
   b. retinal detachment
   c. corneal abrasion
   d. central retinal vein occlusion
   e. central retinal artery occlusion

19. Which of the following correctly matches the electrocardiogram (EKG) wave to its corresponding electrical activity of the heart?
   a. P wave: depolarization of the ventricles
   b. PR interval: depolarization of the atria
   c. QRS complex: repolarization of the ventricles
   d. T wave: first ventricular depolarization to last ventricular repolarization
   e. none of the above

20. Which of the following would be the appropriate diagnostic tool if you needed to rule out epiglottitis?
   a. angiography of the neck
   b. CT scan of the neck
   c. MRI of the neck
   d. X-ray of the neck
   e. ultrasound of the neck

21. Which of the following forms of contraception can last up to ten years?
   a. oral contraceptives
   b. Norplant system
   c. hormone-impregnated vaginal ring
   d. Progestasert IUD
   e. Copper T IUD

22. Which of the following medications is indicated for maintenance therapy of cardiogenic transient ischemic attacks?
   a. tenecteplase
   b. ticlopidine
   c. sulfinpyrazone
   d. dipyridamole
   e. warfarin

23. Which of the following conditions is effectively treated with buproprion?
   a. hypertension
   b. obesity
   c. bulimia nervosa
   d. seasonal affective disorder
   e. body dysmorphic disorder

24. A 44-year-old, obese, African-American female with a history of venous insufficiency and varicose veins presents for a routine office visit. A physical examination of the lower extremities reveals skin that is purple to red in color. Which of the following is the most likely diagnosis?
   a. stasis dermatitis
   b. dyshidrotic eczema
   c. contact dermatitis
   d. neurodermatitis
   e. seborrheic eczema

25. A 62-year-old female patient presents to the emergency department with a four-hour history of "crushing" left-sided chest pain radiating to her left arm and jaw. Which of the following enzymes would most likely be elevated if the source of her pain is a myocardial infarction?
   a. troponin
   b. aspartate transaminase
   c. creatine kinase
   d. creatinine
   e. lactate dehydrogenase

26. A 68-year-old patient with a history of chronic obstructive pulmonary disease (COPD) presents to his primary care physician for a general semiannual checkup. On physical examination, he is found to have a blood pressure of 182/94 and a heart rate of 110 bpm; his past two semiannual blood pressure readings have been 174/88 and 178/90. A recent electrocardiogram and echocardiogram demonstrated no evidence of congestive heart failure. His drug regimen includes inhaled albuterol, inhaled fluticasone, oral atorvastatin, oral hydrochlorothiazide, and oral ramipril. Which of these drugs is most likely to be exacerbating his hypertension and tachycardia?
  a. albuterol
  b. fluticasone
  c. atorvastatin
  d. hydrochlorothiazide
  e. ramipril

27. A 26-year-old female complains of a sudden onset of pain in her left eye with a foreign body sensation. She normally wears contact lenses; however, the pain is not relieved even after she removes the lenses. She denies recent trauma to her eye. A physical exam shows normal visual acuity, benign-appearing eyelids, and mildly injected left conjunctiva without exudates or blood. Her pupils are equal, round, and reactive to light. The blue light with fluorescein exam does not show any lesions. Which of the following is the most likely diagnosis?
  a. chalazion
  b. blepharitis
  c. corneal abrasion
  d. hordeolum
  e. retinal detachment

28. A 44-year-old male with a two-year history of occasional heartburn, which usually occurs once or twice a week, is prescribed omeprazole for relief of his symptoms. Two weeks later, he returns and reports that his symptoms have not improved despite the fact that he takes the drug every time he has an episode. Which of the following is the most likely reason for the failure of his therapy?
  a. incorrect use of the drug
  b. inadequate dose of the drug
  c. insensitivity to the drug
  d. malabsorption of the drug
  e. drug interaction

29. During a regular check-up, a 36-year-old female mentions that her mother was recently diagnosed with osteoporosis. She expresses concerns about her own risk of the disease. Which of the following recommendations is most likely to decrease her chances of developing osteoporosis later in life?
  a. weight-bearing exercise
  b. high-protein diet
  c. low-fat diet
  d. avoidance of hormone replacement therapy
  e. avoidance of oral contraceptive pills

30. A 37-year-old female patient presents to her primary care clinic complaining of a six-day history of redness and irritation in her right eye; she has also noticed some glare in her left eye for the past two days. On further questioning, she recalls that she recently experienced a bout of fever, sore throat, and cough. Her best-corrected visual acuity is 20/40 in the right eye and 20/20 in the left eye. She is otherwise healthy. Which of the following is the most likely cause of the patient's visual disturbance?

a. keratitis

b. conjunctivitis

c. uveitis

d. corneal abrasion

e. acute angle closure

31. A 37-year-old white male presents with chest pressure, dizziness, shortness of breath, and heart palpitations for several weeks. His electrocardiogram is within normal limits. Cholesterol is normal at 190. Troponin levels are normal at 0.2 ng/mL. D-dimer levels are normal at 0.37. Which of the following is the most appropriate diagnostic test?

a. cardiac catheterization to rule out cardiac ischemia

b. myocardial perfusion imaging to rule out cardiac ischemia

c. echocardiogram to rule out cardiac valve abnormalities

d. CT scan of the chest to rule out pulmonary embolism

e. lung ventilation and perfusion scan to rule out pulmonary embolism

32. A 71-year-old man presents to his primary physician with a tremor in his hand that has worsened progressively since he first noticed it approximately two years earlier. The tremor appears to be most significant when he is at rest. On further questioning, he mentions that his wife often complains that his walking speed appears to have deteriorated over the same time period. Physical examination is significant for cogwheel rigidity in the limbs as well as impaired balance when his eyes are closed. Which of the following neurologic structures is most likely to be affected?

a. caudate

b. putamen

c. thalamus

d. hippocampus

e. substantia nigra

33. A 62-year-old male patient with a history of dilated cardiomyopathy presents for a regular follow-up. On physical examination, his blood pressure is found to be 165/105 mmHg, his body mass index is 29 kg/m^2, and his plasma cholesterol level is 5.1 mmol/L. He has not attempted any lifestyle changes for blood pressure control in the past. Which of the following dietary changes is most likely to be beneficial to his prognosis?

a. increased protein content

b. increased fruits and vegetables

c. decreased carbohydrates

d. decreased cholesterol

e. decreased salt

34. A 58-year-old male patient presents to his primary care clinic complaining of increased urinary frequency and urgency. On further questioning, he recalls that he has also experienced urge incontinence, dribbling, and incomplete bladder emptying. These symptoms have been progressively worsening for the past two years. Which of the following investigations is most likely to yield an abnormal result?
   a. urine culture
   b. prostate-specific antigen
   c. urine electrolytes
   d. plasma creatinine
   e. blood urea nitrogen

35. A 28-year-old male patient presents to his primary care clinic with a six-day history of fever, nausea and vomiting, back pain, and headache. His symptoms seemed to have resolved three days earlier, but returned after two days. During the most recent resurgence, he has also experienced dark-colored vomit and epigastric pain. On further questioning, he mentions that he recently returned from a hiking trip in Peru. Physical examination is significant for a body temperature of 38.5°C (101°F) and moderate jaundice. Which of the following is the most likely diagnosis?
   a. hepatitis A
   b. hepatitis B
   c. hepatitis C
   d. yellow fever
   e. hepatocellular carcinoma

36. A 64-year-old male accountant presents with a three-day history of sharp, severe pain in his right big toe with no history of trauma. The pain is temporarily relieved by ibuprofen, but it has been otherwise constant. His past history is significant for hypertension, for which he has been taking hydrochlorothiazide for 12 years and ramipril for three months. He also has a 40-pack-year smoking history. On examination, there is considerable swelling and tenderness in the region of his right first metatarsophalangeal joint. Which of the following is the strongest factor contributing to this episode?
   a. sedentary lifestyle
   b. smoking
   c. ramipril
   d. hydrochlorothiazide
   e. hypertension

37. A 34-year-old female patient presents with a three-month history of unexplained fever. On further questioning, she reports that she has experienced occasional palpitations over the same time period. Abnormalities noted on physical examination include a pulse of 104 bpm and a resting tremor in both hands. Which of the following additional findings would support a diagnosis of Graves' disease rather than thyroid cancer?
   a. night sweats
   b. unintentional weight loss
   c. exophthalmos
   d. low TSH levels
   e. high T4 levels

38. A 54-year-old woman presents with a history of heart palpitations for the past three days. She has no relevant past medical history. Her pulse (120 bpm) is irregularly irregular. Her blood pressure is 130/80. Her physical exam is otherwise unremarkable. An electrocardiogram confirms that the patient has atrial fibrillation. Which one of the following is NOT appropriate as the immediate next step for her new onset atrial fibrillation?
   a. aspirin
   b. electrical cardioversion
   c. metoprolol
   d. heparin
   e. warfarin

39. A 45-year-old woman takes albuterol for her asthma. Which of the following side effects is most consistent with this drug?
   a. oral thrush
   b. lupus
   c. hearing loss
   d. tachycardia
   e. cough

40. A 36-year-old man presents to the emergency department with a one-day history of nausea, loss of appetite, and lower abdominal pain. His pain started in the periumbilical area and traveled to the right lower quadrant (RLQ). He denies other associated symptoms. A physical exam reveals positive tenderness in the RLQ with right thigh extension as well as rebound tenderness. Which of the following is the most likely diagnosis?
   a. gastrointestinal bleed
   b. colon cancer
   c. appendicitis
   d. cholecystitis
   e. pancreatitis

41. Which of the following types of bacteria is most likely to cause pneumonia in a patient with a history of alcohol abuse?
   a. *Legionella pneumophila*
   b. *Klebsiella pneumoniae*
   c. *Mycoplasma pneumoniae*
   d. *Chlamydia pneumoniae*
   e. *Diplococcus pneumoniae*

42. A 66-year-old male patient presents to his primary care clinic for a regular review of some routine blood tests. The tests reveal continued hypercholesterolemia. The patient inquires about the potential long-term consequences of this finding. Which of the following cardiovascular conditions is most strongly associated with hypercholesterolemia?
   a. abdominal aortic aneurysm
   b. giant cell arteritis
   c. Prinzmetal's angina
   d. deep vein thrombosis
   e. pulmonary embolism

43. Which of the following conditions most commonly leads to a Mallory-Weiss tear?
   a. alcohol abuse
   b. cocaine abuse
   c. anorexia nervosa
   d. bulimia nervosa
   e. hiatal hernia

44. A 36-year-old male presents with pain, swelling, and tenderness to palpation in the right ankle. The patient also presents with a fever. A synovial fluid exam is positive for the *Staphylococcus aureus* bacteria. Which of the following is the most likely diagnosis?
   a. septic arthritis
   b. reactive arthritis
   c. calcium pyrophosphate dihydrate disease
   d. gout
   e. osteomyelitis

45. A 39-year-old male, who has just returned from a vacation that involved both airplane travel and scuba diving, presents with severe pain in the inner ear. Which of the following is the most likely diagnosis?
   a. otitis externa
   b. central vertigo
   c. labyrinthitis
   d. barotrauma
   e. tympanic membrane rupture

46. A 45-year-old female presents with muscle weakness in the pelvic girdle and generalized bone pain. She has a history of several fractures stemming from minor traumas. X-rays reveal generalized decrease in bone density with Looser's lines. Blood work reveals vitamin D deficiency and a normal alkaline phosphatase level. Which of the following is the most likely diagnosis?
   a. osteomalacia
   b. rickets
   c. Paget's disease
   d. osteoporosis
   e. osteomyelitis

47. Which of the following types of tumors of the genitourinary system is resistant to radiation therapy?
   a. Wilms' tumor
   b. renal cell carcinoma
   c. nonseminomatous testicular tumor
   d. seminomatous testicular tumor
   e. pheochromocytoma

48. A Wood's light examination is useful to evaluate all of the following EXCEPT
   a. pigment changes.
   b. warts.
   c. ethylene glycol poisoning.
   d. fungal presence.
   e. bacterial presence.

49. Which of the following malignant disorders is a malignancy of plasma cells?
   a. multiple myeloma
   b. chronic lymphocytic leukemia
   c. Hodgkin's lymphoma
   d. acute myelogenous leukemia
   e. polycythemia vera

50. A 42-year-old male patient presents to his primary care clinic with a one-week history of hemoptysis. On further questioning, he reports that he has also experienced dyspnea on mild exertion. Urinalysis detects the presence of red blood cell casts, while blood tests reveal an elevated level of circulating antineutrophil cytoplasmic antibodies (c-ANCA), an antibody that is fairly specific for autoimmune vasculitis. Which of the following is the most appropriate treatment?
   a. antineoplastic chemotherapy
   b. radiotherapy
   c. cyclophosphamide therapy
   d. thrombolytic therapy
   e. antimicrobial therapy

51. A 13-year-old boy is brought to his primary care clinic by his mother because of a two-month history of severe pain in his left thigh that is most significant at the end of an active day. There is no recent history of trauma or illness. Physical examination reveals a tender, non-mobile soft tissue mass over the left femoral shaft with no notable erythema. An X-ray of the leg demonstrates a lytic lesion in the femoral diaphysis with poorly defined boundaries and invasion of neighboring soft tissue. A biopsy of the mass reveals dysplastic cells that are consistent with a sarcoma. Which of the following karyotypic abnormalities is most likely present?

a. trisomy 21
b. 47, XXY karyotype
c. (9,22) translocation
d. (11,22) translocation
e. (8,14) translocation

52. A four-year-old child is brought to the pediatrician by his mother because of a two-day history of right ear pain. For the past five days, he also has experienced an upper respiratory tract infection featuring low-grade fever and a sore throat, but the sore throat has mostly resolved. Physical examination reveals a fever of 38.5°C (101°F) as well as erythema in the middle ear cavity. Which of the following long-term consequences is most likely if no intervention is initiated?

a. sepsis
b. conjunctivitis
c. mastoiditis
d. meningitis
e. facial paralysis

53. A 46-year-old woman presents to her primary care clinic for follow-up after a biopsy of a breast lump. The biopsy reveals a stage 1 invasive ductal carcinoma. Which of the following receptor profiles is associated with the best expected response to pharmaceutical therapy?

a. estrogen receptor positive, progesterone receptor positive, HER2 positive
b. estrogen receptor positive, progesterone receptor positive, HER2 negative
c. estrogen receptor negative, progesterone receptor negative, HER2 positive
d. estrogen receptor negative, progesterone receptor negative, HER2 negative
e. estrogen receptor positive, progesterone receptor negative, HER2 negative

54. A 55-year-old woman presents to the emergency department with acute onset of a severe headache that she describes as "the worst headache that she has ever experienced." The headache first appeared while she was driving to work in the morning and reached its maximum intensity approximately 30 minutes later. She also experienced a bout of vomiting prior to leaving home, as well as considerable neck stiffness that is still present. Which of the following features in a lumbar puncture would be most suggestive of a diagnosis of intracranial hemorrhage over meningitis?

a. turbid cerebrospinal fluid
b. cloudy cerebrospinal fluid
c. bloody cerebrospinal fluid
d. high cerebrospinal fluid pressure
e. low cerebrospinal fluid pressure

55. A 23-year-old patient presents to his primary care clinic with a seven-hour history of a paroxysmal left lower eyelid twitch. He is unable to control the twitch, but he can feel a spasm in his lower eyelid. The episodes last approximately three to four seconds and are sporadic in nature, but occur approximately 20 to 30 times every hour. There is no associated photophobia or deterioration in visual acuity. On further questioning, he reports that he recently finished college and started a new job as a marketing intern; due to his desire to make a positive impression, he has been working long hours and staying up late at night to read industry journals. He usually drinks coffee during his late-night study sessions and his early-morning work hours, but he has not consumed any coffee today. He is otherwise healthy. Which of the following is the most likely cause of his symptoms?
   a. neuropathy
   b. vasospasm
   c. caffeine withdrawal
   d. blepharospasm
   e. stress and sleep deprivation

56. A 22-year-old male with a history of thrombocytopenia presents with petechiae on the skin and mucous membranes. He also complains of abnormal bleeding in the gums. Blood work reveals a decreased platelet count of 40,000/mcL. This patient has been diagnosed with thrombocytopenia and has been prescribed a steroid regimen which has failed. Which of the following treatment options would offer a definitive treatment for his disorder?
   a. increase his dose of prednisone
   b. immunosuppressive therapy
   c. stem cell transplantation
   d. splenectomy
   e. blood transfusion

57. A 43-year-old obese male patient with recently diagnosed noninsulin-dependent diabetes mellitus presents to his primary care clinic for an initial follow-up. His most recent HbA1c level was 6.8% (normal range <6.5%) and his physician has not yet initiated a management plan. Which of the following initial management strategies is most appropriate?
   a. metformin therapy
   b. glyburide therapy
   c. insulin therapy
   d. ACE inhibitor therapy
   e. diet and exercise regimen

58. A 49-year-old Asian man with a history of sleep apnea, tobacco use (15-pack-year), and daily alcohol use is found to have elevated blood pressure during three office visits in the past three months. His blood pressure has been in the 150s systolic and high 80s diastolic. He reports a family history of hypertension as well. He has tried diet and exercise without improvement. Which of the follow medications is the most appropriate treatment for him at this time?
   a. esomeprazole (Nexium)
   b. hydrochlorothiazide (HCTZ)
   c. aspirin
   d. clopidogrel (Plavix)
   e. zolpidem (Ambien)

59. An 83-year-old fair-skinned woman presents to her local family practitioner's office with a skin lesion on her ear. The lesion is difficult to see but is rough to the touch. The lesion is 7.0 mm in diameter. She reports having had similar lesions that were removed with cryotherapy. Which of the following is the most likely diagnosis?
a. melanoma
b. warts
c. discoid lupus
d. acne
e. actinic keratosis

60. A 55-year-old woman presents with acute onset of nausea and severe right flank pain that she describes as "the worst pain that she has ever experienced." The pain is colicky in nature, and she is unable to find a comfortable position. Abdominal X-ray shows a 1.5 cm nonuniform area of radiopacity superior to the right sacroiliac joint at the level of the L2/L3 vertebrae. In addition to acute pain relief, which of the following long-term therapy strategies will be beneficial for the most likely primary abnormality?
a. acidification of urine with L-methionine
b. alkalinization of urine with potassium citrate
c. reduction of uric acid production with allopurinol
d. control of infection with broad-spectrum antibiotics
e. control of infection with narrow-spectrum antibiotics

Section 2
Time: 60 minutes

61. A 73-year-old man presents with worsening of nighttime vision. He has increasing difficulty reading fine prints and road signs, prohibiting him from driving, which greatly affects his quality of life. An eye exam shows bilateral cataract formation. Which of the following is the most appropriate intervention?
a. prescription glasses
b. no intervention is indicated at this time
c. cataract surgery
d. vitamin C and E supplementation
e. eye drops with artificial tears

62. When a three-month-old boy is brought to his local primary care clinic by his mother for regular vaccinations, the clinician notices that he appears to be suffering from mild respiratory distress, including tachypnea and peripheral cyanosis. On further questioning, his mother reports that he occasionally becomes breathless after a few seconds of crying. Examination is significant for a continuous machine-like murmur that is loudest over the left sternal border, immediately inferior to the clavicle. Which of the following is the most likely site of the primary abnormality?
a. ductus arteriosus
b. foramen ovale
c. interventricular foramen
d. aortic valve
e. pulmonary valve

63. A 16-year-old female patient visits her primary care clinic to request a "cervical cancer vaccine." During the initial consultation, she asks about the etiology of cervical cancer. Which of the following subtypes of human papillomavirus are most likely to be carcinogenic?

   a. 6, 11
   b. 6, 18
   c. 11, 16
   d. 11, 18
   e. 16, 18

64. A 38-year-old patient with a nine-year history of systemic lupus erythematosus presents to her primary care clinic complaining of a four-day history of dysuria. Which of the following additional signs and symptoms is most suggestive of glomerular basement membrane disease?

   a. incontinence
   b. hypertension
   c. vaginal bleeding
   d. hematuria
   e. fever

65. A 12-year-old girl is brought to her primary care clinic for investigation of a four-month history of muscle cramps and tingling sensations in her toes. Her height has also been below average for most of her life. Physical examination reveals decreased sensation in her lower extremities. Relevant laboratory findings include decreased levels of calcium and phosphate as well as elevated levels of parathyroid hormone. Which of the following is the most likely diagnosis?

   a. primary hyperparathyroidism
   b. primary hypoparathyroidism
   c. pseudohypoparathyroidism
   d. hypopituitarism
   e. hyperpituitarism

66. A 61-year-old man with a 50-pack-year smoking history is diagnosed with chronic obstructive bronchitis. Which of the following signs or symptoms is LEAST consistent with this diagnosis?

   a. productive cough
   b. dyspnea
   c. clubbing
   d. barrel chest
   e. orthopnea

67. Which of the following radiologic procedures is the gold standard for diagnosing abnormalities of the testicles?

   a. testicular ultrasound
   b. nuclear medicine testicular scan
   c. CT angiogram of the testicles
   d. MRI angiogram of the testicles
   e. X-ray of the pelvis

68. A 78-year-old Asian woman with a history of peptic ulcer disease, previous stroke at age 70, hypertension, and diabetes mellitus has been diagnosed with atrial fibrillation (A-fib). She is complaining of occasional discomfort around her chest area. Which of the following is the most appropriate treatment for her atrial fibrillation?

   a. aspirin
   b. warfarin (Coumadin)
   c. hydrochlorothiazide (HCTZ)
   d. β-blockers
   e. none of the above

69. A 15-year-old boy with a history of mild, intermittent asthma presents to your clinic with acute asthma exacerbation. He ran out of his usual medication a few weeks ago. Which of the following is the most appropriate clinical intervention?

a. short-acting bronchodilator: inhaled beta2-agonist

b. inhaled corticosteroids

c. long-acting bronchodilator: inhaled beta2-agonist

d. oxygen via nasal cannula

e. none of the above

70. A 61-year-old African-American patient presents with a two-day history of worsening left lower quadrant (LLQ) abdominal pain. She reports having chronic constipation. Her physical exam is significant for a 100°F temperature and LLQ tenderness to deep palpation. You suspect that this patient has diverticulitis. Which of the following is the most appropriate prophylactic treatment at this time?

a. ciprofloxacin and metronidazole

b. amoxicillin

c. acetaminophen (Tylenol)

d. oxycodone

e. metronidazole

71. A 63-year-old woman presents complaining of headaches. Her headaches are unilateral and are accompanied with visual disturbances. She also reports some jaw claudication. On examination she has tenderness over her temporal artery. She is suspected to have giant cell arteritis and is scheduled for a biopsy. Which laboratory result would most correlate with this clinical presentation?

a. elevated platelet count

b. reduced platelet count

c. elevated erythrocyte sedimentation rate

d. reduced erythrocyte sedimentation rate

e. reduced interleukin-6

72. A 27-year-old athlete sustained an acute injury while playing football. An X-ray shows a mid-shaft, complete fracture of the left femur. Which of the following is the most appropriate intervention/treatment?

a. splinting and observation

b. splinting, pain management, and observation

c. nonsteroidal anti-inflammatory drugs (NSAIDs)

d. surgical repair with internal fixation

e. physical therapy

73. A 62-year-old HIV negative man with a history of chronic obstructive pulmonary disease (COPD) and poorly controlled type 2 diabetes mellitus presents with a complaint of odynophagia for the past few weeks. He takes daily an inhaled corticosteroid for COPD. Your oral exam shows white plaques on his buccal mucosa, palate, and oropharynx. Which of the following is the most likely diagnosis?

a. thrush

b. tonsillitis

c. gastroesophageal reflux disease (GERD)

d. aphthous ulcers

e. cheilitis

74. A 25-year-old G0 woman presents with a painful left breast lump. She is concerned because the lump seems to have gotten larger and more painful for the past few days since her menstruation started this month. On exam, you find no contour change or nipple discharge from either breast. A firm, smooth, and round mass of 1x2 cm in size is located in the upper outer quadrant of the left breast. Which of the following is the most likely diagnosis?

a. fibroadenoma

b. carcinoma

c. hematoma

d. fibrocystic change

e. fat necrosis

75. A 67-year-old man has recently been diagnosed with benign prostatic hypertrophy (BPH). Which of the following is the most appropriate treatment for his condition?
  a. ciprofloxicin
  b. NSAIDs (nonsteroidal anti-inflammatory drugs)
  c. allopurinol
  d. tamsulosin
  e. fluticasone propionate

76. A 66-year-old Asian man presents with a five-month history of weight loss, night sweats, and dry cough. On exam, the patient is afebrile, slightly malnourished, and has decreased lung sound in the left upper lung field. An X-ray shows apical cavitations in the left upper lung field. Acid-fast bacilli are present on a sputum smear. Which of the following is the most likely diagnosis?
  a. seasonal influenza
  b. pulmonary tuberculosis (TB)
  c. lung cancer
  d. malaria
  e. chronic obstructive pulmonary disease (COPD)

77. A 71-year-old female presents with gross hematuria and flank pain. A physical examination reveals a palpable mass in the affected flank. Laboratory test results and diagnostic studies lead to a diagnosis of localized renal cell carcinoma without metastases. Which of the following treatments is required to adequately treat this disorder?
  a. radiation therapy
  b. chemotherapy
  c. hormonal therapy
  d. radical nephrectomy
  e. cryosurgery

78. A 56-year-old female patient with a five-year history of diabetes mellitus presents to her primary care clinic for a regular review of her management. At the end of the consultation, the patient asks about the purpose of the ophthalmoscopic examination. Which of the following abnormalities that typically leads to diabetic retinopathy is checked for in the ophthalmoscopic examination?
  a. papilledema
  b. optic neuropathy
  c. vascular occlusion
  d. vascular wall compromise
  e. macular degeneration

79. A 47-year-old obese Caucasian female presents with sudden onset of chest tightness radiating to her left arm, along with nausea. A chest X-ray is normal, and an electrocardiogram reveals normal sinus rhythm with ST segment elevation. Troponin level is 0.4. D-dimer level is 0.24. Pulse oximetry is normal at 100% at room air. Blood pressure is 180/80 mmHg. Which of the following is the most appropriate diagnostic study to perform next?
  a. CT scan with contrast of the chest to rule out pulmonary embolism
  b. coronary angiography to evaluate for myocardial infarction
  c. myocardial perfusion scan to evaluate for myocardial infarction
  d. echocardiogram to evaluate cardiac function
  e. CT scan with contrast of the abdomen to rule out aortic dissection

80. A 43-year-old obese female presents with progressive shortness of breath and excessive cough with sputum production. Auscultation of the chest reveals decreased breath sounds, early inspiratory crackles, and prolonged expiration. A chest X-ray reveals hyperinflation and flat diaphragm. Which of the following is the most likely diagnosis?
  a. pneumonia
  b. asthma
  c. bronchiectasis
  d. chronic obstructive pulmonary disease (COPD)
  e. cystic fibrosis

81. A 62-year-old obese male (BMI 32) with past medical history of poorly controlled hypertension, sleep apnea, and 30-pack-year tobacco use presents with bilateral ankle edema, dyspnea, fatigue, and cough. You diagnosed him with congestive heart failure (CHF). He subsequently received medical treatment and has been stable and asymptomatic for the past six months. Which of the following lifestyle modifications would you recommend at this time?
  a. low-salt diet (<2g sodium or <5g of salt per day)
  b. moderate physical activity
  c. tobacco cessation
  d. diet low in fat and high in fruits and vegetables
  e. all of the above

82. In which of the following conditions has the medication ribavirin been proven effective in reducing mortality in children?
  a. Tetralogy of Fallot
  b. epiglottitis
  c. bronchiolitis
  d. hyaline membrane disease
  e. respiratory distress syndrome

83. Which of the following accurately describes the Centor Criteria?
  a. lack of fever, tender anterior cervical adenopathy, productive cough, and pharyngotonsillar exudates
  b. lack of fever, tender anterior cervical adenopathy, lack of cough, and pharyngotonsillar exudates.
  c. fever of greater than 100.4°F, tender anterior cervical adenopathy, lack of cough, and pharyngotonsillar exudates.
  d. fever of greater than 100.4°F, tender anterior cervical adenopathy, productive cough, and pharyngotonsillar exudates.
  e. fever of greater than 100.4°F, no tender anterior cervical adenopathy, non-productive cough, and pharyngotonsillar exudates.

84. A 32-year-old women presents with lethargy and constipation. A diagnosis of hypothyroidism is considered. Which of the following signs or symptoms is most consistent with this diagnosis?
  a. tachycardia
  b. diarrhea
  c. weight gain
  d. diaphoresis
  e. exophthalmos

85. Clomiphene citrate is commonly used for which of the following?
  a. ectopic pregnancy
  b. infertility
  c. oral contraception
  d. transdermal contraception
  e. emergency contraception

86. Which of the following types of stroke is associated with evidence of brain stem dysfunction such as coma, drop attacks, vertigo, nausea, vomiting, and ataxia?
- **a.** stroke involving anterior circulation
- **b.** stroke involving posterior circulation
- **c.** transient ischemic attack (TIA)
- **d.** hemorrhagic stroke
- **e.** thrombotic stroke

87. Light therapy is indicated for treatment of which of the following psychological disorders?
- **a.** obsessive-compulsive disorder (OCD)
- **b.** melancholia
- **c.** seasonal affective disorder (SAD)
- **d.** atypical depression
- **e.** catatonic depression

88. Which of the following mechanisms does the medication minoxidil use to promote hair growth?
- **a.** increasing the number of white blood cells
- **b.** increasing the number of red blood cells
- **c.** vasoconstriction
- **d.** vasodilation
- **e.** inhibiting bacterial growth

89. An 11-month-old boy is brought to the primary care physician by his mother, who is concerned about his reduced exercise tolerance. She reports that he becomes breathless and blue around his lips after crying, eating, or any mild exercise. On further questioning, she mentions that he also has a tendency to squat after he experiences the symptoms. Physical examination is significant for a systolic murmur that is loudest over the superior end of the left sternal border. Which of the following anatomical structures is most likely to be unaffected by this condition?
- **a.** pulmonary valve
- **b.** right ventricular myocardium
- **c.** ascending aorta
- **d.** interventricular septum
- **e.** pulmonary artery

90. A 63-year-old male Japanese immigrant presents with a mild cough productive of pale yellow sputum. He has unintentionally lost 2 kg (4.4 lbs) of weight in the past four months and has also experienced moderate night sweats over the same time period. He has a 25 pack-year smoking history, but he has not smoked for the past 22 years. His FEV_1/FVC ratio is measured to be 71%, and a chest X-ray shows bilateral hilar lymphadenopathy along with an area of opacity in the right apical hemithorax. Which of the following is the most likely diagnosis?
- **a.** pulmonary fibrosis
- **b.** small-cell carcinoma of the lung
- **c.** sarcoidosis
- **d.** tuberculosis
- **e.** chronic obstructive pulmonary disease (COPD)

91. A 48-year-old male patient presents with a three-hour history of vomiting and constant severe epigastric pain that radiates through his abdomen to his back. He has an 18-year history of alcohol abuse, but has been otherwise well. Which of the following enzymes is most likely to be elevated?
   a. aspartate transaminase
   b. alanine transaminase
   c. gamma glutamyl transpeptidase
   d. lipase
   e. gastrin

92. A 22-year-old male presents with a 15-month history of occasional pelvic pain that varies in character and severity but is usually worst in the morning. There are no associated urinary symptoms, and he has no recent history of fevers or systemic infection. He recalls no specific trauma, but he does report that his paternal uncle has Crohn's disease. Physical examination is significant for tenderness in both sacroiliac joints. A pelvic X-ray demonstrates grade 1 sacroiliitis bilaterally. Which of the following is the most likely cause of the inflammation?
   a. trauma
   b. gonococcal arthritis
   c. psoriatic arthritis
   d. ankylosing spondylitis
   e. reactive arthritis

93. Which of the following conditions is commonly treated with diazepam?
   a. barotrauma
   b. acute vertigo
   c. motion sickness
   d. labyrinthitis
   e. presbycusis

94. A 63-year-old female patient presents to her primary care clinic complaining of progressively worsening pain in both knees. The pain is usually most severe in the evening and is exacerbated by walking. Physical examination is significant for antalgic gait and reduced range of movement. Her BMI is measured to be 23 kg/m². An X-ray demonstrates osteophyte formation in both knees. Which of the following lifestyle changes is most likely to be beneficial for improving these symptoms?
   a. weight loss
   b. weight-bearing exercise regimen
   c. exercise regimen focused on swimming
   d. increased dietary calcium
   e. increased sunlight exposure and vitamin D intake

95. A 42-year-old female presents to her primary care physician with a three-month history of amenorrhea and acne. On further questioning, she reports that she has experienced some hirsutism and easy bruising. Her past history includes severe rheumatoid arthritis (for which she is taking methotrexate, hydrocortisone, and naproxen), hypertension (for which she is taking hydrochlorothiazide), and use of an oral contraceptive pill. Physical examination is significant for hypertension, central obesity, peripheral edema, and abdominal striae. Blood tests reveal significant hyperglycemia. Which of the following drugs may be causing her symptoms?
   a. hydrochlorothiazide
   b. hydrocortisone
   c. methotrexate
   d. naproxen
   e. oral contraceptive pill

96. A 42-year-old male is brought to the emergency department by ambulance after he was involved in a motorcycle accident. He is alert and reports that he is experiencing excruciating pain in his lower lumbar spine. A neurologic examination reveals normal motor, sensory, and reflex function in his left leg, but he is unable to move his right leg. Which of the following sensory and reflex findings are likely to be present in his right leg?
  a. hyperactive reflexes, hyperactive sensation
  b. hyperactive reflexes, absent sensation
  c. absent reflexes, hyperactive sensation
  d. absent reflexes, absent sensation
  e. normal reflexes, normal sensation

97. A 53-year-old patient with Crohn's disease develops severe abdominal pain after a routine colonoscopy. An X-ray of his chest shows air under the diaphragm. Which of the following is the most reasonable clinical intervention?
  a. treatment with clarithromycin, amoxicillin, and lansoprazole
  b. IV infusion of infliximab
  c. IV infusion of corticosteroids
  d. immediate CT scan followed by a second colonoscopy
  e. immediate CT scan followed by surgery

98. A 36-year-old woman presents with secondary amenorrhea. A diagnosis of polycystic ovarian syndrome is considered. Which of the following signs or symptoms is NOT consistent with this diagnosis?
  a. BMI of 32
  b. acanthosis nigricans
  c. hirsutism
  d. male pattern baldness
  e. hypotension

99. A 72-year-old patient presents to his primary care clinic with a long history of progressively increasing exertional dyspnea and a productive cough. His past medical history is significant for 55-pack-years of smoking and 18 years of hypertension, which is effectively managed with propranolol and hydrochlorothiazide. Physical examination reveals a respiratory rate of 24, reduced air entry in both lung bases, and a bilateral wheeze. Pulmonary function testing finds an FEV_1/FVC ratio of 64%. Which of the following is most likely to improve this patient's symptoms?
  a. smoking cessation
  b. discontinuation of propranolol
  c. discontinuation of hydrochlorothiazide
  d. daily therapy with inhaled albuterol
  e. daily therapy with inhaled fluticasone

100. A 56-year-old male patient presents to the emergency department complaining of severe chest pain and dyspnea. Physical examination is significant for a blood pressure of 218/155 mmHg. Which of the following further physical examination findings is most suggestive of a diagnosis of malignant hypertension?
  a. irregular heartbeat
  b. hepatomegaly
  c. crackles in lung fields
  d. papilledema
  e. carotid bruit

101. A 23-year-old man is diagnosed with schizophrenia. Which of the following neurotransmitters is most closely associated with this condition?
  a. acetylcholine
  b. dopamine
  c. norepinephrine
  d. serotonin
  e. histamine

102. A 45-year-old woman presents to her physician with an irregular-shaped lesion on her right thigh. The lesion is 2.0 cm in diameter, elevated, asymmetric, and has multiple colors. It is considered to be a melanoma. Which of the following factors best reflects the prognosis of the disease?
  a. elevated erythrocyte sedimentation rate (ESR)
  b. elevated C-reactive protein (CRP)
  c. elevated prostate-specific antigen (PSA)
  d. depth of the lesion on biopsy
  e. vascularity of the lesion on biopsy

103. A 43-year-old woman who is HIV positive presents for a regular checkup. Her CD4 count is noted to be below 200/mm^3. She is considered to be at risk for *Pneumocystis* pneumonia. Which of the following would provide the most appropriate prophylaxis?
  a. ceftriaxone
  b. penicillin
  c. trimethoprim/sulfamethoxazole (TMP-SMX)
  d. vancomycin
  e. doxycycline

104. A chest X-ray reveals a shallow wedge-shaped opacity along the periphery of the lung. Which of the following is indicated by this X-ray?
  a. Hampton's hump
  b. apple core lesion
  c. Codman's triangle
  d. cookie cutter lesion
  e. crescent sign

105. A 44-year-old male with a history of alcoholism presents with epigastric pain that radiates to the back and is relieved when lying in the fetal position. Blood work reveals elevated lipase and amylase levels. Which of the following is the most likely diagnosis?
  a. esophageal varices
  b. acute pancreatitis
  c. chronic pancreatitis
  d. pancreatic neoplasm
  e. cholelithiasis

106. A 36-year-old female presents with proximal muscle weakness, dysphagia, and a heliotrope skin rash. Blood work reveals elevated levels of creatinine phosphokinase and aldolase. Which of the following is the most likely diagnosis?
  a. septic arthritis
  b. reactive arthritis
  c. calcium pyrophosphate dihydrate disease
  d. polymyositis
  e. multiple myeloma

107. A 48-year-old female presents with sudden, acute episodes of vertigo. Which of the following options would you suggest for treatment of this disorder?
  a. scopolamine
  b. meclizine
  c. dimenhydrinate
  d. diazepam
  e. adenosine

108. A follicle-stimulating hormone (FSH) level of 49 IU/mL is classically indicative for which of the following conditions?
  a. pregnancy
  b. ectopic pregnancy
  c. menopause
  d. ovarian cancer
  e. uterine cancer

109. A 52-year-old male patient presents to his primary care clinic for a routine checkup. During the consultation, he mentions that he has experienced occasional heart palpitations with no associated symptoms such as chest pain, dyspnea, or light-headedness. Physical examination is significant for a blood pressure of 100/72 mmHg, and auscultation reveals a click and a high-pitched murmur in late systole. The murmur is loudest at the apex. Which of the following is the most likely diagnosis?

    a. mitral valve stenosis

    b. mitral valve prolapse

    c. pulmonary valve stenosis

    d. pulmonary valve prolapse

    e. multiple valvular defects

110. A 66-year-old man presents to his primary care clinic complaining of lower abdominal discomfort. The pain is constant and is exacerbated by eating. On further questioning, he reports that he has also experienced constipation, lightheadedness, and a low-grade fever. Which of the following aspects of his medical history, if true, would most strongly support a provisional diagnosis of diverticulitis?

    a. recent travel to South America

    b. presence of similar symptoms in other members of his household

    c. past history of an intestinal bleed

    d. recent therapy with clindamycin

    e. recent abdominal surgery

111. A 13-year-old male patient is brought to his primary care clinic by his mother because of a persistent left-sided knee pain that has been present for the past three months. The pain appears to be more significant after his Little League baseball practices, but there is no clear history of significant trauma. On further questioning, she reports that he currently seems to be in the midst of a growth spurt. Physical examination demonstrates an area of soft tissue swelling immediately inferior to the patella in the affected knee. Which of the following is the most likely location of the primary pathologic process?

    a. patella

    b. tibia

    c. fibula

    d. tibialis anterior tendon

    e. patellar tendon

112. A 32-year-old female presents to her primary care clinic hoping to get advice regarding her recent history of depression. She has felt hopeless and amotivated since her four-year-old daughter died in an automobile accident two months earlier. During this time, she has also experienced a loss of appetite (and associated weight loss), general fatigue, persistent insomnia, and recurrent thoughts of suicide. She has no history of drug or alcohol abuse. Which of the following interventions is most appropriate for this patient?

    a. grief counseling

    b. daily fluoxetine

    c. electroconvulsive therapy

    d. nightly temazepam

    e. phototherapy

113. A 64-year-old male patient presents to his primary care clinic for consultation regarding two sun spots on his forehead. Both lesions have been present for a few years and appear to have grown progressively over time. A shave biopsy yields a diagnosis of actinic keratosis. Which of the following is the most likely consequence if the lesions are left untreated?
a. invasion of local tissue
b. development of malignant melanoma
c. development of lentigo maligna
d. development of squamous cell carcinoma
e. development of basal cell carcinoma

114. After a poor outcome during an open heart surgical procedure, you and a colleague are discussing the case in a crowded elevator, where the patient's name was inadvertently mentioned. Which federal regulation has been violated?
a. HIPAA
b. MIPPA
c. Patient Bill of Rights
d. EMTALA
e. Safe Medical Devices Act

115. An 81-year-old female presents with chest pain and shortness of breath. A physical examination and auscultation reveals a low intensity pulse in the carotid arteries. A chest X-ray shows fluid in the lungs. An echocardiogram reveals a calcified, poorly functioning aortic valve. Which of the following is the most likely diagnosis?
a. carotid stenosis
b. pericarditis
c. mitral valve prolapse
d. aortic stenosis
e. congestive heart failure

116. A 20-year-old female complains of unpredictable episodes of dyspnea and palpitations with mild dizziness that is worst when she is in a crowded place. Her symptoms started when she was a teenager and now occur with increased frequency. Each episode lasts for a few minutes and is relieved by deep breathing. Which of the following is the most likely diagnosis?
a. generalized anxiety disorder
b. delusional disorder
c. panic disorder
d. schizoid disorder
e. attention-deficit disorder

117. Pilocarpine is prescribed to treat which of the following conditions by increasing salivary flow?
a. Parkinson's disease
b. Meniere's disease
c. Sjögren's syndrome
d. Hashimoto's disease
e. Wilson's disease

118. Macrocytic anemias are characterized by mean corpuscular volume at which level?
a. 0–50 fL
b. 50–80 fL
c. <80 fL
d. 80–100 fL
e. >100 fL

119. A 47-year-old female who is being treated for gastroesophageal reflux disease (GERD), presents with symptoms of heartburn and regurgitation that are becoming progressively more severe. Histamine blockers have provided no relief of symptoms. Endoscopy reveals severe disease with evidence of erosive gastritis. Which of the following medications would you prescribe to manage this patient's GERD effectively?
   a. antacids
   b. proton pump inhibitors
   c. nitrates
   d. calcium channel blockers
   e. ACE inhibitors

120. A 40-year-old female presents with a throbbing, pulsating headache on the right side of her head. The patient states that her pain is also associated with nausea and light sensitivity. Based on the patient's presentation, which of the following is the most likely diagnosis?
   a. cerebral aneurysm
   b. subarachnoid hemorrhage
   c. cluster headache
   d. migraine headache
   e. tension headache

Section 3
Time: 60 minutes

121. A 39-year-old woman with polycystic ovarian syndrome presents with infertility. She is prescribed clomiphene. Which of the following is the mechanism of action of this drug?
   a. peripheral acting estrogen antagonist
   b. central acting dopamine agonist
   c. peripheral acting estrogen agonist
   d. central acting estrogen partial agonist
   e. peripheral acting progesterone antagonist

122. A 38-year-old male who is a recent immigrant from Nigeria presents complaining of significant exertional dyspnea. He was previously healthy, but his symptoms have progressively deteriorated over the course of the past three months, and he is now unable to walk up a flight of stairs without stopping. His past history is notable for a severe childhood illness in which he experienced persistent fever, sore throat, and arthralgia. Physical examination is notable for a heart murmur and mild pitting edema over the ankles. Which of the following is the most likely nature of the heart murmur?
   a. systolic murmur loudest over the apex
   b. systolic murmur loudest over the superior right sternal border
   c. diastolic murmur loudest over the apex
   d. diastolic murmur loudest over the superior right sternal border
   e. pansystolic murmur loudest over the inferior sternum

123. A 27-year-old man is diagnosed with Crohn's Disease, for which he commences a daily regimen of sulfasalazine along with prednisone to control acute flareups; this controls his symptoms effectively. He returns eight months later with eye pain, photophobia, and red sclerae. Which of the following is the most likely cause of these symptoms?
   a. allergic reaction to sulfasalazine
   b. corticosteroid-induced rash
   c. Cushingoid glaucoma
   d. keratoconjunctivitis
   e. uveitis

124. A 12-year-old male presents with cough, excess sputum, sinus pain, nasal discharge, diarrhea, and abdominal pain. A physical examination reveals clubbing and apical crackles. A high-resolution CT reveals bronchiectasis. A chest X-ray reveals hyperinflation and mucous plugging. Which of the following is the most likely diagnosis?
   a. pneumonia
   b. asthma
   c. bronchiectasis
   d. chronic obstructive pulmonary disease (COPD)
   e. cystic fibrosis

125. Which of the following is a gastrointestinal disorder that is characterized by the twisting of any part of the bowel on itself?
   a. volvulus
   b. celiac disease
   c. Crohn's disease
   d. bowel obstruction
   e. obstipation

126. A 62-year-old male patient presents to his primary care clinic after experiencing an episode of syncope while walking his dog. On further questioning, he reports that he has noticed progressively worsening exertional dyspnea over the past year. Physical examination is significant for a systolic ejection murmur that is loudest over the superior right sternal border. Which of the following investigations is most likely to confirm the diagnosis?
   a. troponin levels
   b. echocardiogram
   c. resting electrocardiogram
   d. exercise stress electrocardiogram
   e. chest X-ray

127. An 18-year old female with history of diarrhea, steatorrhea, weight loss, and weakness has a positive small bowel biopsy for celiac disease. To which of the following treatments must this patient adhere in order to avoid flareups from this disorder?
   a. lactose-free diet
   b. sugar-free diet
   c. gluten-free diet
   d. fat-free diet
   e. fructose-free diet

128. A 34-year-old female patient presents to her primary care clinic complaining of a thick white deposit covering most of her tongue. She first noticed the deposit three days earlier, and it appears to have grown progressively over that time period. Which of the following is the most appropriate treatment for her condition?
   a. intravenous amphotericin B
   b. oral amphotericin B tablets
   c. oral nystatin suspension
   d. oral penicillin tablets
   e. antibacterial mouthwash

129. A 67-year-old man with history of reflux esophagitis, chronic obstructive pulmonary disease (COPD), chronic hypertension, and hyperlipidemia presents to the emergency department complaining of left-sided chest pain for the past six hours. He appears diaphoretic and in acute distress. You suspect acute coronary syndrome. Which of the following laboratory markers are the most cardiac-specific?
   a. ESR
   b. D-dimer
   c. troponin I and T
   d. CK-MM
   e. WBC

130. A two-year-old girl is brought to the emergency department by her mother because of persisting tibial pain two hours after injuring the tibia in a fall. Her past history is significant for two fractures after minimal trauma; one fracture was in the left distal radius, while the other was in the shaft of the right humerus. Physical examination is significant for tenderness over the injured area, a blue-colored tint in the sclerae, and height at the tenth percentile for her age. Which of the following is the most likely basis for this patient's pathological process?
   a. viral infection
   b. calcium deficiency
   c. hyperparathyroidism
   d. autosomal dominant inheritance
   e. X-linked recessive inheritance

131. A 68-year-old man is brought to the emergency department complaining of pressure-like substernal pain for the past two hours. His past medical history includes hypertension, hyperlipidemia, and diabetes mellitus. An electrocardiogram (EKG) shows ST elevations in leads I and aVL. His initial lab result is positive for CK-MB. Your team confirms a diagnosis of acute ST-elevation myocardial infarction (STEMI). You have given him oxygen, morphine for pain, nitroglycerin, and aspirin. Which of the following is the most likely clinical intervention at this time?
   a. continue to observe
   b. electrocardioversion
   c. give a beta-blocker
   d. perform immediate chest compressions
   e. percutaneous coronary intervention (PCI)

132. A 16-year-old African-American teenager with a history of mild, intermittent asthma presents to your clinic with acute asthma exacerbation. He ran out of his usual bronchodilator a few weeks ago. You perform a physical exam. Which of the following is the most likely physical finding?
   a. clear bilateral lung sounds
   b. high-pitched wheezes more pronounced on expiration
   c. body temperature of 102°F
   d. no symptomatic relief after bronchodilator (albuterol) use
   e. none of the above

133. A 42-year-old man complains of frequent acid reflux and has been recently diagnosed with gastroesophageal reflux disease (GERD). His body mass index (BMI) is 36 kg/m², and he smokes one pack of cigarettes daily and drinks socially. Which of the following is the most likely preventative measure(s) you will include in your discussion with this patient?
a. weight loss
b. smoking cessation
c. avoid overeating
d. sitting upright for three hours before lying supine
e. all of the above

134. A 57-year-old post-menopausal woman has recently been diagnosed with osteoporosis on a bone density scan. In addition to increasing weight-bearing exercise, beginning calcium supplementation, and avoiding smoking and drugs that affect bone loss, which of the following is the most appropriate medical treatment?
a. Omega 3 fish oil
b. vitamin E
c. tamsulosin (Flomax)
d. bisphosphonates
e. estrogen replacement therapy

135. A 25-year-old G1 P0 woman who is in her first trimester presents complaining of spotting. On exam, her uterus appears larger than gestational age. You perform an ultrasound exam and see a "snowstorm" appearance. hCG is double the upper limits of normal. Which of the following is the most likely diagnosis?
a. normal pregnancy
b. hydatidiform mole (molar pregnancy)
c. spontaneous abortion
d. atopic pregnancy
e. preterm labor

136. A 68-year-old male presents post-coronary artery bypass graft surgery with pleuritic chest pain, dyspnea, and hemoptysis. An electrocardiogram reveals tachycardia and nonspecific ST-T wave changes. A chest X-ray reveals basilar atelectasis. Auscultation of the chest reveals crackles and accentuation of the pulmonary component of the second heart sound. Which of the following is the most likely diagnosis?
a. myocardial infarction
b. bronchiectasis
c. pulmonary hypertension
d. pulmonary embolism
e. cystic fibrosis

137. A 36-year-old woman, without significant past medical history, presents complaining of recurrent palpitations with chest pain, profuse sweating, and abdominal pain only when she is in a crowded and public place. The symptoms have gotten worse since she lost her daughter to a motor vehicle accident. Which of the following is the most appropriate initial workup for this patient?
a. complete metabolic panel (CMP)
b. complete blood count (CBC)
c. thyroid function tests (TFT)
d. electrocardiogram (ECG)
e. all of the above

138. A four-year-old boy presents with a perioral lesion for the past few days. On exam, there is an area of vesicles surrounded by erythema on the left corner of his mouth. The lesions resemble dew drops on a rose petal. Which of the following is the most likely diagnosis?
a. vitiligo
b. paronychia
c. acne vulgaris
d. impetigo
e. none of the above

139. A 65-year-old female without significant past medical history has her lab results as follows: RBC 4.2 (4.7–6.1 million cells/uL), H/H 10/33 (hemoglobin: 12–15 g/dl; hematocrit: 34–44%). MCV 110 (80–100 fl). MCH 1000 (200–900 ng/ml). Platelet count: 150K (150–400K/uL). Reticulocyte count 0.4% (0.5–2%). Peripheral blood smear shows megalocytes. Which of the following is the most likely diagnosis?
   a. iron deficiency anemia
   b. pernicious anemia
   c. aplastic anemia
   d. G6PD deficiency
   e. sickle cell anemia

140. A 55-year-old female presents with painful kyphosis with a curvature approximately 50 degrees. Which of the following treatment options would you prescribe?
   a. oral corticosteroids
   b. oral anti-inflammatory medications
   c. exercises prescribed for lumbar lordosis and the thoracic spine
   d. application of a Milwaukee brace
   e. surgical correction

141. Which of the following disorders is a Water's view X-ray useful in diagnosing?
   a. nasal fracture
   b. blow-out fracture of the orbital floor
   c. sinusitis
   d. mastoiditis
   e. rhinitis

142. Through which of the following mechanisms does magnesium sulfate work to treat preterm uterine contractions?
   a. decreases estrogen levels
   b. inhibits myometrial contractility mediated by calcium
   c. stimulates β-receptors to relax smooth muscle
   d. increases intracellular magnesium ions
   e. decreases intracelluar calcium ions

143. A 28-year-old male patient presents to his primary care clinic complaining of a one-day history of a sharp stinging sensation in his right eye. He has also experienced photophobia over the same time period. Fluorescein staining demonstrates a 2mm area of increased fluorescein uptake on the inferior aspect of the right cornea. Which of the following is the most likely diagnosis?
   a. keratitis
   b. uveitis
   c. corneal abrasion
   d. entropion
   e. Sjögren's syndrome

144. A 44-year-old female presents with a four-month history of fatigue, depressed mood, and 8 kg (18 lbs) of weight gain. On further questioning, she reports that she seems to have increased sensitivity to cold temperatures. Physical examination reveals a heart rate of 52 bpm and a blood pressure of 95/65 mmHg. Relevant laboratory findings include elevated thyroid-stimulating hormone (TSH) and normal free thyroxine. Which of the following further investigations is most likely to establish the diagnosis?

a. anti-TSH receptor antibody
b. antithyroid peroxidase antibody
c. pituitary MRI
d. pituitary hormones
e. thyroid ultrasound

145. A 38-year-old male presents with a four-day history of cough, purulent sputum, shortness of breath, chest pain, fever, and sweats. Auscultation of the chest reveals altered breath sounds with crackles, dullness to percussion, and bronchial breath sounds over an area of consolidation. A chest X-ray reveals bilateral pleural consolidations. Which of the following is the most likely diagnosis?

a. chronic obstructive pulmonary disease (COPD)
b. acute bronchitis
c. acute epiglottitis
d. tuberculosis
e. pneumonia

146. A 38-year-old female presents to the emergency department with acute onset of dyspnea, hemoptysis, and pain that is exacerbated by breathing. On further questioning, she mentions that she recently returned from a trip to Japan, after which she experienced swelling and pain in her right calf. Which of the following investigations is most likely to help confirm the diagnosis?

a. full blood count
b. chest X-ray
c. CT pulmonary angiogram
d. spirometry
e. methacholine challenge test

147. A 45-year-old man is found to have left ventricular dysfunction after a non-ST-elevation myocardial infarction (NSTEMI). He is given an antihypertensive medication that also decreases remodeling of heart tissue. Which drug fits this description?

a. atropine
b. thiazide
c. nifedipine
d. ramipril
e. prazosin

148. A 54-year-old male patient with pancreatic cancer asks for advice regarding his therapeutic options. He has been told by his oncologist that excision of the cancer would require removal of all tissue supplied by the gastroduodenal artery. Which of the following structures will remain intact after the procedure?

a. gastric antrum
b. gallbladder
c. duodenum
d. jejunum
e. common bile duct

149. A 24-year-old woman with a seven-year history of partial epilepsy presents to her primary care physician for family planning. She is currently taking valproate regularly, but she hopes to become pregnant in the near future and expresses concerns based on some online research that suggested the possibility of neural tube defects with valproate therapy. Which of the following measures is most appropriate?

   a. reassure her that control of her epilepsy with valproate is necessary for the safety of her child
   b. add folate supplementation to the current valproate regimen
   c. reduce dosage of valproate
   d. discontinue valproate during the pregnancy
   e. switch medication to carbamazepine

150. A 16-year-old female volleyball player presents with a five-month history of amenorrhea. On further questioning, she reports that she has been feeling lethargic recently, and her volleyball performance has consequently deteriorated. On physical examination, she is found to have a BMI of 17 kg/m^2 and no other significant signs. Which of the following is the most likely diagnosis?

   a. pregnancy
   b. anorexia nervosa
   c. bulimia nervosa
   d. depression
   e. iron deficiency

151. A 36-year-old man of Irish descent presents with a painless, somewhat shiny red nodule on his forehead. On further questioning, he mentions that he spent four years working as a lifeguard on a beach in Florida after high school, but now works as a restaurant manager. He first noticed the nodule three years ago, but it appears to have grown since then; its current diameter is 1.2 cm. Which of the following is the most likely long-term consequence if the nodule is left untreated?

   a. distant metastasis
   b. local metastasis
   c. local growth of the nodule
   d. local infection
   e. sepsis

152. A 31-year-old man with Marfan syndrome presents with chest pain. He describes the pain as persistent tearing radiating to his back. The patient also has a history of hypertension. On physical examination, the patient is tachycardic (103/min) and tachypneic (23/min). He has radial-radial delay and a systolic murmur radiating to his carotids. A chest X-ray shows widening of the aortic arch. He is referred for immediate surgical intervention. An electrocardiogram shows no specific changes. Which of the following is the most likely diagnosis?

   a. dissection of the proximal aorta
   b. dissection of the distal aorta
   c. abdominal aortic aneurism
   d. ST-elevation myocardial infarction (STEMI)
   e. non-ST-elevation myocardial infarction (NSTEMI)

153. A 32-year-old woman presents for treatment of her diabetes. She is unsure whether she has type 1 or type 2. Which of the following tests would best rule out type 1 diabetes?
  a. elevated C-peptide levels
  b. elevated blood glucose
  c. decreased blood glucose
  d. elevated urine glucose
  e. elevated HbA1c

154. A 42-year-old woman presents with renal failure. She is prescribed furosemide. Which of the following is the site of action of this drug?
  a. thin descending loop
  b. thick ascending loop
  c. proximal convoluted tubule
  d. distal convoluted tubule
  e. cortical collecting duct

155. A 71-year-old woman presents with blisters in her mouth and on her face and axilla. The skin easily peels off when pressure is applied. A diagnosis of pemphigus is considered. Which of the following best represents the pathogenesis of this disease?
  a. IgG against basal lamina
  b. IgG against interepidermal junctions
  c. IgE mediated degranulation
  d. Rheumatoid factor
  e. Anti-dsDNA

156. Which of the following gastrointestinal disorders is commonly treated by decreasing alcohol consumption?
  a. cirrhosis
  b. diverticulitis
  c. chronic pancreatitis
  d. acute cholecystitis
  e. chronic cholecystitis

157. A 40-year-old male presents with facial pain while eating. He also states he feels a click or pop in his jaw while he eats. There is no history of head or facial trauma. He does not take bisphosphonate medications. Which of the following is the most likely diagnosis?
  a. whiplash
  b. extension injury of the cervical spine
  c. temporomandibular joint disorder
  d. rheumatoid spondylitis
  e. jaw osteonecrosis

158. A four-year-old male, brought by his mother, presents with sudden high fever, difficulty swallowing, sore throat, and drooling. A lateral X-ray of the neck shows a so-called "thumb sign." Based on this information, which of the following is the most likely diagnosis?
  a. croup
  b. epiglottitis
  c. esophageal obstruction
  d. tracheal obstruction
  e. acute parotitis

159. A 52-year-old female presents with generalized bone and muscle pain. Blood values reveal markedly elevated serum calcium levels. A nuclear medicine parathyroid exam reveals the presence of a parathyroid adenoma. Which of the following courses of treatment would you prescribe for this disorder?
  a. radiation therapy
  b. chemotherapy
  c. hormonal therapy
  d. surgical removal
  e. oral prednisone

160. A 20-year-old female presents with a history of complaints of signs and symptoms of several diseases and trying to be admitted to the hospital for these diseases by assuming several different names. Full workup including blood work and radiographic study fail to find any clinical explanation for the symptoms she is claiming. Which of the following is the most likely diagnosis?
 a. hypochondriasis
 b. somatization disorder
 c. body dysmorphic disorder
 d. conversion disorder
 e. factitious disorder

161. A 65-year-old male patient presents to his primary care clinic for a regular checkup. He has a four-year history of open-angle glaucoma and increased intraocular pressure, which has been managed with regular timolol eye drops. Physical examination is notable for a blood pressure of 165/105 mmHg and a heart rate of 102 bpm. If a daily regimen of oral atenolol is commenced, which of the following potential effects is most likely to occur as a result of a drug interaction?
 a. increased half-life of atenolol
 b. decreased half-life of atenolol
 c. hepatotoxicity
 d. metabolic alkalosis
 e. heart block

162. A 71-year-old male presents to his primary care clinic complaining of a long history of progressively worsening exertional dyspnea and dry cough. Which of the following additional features in his clinical history, if true, would be most suggestive of pulmonary fibrosis?
 a. 50-pack-year smoking history
 b. history of recurrent pneumonia
 c. history of chronic obstructive pulmonary disease (COPD)
 d. former employment in a shipyard
 e. family history of autoimmune disease

163. A 28-year-old female immigrant from India presents to her primary care clinic for a follow-up after a series of blood tests to investigate her fertility. While her results were mostly normal, a deficiency of Vitamin D was noted. On further questioning, she reports that she avoids sun exposure in order to preserve her complexion. Which of the following potential consequences can be avoided with dietary vitamin D supplementation or increased sunlight exposure in this patient?
 a. osteoporosis
 b. osteoarthritis
 c. osteomalacia
 d. osteopenia
 e. rickets

164. A 24-year-old female presents to her primary care clinic with a four-day history of diffuse lower abdominal pain that is exacerbated with deep inhalation. She has also experienced a fever and a vaginal discharge over the same time period. On further questioning, she reports that she is sexually active with multiple partners and uses the oral contraceptive pill. Her last menstrual period was approximately one week earlier. Physical examination reveals lower abdominal tenderness with no guarding. β-hCG is negative. Which of the following is the most likely diagnosis?
   a. ectopic pregnancy
   b. endometriosis
   c. pelvic inflammatory disease
   d. vaginal candidiasis
   e. bacterial vaginosis

165. A 67-year-old male patient with a ten-year history of diabetes mellitus (type 2) presents to his primary care clinic for a review of glycemic control. Although his condition has been managed with only lifestyle changes thus far, his HbA1c level is measured at 7.4% (normal <6.5%) and his blood pressure is 165/95 mmHg. Urinalysis reveals microalbuminuria and a mild increase in creatinine levels. Which of the following drug regimens is most appropriate for management of this patient's diabetes and hypertension?
   a. metformin and ramipril
   b. metformin and hydrochlorothiazide
   c. glyburide and ramipril
   d. glyburide and hydrochlorothiazide
   e. insulin

166. A three-year-old boy is brought to the emergency department by his mother after a severe arm injury caused by a fall onto his outstretched hand. She reports that she was at work for most of the day, but the boy's father witnessed the accident. Physical examination reveals pain and tenderness over the shaft of the right humerus. Which of the following subsequent actions is most appropriate if child abuse is suspected?
   a. immediately contacting local legal authorities
   b. full body X-ray
   c. right arm X-ray only
   d. genetic screen for osteogenesis imperfecta and von Willebrand's disease
   e. detailed medical history from the boy's father

167. A 62-year-old HIV-negative Asian female presents to your clinic complaining of recent weight loss, fatigue, night sweats, and recurrent cough. You order a chest X-ray and find cavitations in the apex of the right lung. An acid-fast bacilli on smear of sputum is positive for *M. tuberculosis*. Which of the following is the most appropriate treatment?
   a. six-month regimen of isoniazid, rifampin, pyrazinamide, and ethambutol
   b. nine-month regimen of pyrazinamide and ethambutol
   c. twelve-month regimen of isoniazid and rifampin
   d. nine-month regimen of doxycycline, clarithromycin, and metronadizole (Flagyl)
   e. none of the above

168. A 25-year-old male patient presents to his primary care clinic with a three-day history of dysuria and a urethral discharge. He is otherwise well and has no significant past medical history. Which of the following additional findings would be most suggestive of a diagnosis of gonorrhea rather than reactive arthritis?
   a. uveitis
   b. sacroiliitis
   c. knee arthritis
   d. wrist arthritis
   e. fever

169. A 27-year-old male African-American patient presents to the emergency department with acute-onset shortness of breath at rest. He has experienced no chest pain and has no past history of coronary artery disease, hypercholesterolemia, or drug or alcohol abuse. He has recently commenced a regimen of trimethoprim/sulfamethoxazole for a urinary tract infection. Physical examination is significant for scleral icterus, and a urine sample is visibly blood-tinged. Which of the following is the most likely cause of this reaction?
   a. sickle cell disease
   b. sepsis
   c. reaction to trimethoprim/sulfamethoxazole
   d. autoimmune hemolytic anemia
   e. malaria

170. Osteomalacia and rickets are most often caused by a deficiency of which of the following vitamins?
   a. vitamin B6
   b. vitamin B12
   c. vitamin C
   d. vitamin D
   e. vitamin E

171. A 12-year-old male presents with tenderness, redness, and purulent drainage of the penis. The patient also complains of obstructed urinary stream and inability to retract the foreskin over the glans penis. Your diagnosis is phimosis. Which of the following is the proper treatment for symptomatic phimosis?
   a. no treatment required, will resolve when patient gets older
   b. application of steroidal creams
   c. oral antibiotics
   d. circumcision
   e. topical anti-inflammatories

172. A 47-year-old man is infected with hospital-acquired methicillin-resistant Staphylococcus aureus after an appendectomy. He is treated with vancomycin. Which of the following is a possible side effect of this medication?
   a. flushing
   b. aplastic anemia
   c. phototoxicity
   d. pulmonary fibrosis
   e. drug-induced lupus

173. A 37-year-old female patient presents to her primary care clinician with a two-week history of occasional severe pelvic pain accompanied by heavy menstrual bleeding. The pain is exacerbated by tactile pressure, but does not appear to be triggered by any particular stimulus. Physical examination is unremarkable, but gynecologic ultrasonography reveals focal masses in the uterus. Which of the following is the most likely diagnosis?
   a. uterine sarcoma
   b. uterine leiomyomata
   c. endometriosis
   d. endometrial carcinoma
   e. ectopic pregnancy

174. A 36-year-old man presents with severe, unilateral, periorbital headaches lasting from 60 to 90 minutes several times a day over the past six weeks. A physical exam reveals myosis and ptosis. The patient states that lying down makes his headaches worse. Which of the following is the most likely diagnosis?
   a. subarachnoid hemorrhage
   b. cluster headache
   c. migraine headache
   d. tension headache
   e. cerebral aneurysm

175. A 78-year-old male presents with a history of dizziness and loss of consciousness during urination. All lab values are within normal limits, his chest X-ray is normal, and CT scans of his chest, abdomen, and pelvis are all within normal limits. Which of the following is the most likely diagnosis?
   a. septicemia
   b. vasovagal reaction
   c. micturition syncope
   d. orthostatic hypotension
   e. transient ischemic attack

176. A premature infant (31 weeks gestation) is found to have increased work of breathing and a low heart rate after delivery. After emergency intubation, which of the following interventions is most likely to resolve the patient's symptoms?
   a. thoracentesis
   b. intravenous indomethacin
   c. surfactant via endotracheal tube
   d. inhaled albuterol
   e. intravenous antibiotic therapy

177. A newborn infant male presents with cyanosis, acidosis, and tachypnea at birth. An echocardiogram reveals tricuspid regurgitation. Auscultation of the chest reveals a hyperdyanamic apical impulse and a single S1 and S2 sound. Which of the following is the most likely diagnosis?
   a. pulmonary atresia
   b. Tetralogy of Fallot
   c. hypoplastic left heart syndrome
   d. transposition of the great vessels
   e. hyaline membrane disease

178. Which of the following is the preferred radiologic imaging modality in order to differentiate between ischemic and hemorrhagic strokes?
   a. PET scan
   b. CT scan
   c. angiogram
   d. ultrasound
   e. MRI

179. A 77-year-old female patient is brought to her primary care clinic by her son two days after she sustains a fall from standing height in her home. She denies any significant pain related to the trauma, but her son expresses concerns about her risk of future falls. Physical examination is unremarkable. Her current medication regimen includes furosemide for hypertension, atorvastatin for hypercholesterolemia, warfarin for atrial fibrillation, alendronate for osteoporosis, and fluoxetine for mild depression since the passing of her husband eight months earlier. Which of these drugs has the strongest influence on her risk of future falls?
   a. furosemide
   b. atorvastatin
   c. warfarin
   d. alendronate
   e. fluoxetine

180. A 56-year-old woman with a 40-pack-year cigarette smoking history presents for a regular checkup. She mentions that she has a mild chronic productive cough and occasional exertional dyspnea, but she is not currently in respiratory distress. On spirometry, her FEV_1/FVC ratio is found to be 65% (normal range 70%–80%). Which of the following actions is most likely to improve her long-term prognosis independently with regard to respiratory function?
   a. smoking cessation
   b. aerobic exercise program
   c. bronchodilator therapy
   d. inhaled corticosteroid therapy
   e. chemotherapy

Section 4
Time: 60 minutes

181. A 42-year-old woman has drug-induced lupus. Which of the following antibodies is expected to be present in her blood?
   a. anti-dsDNA
   b. anti-centromere
   c. anti-streptolysin O
   d. anti-IgM
   e. anti-histone

182. The medication ursodiol is an effective treatment for which of the following gastrointestinal disorders?
   a. gallstones
   b. diverticulitis
   c. ulcerative colitis
   d. pancreatitis
   e. hepatitis

183. A nine-year-old boy is brought to his primary care clinic by his mother with concerns about his short stature. Physical examination is significant for height at the fifth percentile for his age. Additionally, he is found to have a bitemporal hemianopia. Which of the following investigations is most likely to provide a diagnosis?
   a. slit lamp examination
   b. MRI of the pituitary
   c. pituitary hormone levels
   d. nutritional assessment
   e. inflammatory markers

184. A 36-year-old pregnant female at 23 weeks gestation presents to the emergency department in labor. Her contractions are approximately 10 minutes apart, and she has noticed a watery discharge from her vagina. Gynecologic examination reveals cervical dilation and effacement. Which of the following is the most likely prognosis of the infant?

   a. normal growth with no disability

   b. mild to moderate disability with full life expectancy

   c. severe disability with full life expectancy

   d. life expectancy of one to six years

   e. life expectancy of less than one year

185. A two-year-old boy is brought to his primary care clinic by his mother for travel vaccinations. He appears mostly healthy, but excessive bruising is noticed in multiple areas on his upper and lower limbs. His mother reports that he tends to bruise easily with minimal trauma. A complete blood count shows normal levels of platelets; coagulation studies reveal normal prothrombin time, increased activated partial thromboplastin time, and increased bleeding time. Which of the following is the most likely diagnosis?

   a. hemophilia A

   b. hemophilia B

   c. von Willebrand's disease

   d. vitamin K deficiency

   e. child abuse

186. A 34-year-old female immigrant from Thailand presents to her primary care clinic with a three-month history of a progressive cough productive of yellow sputum. On further questioning, she recalls that she has also experienced night sweats and 5 kg (11 lbs) of weight loss over the same time period. Physical examination reveals decreased breath sounds in the left upper lung lobe. A chest X-ray shows a solitary pulmonary nodule in the left upper hemithorax. Which of the following microbiological tests is most appropriate?

   a. sputum Gram stain

   b. sputum coagulase test

   c. sputum acid fast stain

   d. blood culture

   e. hilar lymph node biopsy and culture

187. A seven-year-old overweight female patient is brought to the emergency department with acute onset of dyspnea with no associated cough or fever. On further questioning, her parents report that she has a history of atopic eczema, which has been treated with topical hydrocortisone. Examination is significant for an elevated respiratory rate and a bilateral wheeze. After treatment with inhaled albuterol, her symptoms improve markedly. Which of the following forms of regular therapy is most likely to prevent any future episodes?

   a. daily inhaled albuterol

   b. daily inhaled fluticasone and salmeterol

   c. daily oral prednisone

   d. daily oral antihistamines

   e. weight loss

188. A 55-year-old woman is given a regimen of amiodarone for management of a tachyarrhythmia that is nonresponsive to other forms of therapy. Which of the following investigations should be monitored regularly in order to detect early signs of potential amiodarone-related toxicity?
- **a.** full blood count
- **b.** blood urea nitrogen and creatinine levels
- **c.** plasma electrolyte levels
- **d.** liver enzyme levels
- **e.** pancreatic enzyme levels

189. A pediatric X-ray reveals a so-called rachitic rosary abnormality. Which of the following is this abnormality associated with?
- **a.** cardiomyopathy
- **b.** hyaline membrane disease
- **c.** rickets
- **d.** croup
- **e.** epiglottitis

190. A 31-year-old woman presents with pelvic inflammatory disease (PID). Which of the following is the most common cause of this condition?
- **a.** autoimmune disease
- **b.** radiation exposure
- **c.** HPV infection
- **d.** chlamydia infection
- **e.** cardiovascular compromise

191. A nine-year-old boy is brought to the emergency department by his mother after he experiences a fall onto his outstretched hand. If there is a fracture in his forearm, which of the following is the most likely site?
- **a.** distal radius
- **b.** distal ulna
- **c.** proximal radius
- **d.** proximal ulna
- **e.** carpal bones

192. A patient asks you about the function of vitamin D. Which of the following is the best response?
- **a.** It helps you to stop bleeding.
- **b.** It maintains your vision.
- **c.** It strengthens your bones.
- **d.** It helps your body to use fat.
- **e.** It helps your body to use sugars.

193. A-38 year-old Caucasian woman presents to her primary care physician with a painless dark brown lesion on her left forearm that has been increasing in size over the past three years. She has noticed no other signs or symptoms. Physical examination reveals an asymmetric lesion with irregular borders, a nonuniform color profile, and a diameter of approximately 13mm. Dermatoscopic inspection shows a clear light blue film over an irregular network of small brown lumps. Which of the following is the most likely diagnosis?
- **a.** basal cell carcinoma
- **b.** squamous cell carcinoma
- **c.** melanoma
- **d.** seborrheic keratosis
- **e.** melanocytic nevus

194. A 64-year-old female presents with progressive deterioration in her peripheral visual fields and no history of eye pain. Her intraocular pressure is measured to be 25 mmHg, and she is found to have an enlarged optic cup on fundoscopy. What is the most likely location of the primary abnormality?
- **a.** anterior capsule
- **b.** macula
- **c.** Canal of Schlemm
- **d.** retina
- **e.** optic nerve

195. A 52-year-old male patient is brought to the emergency department by his wife because he appears to have developed disorientation to place and time. She reports that he has a long history of alcoholism. Which of the following further history or physical examination findings would be most suggestive of vitamin B3 deficiency?
a. dysphasia
b. confusion
c. peripheral rash
d. peripheral neuropathy
e. pallor

196. A 50-year-old gentleman presents with complaints of memory problems. He has the appearance of being agitated. A physical examination shows his attention span and concentration to be normal. Which of the following is the most likely diagnosis?
a. pseudodementia
b. frontotemporal dementia
c. vascular dementia
d. Alzheimer's disease
e. Huntington's disease

197. A 36-year-old man without significant past medical history presents to the emergency department complaining of mild dyspnea and worsening chest pain for the past few days. He recalls a recent upper respiratory infection that "went away." A physical exam is negative for heart murmurs but significant for pleuritic chest pain around the substernal area with pericardial friction rub. Which of the following is the most likely diagnosis?
a. mitral regurgitation
b. gastroesophageal reflux disease (GERD)
c. aortic stenosis
d. acute pericarditis
e. cor pulmonale (pulmonary heart disease)

198. A 45-year-old man who has a family history of coronary arterial disease and a personal history of hypertension, hyperlipidemia, and obesity (BMI of 34) presents to your clinic. Which of the following is the most appropriate health maintenance measure for this patient?
a. diet low in saturated fat and high in fiber
b. physical exercise
c. home blood pressure monitoring
d. weight loss and BMI reduction to less than 25
e. all of the above

199. A 66-year-old man presents to the emergency department complaining of substernal pressurelike chest pain and lightheadedness for the past two hours. He appears diaphoretic and weak. A physical exam shows blood pressure of 144/86, respiration of 23, pulse of 63 bpm, and oxygen saturation of 97%. An electrocardiogram (EKG) shows normal sinus rhythm with ST elevation in lead V2. Which of the following is the most likely diagnosis?
a. gastroesophageal reflux disease (GERD)
b. anxiety attack
c. aortic stenosis
d. pulmonary embolism
e. myocardial infarction

200. A 17-year-old high school football player presents to his primary care clinic with pain and swelling in his right knee three days after an injury. The injury was caused by trauma to the lateral aspect of the knee. His gait is antalgic, and he has reduced weight bearing in his affected knee. Which of the following clinical tests is most likely to be normal?

a. anterior drawer (testing anterior cruciate ligament)

b. posterior drawer (testing posterior cruciate ligament)

c. Apley grind test for medial meniscus

d. Apley grind test for lateral meniscus

e. range of motion

201. A 12-year-old girl is brought into the clinic after a recent throat infection. Her parents complain that she has had uncontrollable dance-like movements for the past few days. During the physical examination, she is noted to have subcutaneous nodules and a systolic heart murmur. Her blood titers are positive for anti-streptolysin O. Which of the following is the most likely diagnosis?

a. Dressler's syndrome

b. systemic lupus erythematosus (SLE)

c. rheumatic fever

d. sarcoidosis

e. group B strep infection

202. A 17-year-old patient presents with an acute asthma attack. You measure her responsiveness to treatment with spirometry before and after a short-acting bronchodilator treatment. Which of the following is the most likely outcome if the patient responds well to the bronchodilator?

a. no change in FEV_1/FVC after treatment

b. a decrease in FEV_1/FVC after treatment

c. an increase in FEV_1/FVC after treatment

d. a decrease in FEV_1 after treatment

e. no change in FEV_1 after treatment

203. A 57-year-old post-menopausal woman has recently been diagnosed with osteoporosis on a bone density scan. In addition to prescribing a bisphosphonate, which of the following is the most appropriate health maintenance measure(s) you should recommend to the patient?

a. increase calcium supplementation

b. add weight-bearing exercises

c. avoid smoking

d. increase vitamin D supplementation

e. all of the above

204. A 72-year-old female presents with shortness of breath, retrosternal chest pain, fatigue, and cyanosis. Auscultation of the chest reveals a systolic ejection click. A chest X-ray reveals enlarged pulmonary arteries. An ultrasound of the abdomen reveals the presence of ascites. Which of the following is the most likely diagnosis?

a. congestive heart failure

b. bronchiectasis

c. pulmonary hypertension

d. pulmonary embolism

e. cystic fibrosis

205. A G2 P1001 woman in her second trimester presents with an acute right upper quadrant (RUQ) pain that radiates to her right shoulder area. She reports intolerance to fatty foods. She appears jaundiced. Her lab test shows increased liver enzymes, bilirubin, amylase, and lipase. You diagnose her with gallstone pancreatitis. Which of the following is the most appropriate treatment?

    a. avoidance of fatty foods

    b. ciprofloxicin

    c. open cholecystectomy

    d. laparoscopic cholecystectomy

    e. appendectomy

206. A 46-year-old woman is found to have a palpable, firm nodule on her left thyroid gland. A thyroid ultrasound confirms a solid nodule. A fine needle aspiration (FNA) biopsy of the nodule shows papillary carcinoma. Which of the following is the most appropriate treatment for this patient?

    a. levothyroxin

    b. propylthiouracil

    c. radioactive iodine therapy

    d. subtotal thyroidectomy

    e. observation for now

207. A 36-year-old woman complains of easy fatigability for the past year. Pronounced fatigue is worst after activity and relieved by rest. She reports occasional shortness of breath without any triggers and also complains of some joint stiffness. On exam, you notice ptosis of both eyelids. Lab work is otherwise normal except for positive blood acetylcholine antibody. Repetitive nerve stimulation test shows decreased muscle action potential. Which of the following is the most likely diagnosis?

    a. hypothyroidism

    b. hyperthyroidism

    c. Guillain-Barré syndrome (GBS)

    d. myasthenia gravis

    e. asthma

208. A 32-year-old man is given alprazolam (Xanax) for his generalized anxiety disorder. Which of the following is the most likely mechanism of action of alprazolam?

    a. dopamine antagonist

    b. GABA (gamma-amino butyric acid) receptors agonist

    c. inhibits GABA receptors

    d. inhibits acetylcholinesterase

    e. SSRI (selective serotonin receptor inhibitor)

209. A 19-year-old female presents with itchy eyelids and burning eyes. A physical examination of the eyes reveals red eyelid margins, swollen eyelids, and crust formation in the eyelashes. Which of the following is the most likely diagnosis?

    a. chalazion

    b. blepharitis

    c. glaucoma

    d. cataracts

    e. orbital cellulitis

210. A 63-year-old Caucasian man presents with a nonhealing, ulcerated lesion on his left cheek for "many months." On exam, the lesion appears to be 0.7 x 0.4 cm in size, a pearly papule with central erosion, and is surrounded by a few telangiectatic vessels. Which of the following is the most appropriate intervention for this patient?
  a. a biopsy with complete excision
  b. electrodesiccation
  c. continue observation
  d. topical antibiotic ointment
  e. topical corticosteroid ointment

211. A 66-year-old female patient presents to her primary care clinic because of a one-week history of lightheadedness. On further questioning, she recalls a few episodes of palpitations during the same time period. Physical examination is significant for a heart rate of 122 bpm with an irregularly irregular pulse. Which of the following is the most likely long-term consequence if her condition is left untreated?
  a. pulmonary embolism
  b. cerebrovascular attack
  c. myocardial infarction
  d. heart block
  e. aortic stenosis

212. A 25-year-old female without any significant past medical history presents with an anemia. Her RBC is within normal limits. H/H: 11/33 (hemoglobin: 12–15 g/dl; hematocrit: 34–44%), MCV 75:(80–100 fl), MCH: 200 (200–900 ng/ml). Which of the following is the most appropriate treatment?
  a. vitamin B12 injections
  b. folic acid supplement
  c. iron supplement
  d. vegetarian diet
  e. no treatment is necessary

213. Which of the following types of lung neoplasms respond best to chemotherapy?
  a. chondroadenoma
  b. solitary pulmonary nodule
  c. small cell carcinoma
  d. non-small cell carcinoma
  e. carcinoid tumor

214. A 16-year-old female presents with dizziness and nausea without loss of consciousness. The patient was active all day at a tennis tournament. No chest X-ray abnormalities, CT scan abnormalities, or blood work abnormalities are found. Which of the following is the most likely diagnosis?
  a. orthostatic hypotension
  b. adrenal insufficiency
  c. vasovagal reaction
  d. micturition syncope
  e. septicemia

215. Which of the following sexually transmitted diseases is effectively treated with ceftriaxone in both men and women?
  a. chlamydia
  b. syphilis
  c. gonorrhea
  d. genital warts
  e. HIV

216. A 35-year-old male presents with pain in the inner ear after an airplane flight. You diagnose this patient with barotrauma. Which of the following practices would you advise this patient to perform during an airplane flight?
  a. take scopolamine prior to takeoff
  b. place his head between his legs prior to takeoff
  c. recline his seat prior to takeoff
  d. yawn or swallow when he feels pressure begin to increase
  e. take diuretics the day prior to eliminate mucosal edema

217. Which of the following medications is used to reduce the damage caused by an acute ischemic stroke?
a. heparin
b. warfarin
c. alteplase
d. reteplase
e. tenecteplase

218. A two-month-old boy is brought to his family physician by his mother for his regular vaccinations. Prior to administering an intramuscular injection in the thigh, the clinician notices that his legs appear excessively cold and mildly pale. On physical examination, his femoral pulses are found to be delayed and weak bilaterally. If left untreated, which of the following is the most likely long-term consequence of this patient's condition?
a. Turner syndrome
b. left ventricular hypertrophy
c. dilated cardiomyopathy
d. peripheral neuropathy
e. pulmonary embolism

219. A 64-year-old male presents to his primary care clinic with a two-day history of exertional dyspnea and a cough productive of a pink frothy fluid. He also reports that he has been using three pillows at night in an effort to control paroxysmal nocturnal dyspnea. His past history is significant for severe poorly-controlled hypertension and a 40-pack-year history of smoking. Which of the following physical examination findings is most suggestive of pulmonary edema?
a. dullness to percussion
b. hyperresonance to percussion
c. bilateral inspiratory wheeze on auscultation
d. bilateral inspiratory crackles on auscultation
e. bilateral reduced air entry on auscultation

220. An 18-year-old woman presents with a two-day history of cough, rhinorrhea, and pain over the maxillary sinus. A diagnosis of acute viral sinusitis is made. Which of the following pharmaceutical therapies is NOT appropriate?
a. pseudoephedrine nasal spray
b. saline nasal spray
c. oxymetazoline hydrochloride nasal spray
d. guaifenesin
e. amoxicillin

221. A 73-year-old woman presents with a two-week history of lower back pain that is exacerbated by activity and does not radiate to the legs. She does not recall a particular traumatic incident that may have caused the pain. Her last DXA scan was eight years ago, at which point her T-score was –1.7. Which of the following additional findings would be adequate to establish a diagnosis of osteoporosis?
a. T-score of –2.1
b. hypocalcemia
c. vitamin D deficiency
d. hyperparathyroidism
e. vertebral stress fracture on X-ray

222. A 28-year-old heterosexual male presents to a public sexual health clinic with concerns about four small, soft painless lesions on his penis. He reports that he first noticed the lesions approximately three days prior to the consultation. On examination, he is found to have small white warts on the dorsal surface of the penis. Which of the following interventions is most likely to be beneficial?
a. IV antibiotic therapy
b. topical antibiotic therapy
c. chemotherapy
d. cryotherapy
e. topical steroid therapy

223. A 57-year-old male patient is brought to the emergency department by his wife after experiencing a convulsive seizure soon after waking up in the morning. He now appears confused and agitated; his wife reports that he has a history of alcohol abuse, and although he had not consumed any alcohol since waking up, he normally consumes approximately one 12-pack of beer every day. He is otherwise healthy and has no past history of head trauma or epilepsy. A physical examination is significant for tachycardia and a mild resting tremor. Which of the following drugs is most likely to benefit this patient?

   a. lithium

   b. clozapine

   c. carbamazepine

   d. diazepam

   e. phenytoin

224. A 39-year-old male presents to his primary care physician complaining of markedly increased urinary frequency. He denies any history of dysuria, hematuria, or urge incontinence. On further questioning, he reports that he has a history of bipolar disorder and is currently taking lithium carbonate and lamotrigine. He is also currently taking hydrochlorothiazide for management of hypertension. Which of the following is the most likely cause of his symptoms?

   a. benign prostatic hyperplasia

   b. nephrogenic diabetes insipidus

   c. neurogenic diabetes insipidus

   d. hyperglycemia

   e. hypernatremia

225. A 23-year-woman who is a smoker presents for preoperative assessment eight weeks prior to an elective surgery. During the assessment the anaesthesiologist suggests that the patient should stop smoking as it improves certain operative outcomes. Which one of these outcomes is NOT improved?

   a. wound healing

   b. risk of infection

   c. CO blood concentrations

   d. peripheral oxygenation

   e. risk of malignant hyperthermia

226. A 61-year-old female with hepatic encephalopathy is given lactulose. Which of the following is the main reason for prescription of this medication?

   a. aid removal of nitrogenous waste products

   b. decrease hepatic blood flow

   c. prevent constipation

   d. reduce acidity of urine

   e. restore thiamine levels

227. A 58-year-old women presents with hot flashes. Menopause is considered as a possible explanation. Which of the following changes in hormone levels would be most consistent with menopause?

   a. rise in estriol

   b. rise in progesterone

   c. drop in follicle-stimulating hormone (FSH)

   d. drop in lutenizing hormone (LH)

   e. rise in follicle-stimulating hormone (FSH)

228. A 42-year-old male presents to the emergency room with a tension pneumothorax. Initial blood pressure is 150/100 mmHg. Prior to decompression with a large-bore needle, the patient's blood pressure falls to 80/40 mmHg, heart rate rises to 150 bpm, and mental status becomes altered. Based on the presentation and the patient's condition, which of the following is the most likely diagnosis?
   a. obstructive shock
   b. cardiogenic shock
   c. hypovolemic shock
   d. septic shock
   e. neurogenic shock

229. A 26-year-old male with type 1 diabetes presents with tiredness, lethargy, and confusion. He has had a recent episode of unresolved pneumonia. On examination, he is tachycardic, hypotensive, and febrile. He has an acetone breath, decreased reflexes, and decreased skin turgor. Urinalysis reveals the presence of glucose and ketone bodies. An arterial blood gas shows a metabolic acidosis with an anion gap. Which of the following clinical interventions would NOT be appropriate?
   a. insulin infusion
   b. glucose infusion
   c. furosemide
   d. K$^+$ correction
   e. antibiotics

230. A 25-year-old female presents with redness, inflammation, burning, and small eruptions around the mouth. Which of the following is the most likely diagnosis?
   a. seborrheic keratosis
   b. seborrheic dermatitis
   c. perioral dermatitis
   d. cellulitis
   e. erythema multiforme

231. A 62-year-old male patient sustains a myocardial infarction and dies instantly. His past medical history is significant for marked coronary atherosclerosis. Which of the following arteries is the most likely location of the infarction?
   a. right main coronary artery
   b. right marginal artery
   c. posterior interventricular artery
   d. left circumflex artery
   e. left anterior descending artery

232. A 54-year-old woman presents to her primary care clinic complaining of a long progressive history of heartburn. Recently, her symptoms have become increasingly severe and are particularly pronounced at night. She is currently taking warfarin for management of atrial fibrillation. Which of the following gastric acid suppressants is safest to use in this patient?
   a. omeprazole
   b. esomeprazole
   c. lansoprazole
   d. pantoprazole
   e. cimetidine

233. A five-year-old girl of Korean ancestry is brought to her pediatrician by her mother because of a six-day history of high fever and excessive irritability. Physical examination reveals bilateral erythema and edema of the fingertips, cervical lymphadenopathy, and a polymorphous rash over the lower trunk, groin, and upper legs. Which of the following ophthalmological findings is most likely if this patient's presentation is caused by mucocutaneous lymph node syndrome (Kawasaki disease)?
   a. reduced visual acuity
   b. diminished visual fields
   c. eye pain
   d. conjunctival injection
   e. diplopia

234. A 16-year-old girl presents to her primary care clinic because of absence of menarche. Physical examination reveals short stature and mild webbing of the neck. She has small breast buds and normal female external genitalia. Her BMI is 24 kg/m^2. A pelvic CT scan reveals the presence of a small uterus and ovaries. Which of the following additional investigations is most likely to help confirm a diagnosis?

a. chromosomal karyotype
b. inflammatory markers
c. pituitary MRI
d. blood glucose test
e. IQ test

235. A 27-year-old male car salesman presents to his primary care clinic along with his wife, who reports that she has noticed a significant change in his behavior over the past eight months. He has been neglecting his hygiene and has lost interest in social interaction, which has also caused significant deterioration of his sales performance. He has also developed a fear that his coworkers are trying to steal all of his sales, and some colleagues have noticed him holding conversations with imaginary customers. He denies any history of substance abuse. Which of the following interventions is most likely to be beneficial?

a. cognitive behavioral therapy alone
b. cognitive behavioral therapy along with risperidone therapy
c. cognitive behavioral therapy along with fluoxetine therapy
d. cognitive behavioral therapy along with methylphenidate therapy
e. cognitive behavioral therapy along with lithium therapy

236. An 85-year-old female patient is brought to her primary care clinic by a community nurse for a regular checkup. She began living in a full-time aged care facility two months earlier. During the consultation, she complains of a progressive history of lethargy and weakness. Physical examination reveals a blood pressure of 95/65 mmHg with a 15 mmHg postural drop, a resting heart rate of 110 bpm, and 2 kg (4.4 lbs) of weight loss since her last visit three months earlier. Her most recent blood test, which was conducted one week earlier, reveals a plasma sodium level of 152 mEq/L (normal 135–145 mEq/L); creatinine and other electrolytes were normal. Which of the following is the most likely diagnosis?

a. diabetes insipidus
b. diabetes mellitus
c. kidney failure
d. Cushing's syndrome
e. hypovolemic hypernatremia

237. A newborn male infant presents with extreme cyanosis, polycythemia, hyperpnea, and agitation. A physical examination reveals clubbing of the fingers and toes. Auscultation reveals right ventricle impulse at left lower sternal border. Which of the following is the most likely diagnosis?

a. pulmonary atresia
b. Tetralogy of Fallot
c. hypoplastic left heart syndrome
d. transposition of the great vessels
e. hyaline membrane disease

238. Maintenance therapy of chronic asthma is commonly achieved by administration of which of the following medications?
   a. antibiotics
   b. anticholinergics
   c. inhaled corticosteroids
   d. β-adrenergic agonists
   e. diuretics

239. A 51-year-old Caucasian man with a 22-year history of gastroesophageal reflux disease (GERD) presents with dysphagia. On endoscopy, a dark-colored mass is seen in the lower esophagus, immediately superior to the lower esophageal sphincter. Which of the following is the most likely diagnosis?
   a. esophageal adenocarcinoma
   b. esophageal squamous cell carcinoma
   c. precancerous Barrett's esophagus
   d. infectious esophagitis
   e. autoimmune esophagitis

240. A 44-year-old male presents in November stating he has been lethargic and depressed and has had a lack of interest in any activities for the past three to four weeks. He states this happens to him every year around this time. Based on the patient's history and presentation, which of the following is the most likely diagnosis?
   a. melancholia
   b. seasonal affective disorder
   c. atypical depression
   d. catatonic depression
   e. malingering

Section 5
Time: 60 minutes

241. A 64-year-old male visits his primary care physician complaining of a three-month history of gradually increasing constant right-sided chest pain and dyspnea. His symptoms are generally exacerbated by inhalation, and the severity generally varies from day to day. He has a 46-pack-year smoking history and spent 30 years as a shipyard worker. Physical examination is significant for reduced air entry and dullness to percussion over the right lung base. Pulmonary function testing demonstrates an FEV_1/FVC ratio of 82%. A chest CT shows right-sided pleural thickening and significantly decreased size of the air space in the right lung. Which of the following is the most likely diagnosis?
   a. squamous cell carcinoma
   b. mesothelioma
   c. asbestosis
   d. interstitial pneumonia
   e. emphysema

242. A 53-year-old man with a two-year history of non-insulin-dependent diabetes mellitus comes in for a regular checkup, at which time his blood pressure is measured to be 175/105. At his past three semiannual checkups, his blood pressure was recorded as 155/96, 163/102, and 168/103. As a result of recommendations at the last consultation, he has increased his exercise and improved his diet; consequently, he has lost approximately 5 kg (11 lb) in the past year and requires no antidiabetic medication. Which of the following is the most appropriate intervention to help control his hypertension at this point?
   a. further lifestyle changes
   b. ramipril
   c. atenolol
   d. hydrochlorothiazide
   e. irbesartan

243. Maintenance therapy of hypochromic micro-cytic anemia can be achieved by administration of which of the following?
a. folic acid
b. ferrous sulfate
c. erythropoietin
d. vitamin B12
e. vitamin E

244. A 30-year-old female in her eighteenth week of pregnancy presents with vaginal bleeding. A gynecological exam reveals an open cervix. Which of the following is the most likely diagnosis?
a. placenta previa
b. spontaneous abortion
c. ectopic pregnancy
d. gestational trophoblastic disease
e. uterine cancer

245. A hiatal hernia is most effectively diagnosed by which of the following diagnostic procedures?
a. chest X-ray
b. barium swallow
c. CT scan of the chest
d. endoscopy
e. esophageal transit study

246. An 18-year-old male presents with a chronic, non-tender mass on the right side of the scro-tum. The lesion has the consistency of a "bag of worms," increases in size when the Valsalva maneuver is performed, decreases with eleva-tion of the testicles, and is appreciated upon physical examination. Which of the following is the most likely diagnosis?
a. epididymitis
b. varicocele
c. hydrocele
d. spermatocele
e. testicular torsion

247. A 34-year-old female immigrant from India presents to her primary care clinic complain-ing of ringing in her ears. Her symptoms are fairly constant but are exacerbated by changes in position. There is no history of vertigo or barotrauma. On further questioning, she reports that she is currently undergoing a standard treatment regimen for tuberculosis, which includes isoniazid, rifampicin, strepto-mycin, ethambutol, and pyrazinamide. Which of these drugs is most likely to be causing her presenting symptoms?
a. isoniazid
b. rifampicin
c. streptomycin
d. ethambutol
e. pyrazinamide

248. A 26-year-old female patient presents to her primary care clinic with a six-hour history of severe left calf pain. She explains that her calf has been swollen and mildly tender since she returned from a trip to Japan two days earlier. Her past medical history is significant only for the use of oral contraceptives for the past eight years. Physical examination reveals right-sided calf tenderness. Which of the fol-lowing interventions is most appropriate?
a. compression stockings
b. thrombolytic therapy
c. anticoagulant therapy
d. surgical insertion of an inferior vena cava filter
e. massage and physiotherapy

249. An otherwise healthy 37-year-old female patient presents with a two-day history of progressive limb weakness starting in the lower extremities and progressing upward. On further questioning, she mentions that she experienced a two-day bout of bloody diarrhea three weeks earlier. All reflexes are absent in the lower limbs and are markedly reduced in the upper limbs. Which of the following is the most likely diagnosis?
a. myasthenia gravis
b. Guillain-Barré syndrome
c. cerebrovascular infarction
d. upper motor neuron disease
e. conversion disorder

250. A 27-year-old male patient presents to his primary care clinic complaining of a one-month history of muscle pain and weakness. He was prompted to visit the clinic after experiencing a bout of nausea and vomiting the previous evening. Physical examination is significant for a blood pressure of 102/64 and mild hyperpigmentation of the skin; on further questioning, he reports that his skin appears to be more tan than usual, but he has not actively sought a tan. Blood electrolyte testing reveals hyponatremia and hyperkalemia. Which of the following additional investigations may help to confirm a diagnosis?
a. ACTH stimulation test
b. dexamethasone suppression test
c. plasma glucose
d. urine dipstick
e. serum creatinine levels

251. A 38-year-old patient with a history of alcoholism presents to his primary care clinic complaining of a four-day history of fever and a cough productive of yellow-green sputum. If his symptoms are caused by a lobar pneumonia, which of the following lobes is most likely affected?
a. right upper lobe
b. right middle lobe
c. left upper lobe
d. left lower lobe
e. lingula

252. A 42-year-old woman visits her primary physician because of a two-month history of sporadic fatigue and fevers around 38°C (100°F). On further questioning, she reports generalized muscle pain, occasional abdominal pain, frequent headaches, and approximately 5 kg (11 lb) weight loss over approximately the same time period. Physical examination is significant for a fever of 37.5°C (99°F), but investigations reveal an elevated erythrocyte sedimentation rate. Which of these features is most suggestive of a diagnosis of polyarteritis nodosa rather than giant cell arteritis?
a. age
b. erythrocyte sedimentation rate
c. muscle pain
d. headaches
e. fever

253. A 58-year-old man with a history of poorly controlled hypertension and type II diabetes presents to the emergency department complaining of "the worst headache of his life" for the past one hour. Physical exam shows nuchal rigidity. A neurological exam is without deficits at this time. His blood pressure is 140/89. A brain CT confirms subarachnoid hemorrhage. An angiography shows multiple intracranial aneurysms. After admission to the intense care unit (ICU), which of the following is the most appropriate treatment for this patient?
a. confine patient to bed and avoid exertion
b. symptomatic treatment for headaches
c. phenytoin to prevent seizures
d. surgical clipping of the aneurysm base
e. all of the above

254. A 55-year-old Asian woman with a history of glucose intolerance is recalled for abnormal lab results. Her HgA1c three months ago was 7.0. After five pounds of weight lost with diet and exercise, her repeat HgA1c is 7.2. Which of the following is the most appropriate treatment option for this patient?
a. continue diet and exercise
b. furosemide
c. metoprolol
d. metformin
e. levothyroxin

255. A nine-year-old female patient is brought to the emergency department by her parents because of fever, vomiting, and lower abdominal pain. Which of the following physical examination findings would suggest a diagnosis of appendicitis rather than gastroenteritis?
a. rebound tenderness in the right lower quadrant
b. inguinal lymphadenopathy
c. tender mass on digital rectal examination
d. abdominal distention
e. hypotension

256. Non-small cell carcinoma of the lung is most effectively treated by which of the following options?
a. cryotherapy
b. chemotherapy
c. radiation therapy
d. hormonal therapy
e. surgery

257. A 52-year-old woman presents with acute left eye pain, decreased visual acuity, and mild headache. She sees a "halo" around lights. Physical exam shows injected left conjunctiva and corneal cloudiness. You see cupping of optic nerves with an otoscope. Her intraocular pressure is 31 mmHg (normal ranges: 8 to 21 mmHg). Which of the following is the most likely diagnosis?
a. cataract
b. angle-closure glaucoma
c. retinal detachment
d. conjunctivitis
e. corneal abrasion

258. A 72-year-old obese male with a past medical history of poorly controlled hypertension, sleep apnea, and 30-pack-year tobacco use presents with bilateral ankle edema, dyspnea, fatigue, and cough. You diagnose him with congestive heart failure (CHF). Which of the following is the most appropriate initial treatment for symptomatic relief?
a. antitussives
b. esomeprazole
c. thiazide diuretics
d. aspirin
e. clopidogrel

259. A 12-year-old Caucasian male has recently been diagnosed with cystic fibrosis. Which of the following laboratory tests is the most appropriate for this condition?
   a. ceruloplasmin
   b. troponin T
   c. chest X-ray
   d. electrocardiogram (EKG)
   e. quantitative pilocarpine iontophoreses sweat test

260. A 25-year-old woman presents to the emergency department with a two-day history of nausea, loss of appetite, and lower abdominal pain. Her pain started in the periumbilical area and traveled to the right lower quadrant (RLQ). She denies other associated symptoms. A physical exam reveals positive tenderness in the RLQ with right thigh extension. There is abdominal discoloration or pain in the RLQ when palpating the left lower quadrant (LLQ). An abdominal CAT scan confirms appendicitis. Which of the following is the correct physical sign revealed by the physical exam?
   a. Rovsing's sign
   b. Collen's sign
   c. Obturator sign
   d. Psoas sign
   e. Grey-Turner's sign

261. Which of the following is the correct sequence through a complete circuit of the cardiovascular system?
   a. oxygenated blood fills the left ventricle → blood is ejected into the aorta → cardiac output is circulated among various organs → blood flow from the organs is collected in the veins → venous return to the right atrium → blood fills the right ventricle → blood is ejected into the pulmonary artery → blood flow from the lungs is returned to the heart via the pulmonary vein
   b. blood flow from the organs is collected in the veins → oxygenated blood fills the left ventricle → blood flow from the lungs is returned to the heart via the pulmonary vein → venous return to the right atrium → blood fills the right ventricle → blood is ejected into the pulmonary artery → blood is ejected into the aorta
   c. blood is ejected into the aorta → cardiac output is circulated among various organs → blood flow from the organs is collected in the veins → venous return to the right atrium → blood fills the right ventricle → blood is ejected into the pulmonary artery → oxygenated blood fills the left ventricle → blood flow from the lungs is returned to the heart via the pulmonary vein
   d. oxygenated blood fills the left ventricle → blood flow from the lungs is returned to the heart via the pulmonary vein → venous return to the right atrium → blood fills the right ventricle → blood flow from the organs is collected in the veins → blood is ejected into the aorta → blood is ejected into the pulmonary artery → cardiac output is circulated among various organs
   e. none of the above

262. A 66-year-old man with a history of hypertension presents with pain in his left toe for the past two days. On exam, you find a tender, red, and warm swelling on the first metatarsal phalangeal joint of his left foot. Which of the following is the most likely diagnostic finding that confirms a diagnosis of true gout?

a. joint aspiration showing negatively birefringent, needle-shaped crystals

b. joint aspiration showing rhomboidal, positively birefringent crystals

c. joint aspiration positive for *S. aureus*

d. X-ray showing a hairline fracture of the first metatarsal phalangeal joint

e. none of the above

263. An 18-year-old G0 woman presents with a three-month history of amenorrhea. She is tested negative for pregnancy. Her pelvic exam does not show any obstruction of the genital tract. You have also ruled out central nervous system tumors. Her FSH and LH are slightly increased. Which of the following is the most appropriate treatment for this patient?

a. oral contraceptives

b. oxytocin

c. laparoscopic surgery

d. spironolactone

e. levothyroxine

264. A 66-year-old man complains of increasing frequency of nighttime urination. He reports having weak stream and urinary urgency. He denies hematuria, dysuria, or pyuria. His urinalysis is within normal limits. Which of the following is the most likely diagnosis?

a. urinary tract infection

b. testicular torsion

c. urinary incontinence

d. benign prostatic hyperplasia (BPH)

e. pyelonephritis

265. In addition to drainage, which of the following is required for proper treatment of malignant pleural effusions after they have been drained of fluid?

a. pericardiocentesis

b. thoracentesis

c. paracentesis

d. pleurodesis

e. amniocentesis

266. A 63-year-old Caucasian man presents with a nonhealing, ulcerated lesion on his left cheek for a many months. A biopsy confirms the lesion to be basal cell carcinoma (BCC). This lesion is subsequently completely excised. Which of the following is the most appropriate for patient education?

a. close follow-up for detection of new lesions

b. sun protection measures

c. caution against tanning bed use

d. all of the above

e. none of the above

267. A 38-year-old African-American male presents with dizziness and nausea when moving from a sitting to a standing position. You have diagnosed him with orthostatic hypotension. Which of the following is the most appropriate clinical intervention?

a. prescribe calcium channel blockers

b. prescribe ACE inhibitors

c. prescribe beta blockers

d. decrease dietary intake of water, caffeine, and salt

e. increase dietary intake of water, caffeine, and salt

268. A 56-year-old African-American male presents with sudden onset of crushing substernal chest pain, shortness of breath, and hemoptysis. He underwent coronary artery bypass graft surgery two weeks ago. An electrocardiogram reveals sinus tachycardia at a rate of 127 bpm with no ST segment abnormality. Pulse oximetry reveals a level of 84% on room air. Troponin level is >0.1 ng. D-dimer level is 7.80 mg/L. BUN is 38 mg/dl. Creatinine is 2.2 mg/dl. GFR is 52 ml/min. Which of the following is the most appropriate diagnostic study to perform next?

a. lung ventilation and perfusion scan to rule out pulmonary embolism

b. CT scan with contrast of the chest to rule out pulmonary embolism

c. myocardial perfusion scan to rule out acute myocardial infarction

d. CT scan with contrast of the abdomen to rule out aortic dissection

e. cardiac catheterization to assess myocardial ischemia

269. A 40-year-old Caucasian female who is undergoing treatment for an inner ear infection presents with increased temperature and drainage from the affected ear along with pain, redness, and swelling around the affected ear. Your clinical diagnosis for this patient is mastoiditis. What course of treatment would you prescribe?

a. intravenous antibiotics

b. antibiotic therapy combined with corticosteroids

c. antibiotic therapy combined with anti-inflammatory agents

d. biopsy of affected ear

e. mastoidectomy

270. A 23-year-old female presents with a history of weight loss, fatigue, and abnormal skin color. Thyroid hormone levels are within normal limits. Her chest X-ray is normal. CT scan and ultrasound exams of the abdomen both reveal abnormalities to the adrenal glands. Serum cortisol levels are 4.2 mcg/dl. Serum potassium level is 5.5 mEq/L. Serum sodium level is 120 mEq/L. Which of the following is the most likely diagnosis?

a. pheochromocytoma

b. Wilson's disease

c. Graves' disease

d. Addison's disease

e. Huntington's disease

271. A 68-year-old male patient with a history of congestive heart failure and chronic obstructive pulmonary disease (COPD) presents to his primary care clinic for a regular review. On physical examination, his blood pressure is found to be 155/104; this is his third consecutive high blood pressure reading. He is currently taking digoxin, which his cardiologist has considered discontinuing because of his borderline low potassium levels. Which of the following antihypertensive drugs is most appropriate for treatment of this patient's hypertension?

a. hydrochlorothiazide

b. furosemide

c. propranolol

d. timolol

e. amiloride

272. Stroke therapy with recombinant tissue plasminogen activator is most effective when administered within how long after the initial onset of symptoms?
   a. three hours
   b. six hours
   c. twelve hours
   d. eighteen hours
   e. twenty-four hours

273. Which of the following types of medication is contraindicated by the amino acid tyramine?
   a. ACE inhibitors
   b. SSRIs
   c. DMARDs
   d. NSAIDs
   e. MAOIs

274. A 63-year-old woman presents to her primary physician with a two-year history of pain and stiffness in her wrists and knuckles. On further questioning, she reports that her symptoms are most severe early in the morning and generally improve over the course of the day. History and physical examination reveal bilateral tenderness in the carpometacarpal joints, the metacarpophalangeal joints, and the proximal interphalangeal joints. Which of the following is the most likely diagnosis?
   a. osteoarthritis
   b. rheumatoid arthritis
   c. carpal tunnel syndrome
   d. scleroderma
   e. peripheral neuropathy

275. A 38-year-old female patient presents with a three-day history of generalized abdominal pain accompanied by a low-grade fever and nonbloody diarrhea. Clinical examination reveals rebound tenderness in the abdomen, and a CT scan shows colonic wall thickening. A complete blood count finds an elevated white blood cell count (13.5×10^9/L). On further questioning, she mentions that she recently took a course of ciprofloxacin for a urinary tract infection. Which of the following is the most likely diagnosis?
   a. colorectal carcinoma
   b. colorectal adenoma
   c. ischemic colitis
   d. pseudomembranous colitis
   e. ulcerative colitis

276. A 37-year-old female patient presents to her primary care physician complaining of multiple episodes of dizziness. On further questioning, she explains that she experiences a distinct sensation that her own position is fairly stationary while her surroundings are spinning around her. The episodes last a few seconds and are generally associated with standing up from a seated position. The problem is most severe when she gets up from bed or turns her head at a certain angle. Which of the following additional signs or symptoms is most likely to be present?
   a. orthostastic hypotension
   b. emesis
   c. presyncope
   d. otitis media
   e. nausea

277. An 18-year-old female presents to her primary care physician because she has never experienced a period. On physical examination, her breast tissue appears normal, but she is found to have no pubic or axillary hair. Which of the following is most likely to be found on a blood test?

a. normal testosterone, normal dihydrotestosterone

b. low testosterone, low dihydrotestosterone

c. normal testosterone, low dihydrotestosterone

d. low testosterone, normal dihydrotestosterone

e. normal testosterone, high dihydrotestosterone

278. A 12-year-old boy is brought to his primary care physician with a three-day history of exertional dyspnea. He has been otherwise healthy until this point. Physical examination reveals peripheral edema, while a urine dipstick finds moderate proteinuria with no glucose, red blood cells, or white blood cells. A blood test is significant for hyponatremia, hypokalemia, hypoalbuminemia, and hypercholesterolemia. Which of the following is the most effective intervention?

a. systemic corticosteroids

b. broad-spectrum antibiotics

c. plasmapheresis

d. hemodialysis

e. antineoplastic chemotherapy

279. A 23-year-old male patient presents to his primary care clinic complaining of an erythematous rash covering the dorsal aspect of both of his arms. He recently underwent oral surgery under general anesthetic for removal of wisdom teeth, and he is currently taking a regimen of cephalexin for prophylaxis as well as oxycodone for pain. Which of the following is the most likely cause of the rash?

a. allergy to cephalexin

b. allergy to anesthetic

c. allergy to oxycodone

d. infectious dermatitis

e. autoimmune disorder

280. A two-year-old male patient with hereditary spherocytosis undergoes a splenectomy. The procedure goes smoothly, and his anemia and jaundice resolve quickly. However, his mother brings him back to the primary care physician because of recurrent episodes of food poisoning associated with vomiting, fever, and lethargy. Which of the following pathogens is the most likely cause of his infections?

a. *Escherichia coli*

b. *Shigella spp.*

c. *Entamoeba histolytica*

d. *Clostridium spp.*

e. *Salmonella typhi*

281. A 26-year-old female with multiple track marks on her arms presents to the emergency department with fever and drowsiness. On examination, she has a pulse of 105/min, a blood pressure of 93/60 mmHg, and a temperature of 40°C (104°F). Auscultation of the heart reveals a murmur. Which of the following murmurs is most consistent with the clinical picture?

   a. aortic regurgitation
   b. aortic stenosis
   c. mitral regurgitation
   d. tricuspid regurgitation
   e. pulmonary stenosis

282. A 47-year-old man presents with conductive hearing loss due to waxy buildup in his ears. After his ears have been syringed, he asks if there is anything he can do to prevent any further buildup of wax. Which of the following suggestions is NOT appropriate?

   a. regular cleaning of ear canal with cotton swab
   b. regular checkups with a primary care physician
   c. regular cleaning of the auricle
   d. use of commercial ear drops
   e. decreased use of ear buds

283. A 73-year-old woman is brought in by ambulance after a syncopal episode preceded by slurring of speech, which occurred less than an hour ago. She has a recorded history of hypertension, diabetes, hypercholesterolemia, and intermittent atrial fibrillation. She is known to be uncompliant with medication and has had several episodes of transient ischemic attacks in the past. A diagnosis of stroke is considered. A noncontrast CT is used to rule out any intracranial hemorrhage. On examination she has an irregular pulse with a rate of 90/min. Her blood pressure is 161/90. Which of the following is NOT an appropriate clinical intervention for this patient?

   a. anticoagulation
   b. CT brain angiogram
   c. blood pressure management
   d. deep vein thrombosis (DVT) prophylaxis
   e. lipid-lowering therapy

284. A 42-year-old man presents with tiredness, lethargy, and depression. He denies any previous mental illness or suicide ideation. In addition to a full history and examination, a series of blood tests are ordered. Which of following laboratory tests would NOT be useful in working up his condition?

   a. full blood count
   b. B12/folate
   c. thyroid-stimulating hormone (TSH)
   d. blood toxicology screen
   e. C-reactive protein (CRP)

285. A 38-year-old male presents with difficult, painful swallowing. An endoscopy is performed and reveals large deep ulcers. A culture is positive for the cytomegalovirus. Which of the following is the most likely diagnosis?
   a. esophageal varices
   b. esophageal neoplasm
   c. infectious esophagitis
   d. esophageal dysmotility
   e. reflux esophagitis

286. A 32-year-old woman presents with progressively worsening tiredness and lethargy. The patient started a vegetarian diet last year. She denies having any depression and has not noticed a change in her menstrual cycle. A blood test confirms a reduced ferritin level. Which of the following signs or symptoms is NOT consistent with the patient's diagnosis?
   a. tachycardia
   b. shortness of breath
   c. pica
   d. melena
   e. Romberg's sign

287. A 21-year-old male presents to the primary care clinic complaining of occasional crushing left-sided chest pain. The pain radiates to his left arm, usually appears during exercise, and is alleviated by rest. On further questioning, he recalls that his father and grandfather both died of myocardial infarctions before age 40. Physical examination is significant for bilateral xanthelasmata. Which of the following proteins is most likely deficient in this patient?
   a. LDL receptor
   b. VLDL receptor
   c. HDL receptor
   d. chloride channel
   e. transferrin receptor

288. A 41-year-old male patient presents to his primary care clinic on account of a recent episode of bloody vomiting. On further questioning, he reports that he experienced several episodes of vomiting in the past month after a few incidents of binge drinking. Which of the following investigations is most useful for diagnosis of an esophageal tear?
   a. barium swallow
   b. chest X-ray
   c. chest CT
   d. full blood count
   e. endoscopy

289. A 42-year-old male patient presents to his primary care clinic with a two-day history of left hip pain that is exacerbated by weight bearing. He recalls no incidents of trauma to the affected area. Physical examination is significant for tenderness and reduced range of motion in all directions at the left hip, while the right hip is normal. A hip X-ray reveals sclerosis and reduced bone density at the femoral head. Which of the following clinical history findings, if true, would be most suggestive of a diagnosis of avascular necrosis rather than osteoarthritis or osteoporosis?
   a. acute onset
   b. positive family history
   c. increased pain with weight bearing
   d. lessening of symptoms over the course of the day
   e. multiple joint/bone involvement

290. Which of the following is the most appropriate course of treatment for penetrating trauma of the eye?
  a. Do not remove object. Place an eye patch over the eye, tell the patient to follow up with an ophthalmologist, and send the patient home.
  b. Do not remove object. Arrange for the patient to be transported to the nearest emergency room for consultation with an ophthalmologist.
  c. Surgically remove the object, place an eye patch over the eye, prescribe eye drops, and send the patient home.
  d. Surgically remove the object, place an eye patch over the eye, tell the patient to follow up with an ophthalmologist, and send the patient home.
  e. Surgically remove the object and arrange for the patient to be transported to nearest emergency room for ophthalmology consultation.

291. A 22-year-old female patient presents to her primary care clinic for a routine pap smear. During the consultation, she admits to using cannabis one to two times on most weekends for the past two years. She usually consumes the drug by smoking from a pipe with her friends. She is interested in the potential health consequences of this cannabis use. Which of the following conditions is more prevalent in cannabis users?
  a. chronic obstructive pulmonary disease (COPD)
  b. asthma
  c. schizophrenia
  d. major depressive disorder
  e. lung cancer

292. Which of the following radiographic procedures allows you to differentiate croup from epiglottitis?
  a. posteroanterior neck radiograph
  b. lateral neck radiograph
  c. CT scan of the neck
  d. MRI scan of the neck
  e. ultrasound of the neck

293. A 34-year-old male with a history of chlamydial urethritis develops asymmetric arthritis in his knee and ankle. His physical examination reveals inflammation of the foreskin of the penis and conjunctivitis. Which of the following is the most likely diagnosis?
  a. septic arthritis
  b. rheumatoid arthritis
  c. psoriatic arthritis
  d. reactive arthritis
  e. scleroderma

294. A 28-year-old female presents to the primary care clinic for help with family planning. She is concerned because she has been unable to become pregnant despite trying since she was married 12 months earlier. She is reluctant to discuss her sexual history, but on further questioning, she reports that her first sexual encounter occurred on her wedding night; prior to this, she had been abstinent for religious and cultural reasons. Since then, she has experienced pain on vaginal penetration, and her husband usually has to withdraw after a short period. She also experiences similar pain when attempting to insert tampons, and consequently prefers not to use them. Which of the following is the most appropriate initial therapeutic strategy?
  a. pain relief
  b. surgical correction
  c. psychological support
  d. antibiotic therapy
  e. antifungal therapy

295. A 27-year-old male presents with recent onset of male pattern baldness. His area of hair loss is relatively small. The patient's history shows that other men in his family also suffered from early onset of male pattern baldness. Which of the following is the safest, most effective treatment to slow the progression of this patient's male pattern baldness?
a. finasteride
b. vitamin A
c. minoxidil
d. topical steroid creams
e. topical antibiotic creams

296. Prior to a surgical procedure in which a patient's right leg is to be amputated, the surgical team is obligated to take a moment and confirm the exact procedure and the location of the procedure. Which of the following is the proper term for this confirmation?
a. HIPAA
b. time out
c. Safe Medical Devices Act
d. Patient's Bill of Rights
e. EMTALA

297. A 26-year-old female, in her third pregnancy, presents for a routine visit and states that after this child is delivered, she does not want any more children and wants surgical intervention as a guarantee. Given the patient's age, which of the following surgical procedures is reversible if she changes her mind later in life?
a. oophorectomy
b. tubal ligation
c. hysterectomy
d. orchiectomy
e. salpingectomy

298. A 12-year-old boy, recently diagnosed with mumps, presents with fever, tachycardia, testicular swelling, and tenderness. You diagnose him with orchitis secondary to the mumps virus. Which of the following treatments is recommended for treatment of this disorder?
a. ice packs and analgesics
b. ceftriaxone
c. doxycycline
d. ciproflaxin
e. trimethoprim/sulfamethoxazole

299. A 35-year-old female patient presents to her primary care clinic complaining of a two-month history of mild dryness in her eyes and her mouth. Physical examination is significant for bilateral parotid gland enlargement and no corneal abrasions. An autoimmune screen reveals elevated levels of rheumatoid factor. Which of the following long-term treatment regimens is most appropriate at this stage?
a. fluid replacement when necessary
b. artificial tears and saliva
c. oral corticosteroid therapy
d. oral methotrexate therapy
e. oral desmopressin therapy

300. Which of the following medications is the most appropriate treatment for gonorrhea in men and women?
a. penicillin
b. mebendazole
c. ceftriaxone
d. chloroquine
e. ciprofloxacin

Answers and Explanations

Section 1

1. **d.** Patients with esophageal dysmotility (choice **d**) classically present with difficulty swallowing or complaints of food not going down properly. Barium swallow is commonly performed; it can reveal both motor and structural abnormalities of the esophagus. Achalasia, a global esophageal motor disorder, is characterized by the esophagus resembling a parrot's beak because of a dilated esophagus tapering to the distal obstruction. Choices **a**, **b**, and **c** are all incorrect because each of these disorders can only be diagnosed via an endoscopy procedure. Choice **e**, reflux esophagitis, can be diagnosed via barium swallow; however, the presence of a parrot's beak should indicate esophageal dysmotility.
   Task Area: Formulating Most Likely Diagnosis
   Organ System: Gastrointestinal/Nutritional

2. **d.** Kayser-Fleischer rings (choice **d**) are pathognomonic for Wilson disease, not schizophrenia. Disorganized speech (choice **a**), disorganized thought (choice **b**), and flat affect (choice **e**) are all common in schizophrenia. Agraphesthesia (choice **c**), the inability to recognize letters or numbers traced on the skin, can also occur in schizophrenia.
   Task Area: History Taking and Performing Physical Examinations
   Organ System: Psychiatry/Behavioral Science

3. **c.** This patient appears to have an incisional hernia, a common complication of abdominal surgery. When an incisional hernia is detected, it is important to refer the patient back to the surgeon for follow-up. In most cases, the hernia must be repaired surgically (choice **c**) by insertion of a mesh to block the protrusion. Abdominal strength training (choice **a**) may prevent a hernia, but is not likely to be useful for an existing hernia. Regular review (choice **b**) alone is unlikely to yield any benefit. Antibiotic therapy (choice **d**) may be helpful if there are signs of an infection. Drainage of the lesion (choice **e**) would be useful in the case of a cyst or an abscess, but this patient's recent history of abdominal surgery is suggestive of an incisional hernia.
   Task Area: Clinical Intervention
   Organ System: Gastrointestinal/Nutritional

4. **d.** The correct answer is choice **d**, mitral regurgitation, given the characteristic pansystolic murmur. Choice **a**, aortic stenosis, is incorrect because aortic stenosis is usually associated with harsh systolic murmur that radiates to the neck. Choice **b**, mitral stenosis, is incorrect because mitral stenosis is usually associated with prominent S1 heart sound and an opening snap. Choice **c**, chronic obstructive pulmonary disease (COPD), is incorrect because abnormal heart sounds are not a typical finding in COPD patients without cardiac involvement. Choice **e**, first-degree heart block, is incorrect because first-degree heart block usually presents with diminished S1 heart sound.
   Task Area: History Taking and Performing Physical Examinations
   Organ System: Cardiovascular

5. d. The correct answer is choice **d**, cystic fibrosis, given the positive sweat test. Cystic fibrosis is a hereditary disorder caused by abnormalities in a membrane chloride channel. Choice **a**, acute asthma exacerbation, is incorrect because asthma patients should not test positive for sweat test. Choice **b**, pneumonia, is incorrect because of the positive sweat test, and there is no mention of fever. Choice **c**, pulmonary tuberculosis, is incorrect because of the reasons mentioned above. Choice **e**, chronic obstructive pulmonary disease (COPD), is incorrect because it typically affects older patients with a history of tobacco use, and they do not test positive for sweat test.

Task Area: Formulating Most Likely Diagnosis
Organ System: Pulmonary

6. d. Atorvastatin (choice **d**), an HMG-CoA reductase inhibitor, is a very widely used lipid-lowering drug. It is generally very effective, but it occasionally causes myalgia and, in more severe cases, rhabdomyolysis (the breakdown of muscle fibers leading to the release of nephrotoxic myoglobin particles into the bloodstream). This myalgia is often accompanied by elevated levels of creatine kinase. Polymyalgia rheumatica (choice **a**) and fibromyalgia (choice **b**) are also possible causes of myalgia, but they are far less likely than iatrogenic causes in a patient who is taking atorvastatin. Trauma (choice **c**) is generally more localized and is unlikely to cause pain that persists for six months. Furosemide (choice **e**) may cause myalgia due to hypokalemia, but this option is incorrect because the patient's potassium levels are normal.

Task Area: Pharmaceutical Therapeutics
Organ System: Cardiovascular

7. c. Polycystic ovarian syndrome (choice **c**) is the most common cause of androgen excess and hirsutism. Patients may present with hirsutism, infertility, truncal obesity, irregular menstruation, and skin discoloration. Choice **a**, ovarian cysts, should be excluded based on symptoms because ovarian cysts can cause abdominal pain, pelvic pain, and menstrual irregularities; ovarian cysts do not cause excessive hair growth and acne. Choice **b**, ovarian cancer, should also be excluded based on symptoms because ovarian cancer causes bloating, abdominal pain, pelvic pain, and vaginal bleeding, but does not cause excessive hair growth and acne. Choice **d**, endometrial cancer, should be excluded based on symptoms because endometrial cancer may cause vaginal bleeding, abdominal pain, pelvic pain, and clear or white vaginal discharge. Endometrial cancer does not cause excessive hair growth and acne. Choice **e**, endometriosis, should be excluded because this disorder is associated with lower abdominal and pelvic pain. Endometriosis does not cause excessive hair growth and acne.

Task Area: History Taking and Performing Physical Examinations
Organ System: Reproductive

8. c. The correct answer is choice **c**, acute gout. The birefringent, needle-shaped crystals are diagnostic for gout. Choice **a**, septic joint, is incorrect because a joint aspirate for septic joint will be positive for presence of bacteria. Choice **b**, pseudogout, is incorrect because the joint aspirate will show positively birefringent crystals. Choices **d**, osteoarthritis of the foot, and **e**, fracture of the first toe, are incorrect because they are inconsistent with the joint aspiration findings.

Task Area: Formulating Most Likely Diagnosis
Organ System: Musculoskeletal

9. b. Bactrim (choice **b**) is a combination of sulfamethoxazole and trimethoprim and is commonly prescribed for treatment of confirmed pneumocystis pneumonia, for prevention against occurrence of pneumocystis pneumonia in immunosuppressed patients, and for the treatment of many other infections. Choice **a**, Zithromax, is another name for azithromycin. Choice **c**, Cipro, is scientifically known as ciproflaxin. Choices **d**, penicillin, and **e**, erythromycin, are generally referred to only by those names.

Task Area: Pharmaceutical Therapeutics
Organ System: Pulmonary

10. e. The correct answer is choice **e**, all of the above. All of the options are important to address the health and emotional needs of a victim of sexual violence.

Task Area: Health Maintenance
Organ System: Reproductive

11. e. Cystic fibrosis is a chronic inherited disease affecting exocrine gland function. It is characterized by several systemic complications, including recurrent respiratory infections. From an early age, affected patients' lungs are colonized by pneumonia-causing bacteria, the most common of which is *Pseudomonas aeruginosa* (choice **e**). The bacteria generally develop antibiotic resistance over time and can be very challenging to combat. Choices **a**, **b**, **c**, and **d** are other common pneumonia-causing bacteria; however, they are all less common than *Pseudomonas* in patients with cystic fibrosis.

Task Area: Applying Basic Science Concepts
Organ System: Pulmonary

12. c. Choice **c**, Cushing's syndrome, is the correct answer. Choice **a**, hyperthyroidism, and choice **b**, hypothyroidism, are incorrect because there is no mention of an abnormal TSH level. Choice **d**, Paget's disease, is incorrect because it is a bone disease that is inconsistent with the lab findings in this case. Choice **e**, obesity, is incorrect because obesity alone will not test positive for the excessive cortisol level.

Task Area: Formulating Most Likely Diagnosis
Organ System: Endocrine

13. d. Celiac symptoms get worse with the ingestion of gluten (choice **d**). Colicky abdominal pain (choice **a**) and foul-smelling stools (choice **b**) are nonspecific symptoms for malabsorption disease. Nosebleeds (choice **e**) are usually not related to gastrointestinal syndromes. Perianal bleeding (choice **c**) is indicative of a distal gastrointestinal disease.

Task Area: History Taking and Performing Physical Examinations
Organ System: Gastrointestinal/Nutritional

14. e. This patient's clinical presentation is typical for migraine attacks. The correct answer is choice **e**, all of the above. Any of the choices can be used to treat acute migraine attacks.

Task Area: Pharmaceutical Therapeutics
Organ System: Neurologic

15. d. The correct answer is choice **d**, acute glomerulonephritis, which is the only condition where red cell casts are present. All other choices are incorrect, although they are valid differential diagnoses of acute renal failure.

Task Area: Using Laboratory and Diagnostic Studies
Organ System: Genitourinary

16. c. Bronchiectasis (choice **c**) is characterized by chronic purulent sputum that is often foul smelling, hemoptysis, chronic cough, and recurrent pneumonia. A physical examination will reveal localized chest crackles and clubbing of the fingernails. A high resolution CT scan will reveal dilated tortuous airways. A chest X-ray can reveal crowded bronchial markings and basal cystic spaces, tram-track lung markings, honeycombing, and atelectasis. Choice **a**, pneumonia, might be a consideration based on the patient's history; however, the presence of additional symptoms such as foul-smelling sputum, hemoptysis, and clubbing of the fingernails should rule this out. Choice **b**, asthma, is incorrect because of the presence of foul-smelling sputum and hemoptysis. The presence of foul-smelling sputum and hemoptysis should also rule out choice **d**, chronic obstructive pulmonary disease (COPD). The age of the patient should rule out choice **e**, cystic fibrosis, as cystic fibrosis is diagnosed in childhood or adolescence.

Task Area: Formulating Most Likely Diagnosis
Organ System: Pulmonary

17. e. The correct answer is choice **e**, sleep patterns. Studies have shown that patients with fibromyalgia have low levels of serotonin and disturbed sleep patterns, which lead to fatigue and increased pain. SSRIs function to regulate serotonin levels and sleep patterns, thus alleviating symptoms associated with fibromyalgia. Choices **a**, **b**, **c**, and **d** are all incorrect because SSRIs are effective in regulating levels of serotonin which, in turn, will regulate sleep patterns, thus alleviating the symptoms associated with fibromyalgia.

Task Area: Pharmaceutical Therapeutics
Organ System: Musculoskeletal

18. c. A corneal abrasion (choice **c**) can cause pain, sensations of a foreign body, tearing, photophobia, and blepharospasm. Corneal abrasions are normally caused by minor trauma from a fingernail, contact lens, eyelash, or some other small foreign body. Choice **a**, orbital cellulitis, is incorrect because this condition is accompanied by fever and decreased vision, which this patient does not report experiencing. Choice **b**, retinal detachment, is incorrect because this disorder is accompanied by visual disturbances such as floaters, flashing lights, and partial blindness. Choice **d**, central retinal vein occlusion, is incorrect because this disorder is characterized by sudden, painless, blurred vision or loss of vision. Choice **e**, central retinal artery occlusion, is incorrect because this disorder is characterized by sudden, painless, marked loss of vision.

Task Area: History Taking and Performing Examinations
Organ System: EENT (Eye, Ear, Nose, and Throat)

19. e. The correct answer is choice **e**, none of the above. Choice **a**, P wave: depolarization of the ventricles, is incorrect because the P wave represents depolarization of the atria, not the ventricles. Choice **b**, PR interval: depolarization of the atria, is incorrect because the PR interval represents the initial depolarization of the atria to the initial depolarization of the ventricles. Choice **c**, QRS complex: repolarization of the ventricles, is incorrect because the QRS complex represents the depolarization, not repolarization, of the ventricles. Choice **d**, T wave: first ventricular depolarization to last ventricular repolarization, is incorrect because the T wave represents the repolarization of the ventricles.

Task Area: Applying Basic Science Concepts
Organ System: Cardiovascular

20. **d.** A lateral soft tissue X-ray of the neck (choice **d**) shows a classic thumb sign if epiglottitis is present. Choice **a**, angiography of the neck, would not be considered because it is an invasive procedure that would not assist you in the diagnosis of this condition. Choice **b**, CT scan of the neck; choice **c**, MRI of the neck; and choice **e**, ultrasound of the neck, are all viable choices in order to diagnose epiglottitis. However, it is easier, quicker, and less invasive for the patient to perform a simple X-ray to make your diagnosis.

Task Area: Using Laboratory and Diagnostic Studies

Organ System: EENT (Eye, Ear, Nose, and Throat)

21. **e.** The Copper T intrauterine device (choice **e**) can be an effective form of contraception for up to ten years. This device reduces the viability and number of sperm that reach the egg and also decreases the movement and number of eggs that reach the uterus. The continuous release of copper from the coils and sleeves of the device enhances the contraceptive effect. Choice **a**, oral contraceptives, need to be taken on a daily basis in order to be effective. Choice **b**, the Norplant system, was effective for five years, but it has since been taken off the market in the United States as a form of contraception. Choice **c**, hormone-implanted vaginal ring, such as the Nuvaring, must be implanted once every month. Choice **d**, the Progestasert IUD, must be replaced every 8 to 24 months.

Task Area: Clinical Intervention

Organ System: Reproductive

22. **e.** The correct answer is choice **e**, warfarin. While patients are hospitalized after a cardiogenic transient ischemic attack, anticoagulation is required with intravenous heparin. A long-term maintenance regimen postcardiogenic transient ischemic attack is obtained through the use of warfarin. Choice **a**, tenecteplase, is not used for maintenance therapy for transient ischemic attacks; it is used to reduce mortality from acute myocardial infarctions. Choice **b**, ticlopidine, should only be used if other medications fail because it can cause a decrease in white blood cells, which can leave patients susceptible to infections. Choice **c**, sulfinpyrazone, will be of no use in this situation, as it is used to treat gouty arthritis. Choice **d**, dipyridamole, is used primarily in conjunction with other medications to reduce blood clot formation after heart valve replacement surgery.

Task Area: Health Maintenance

Organ System: Neurologic

23. d. The correct answer is choice **d**, seasonal affective disorder. Buproprion, commonly marketed as Wellbutrin, is an antidepressive medication that is used to treat seasonal affective disorder (SAD), a form of depression that occurs in the fall and winter, and also as a smoking cessation aid as well as in treatment of other psychological disorders Buproprian is not used to treat hypertension (choice **a**), which is treated with a variety of medications such as diuretics, beta blockers, and calcium channel blockers. Choice **b**, obesity, is incorrect due to the fact that buproprion is not an FDA approved medication for treatment of obesity. Choice **c**, bulimia nervosa, is commonly treated with drugs such as Prozac, Topamax, and Effexor. Buproprian is not used to treat body dysmorphic disorder (choice **e**), which is a form of obsessive compulsive disorder that is commonly treated with cognitive behavioral therapy.

Task Area: Pharmaceutical Therapeutics
Organ System: Psychiatry/Behavioral Science

24. a. Stasis dermatitis (choice **a**) occurs as a direct result of venous insufficiency. Disturbed function of the one-way valvular system in the deep venous plexus of the legs results in backflow of blood from the deep venous system to the superficial venous system, with accompanying venous hypertension. This condition is characterized by light brown or purplish-red discoloration of the lower legs due to a backup of blood in the lower extremities. Individuals with varicose veins are particularly susceptible to this disorder. Choice **b**, dyshidrotic eczema, is characterized by severe itching on the palms of the hands and sometimes the soles of the feet. Choice **c**, contact dermatitis, is an incorrect diagnosis because there is no history of contact with an allergen or evidence of bumps, red rash, or blisters on the skin. Choice **d**, neurodermatitis, normally appears as scratch marks in the skin caused by the patient's repeated scratching of the skin surface. Choice **e**, seborrheic eczema, is incorrect because this disorder is characterized by yellow, oily, scaly patches of skin on the scalp, face, and ears, and occasionally other parts of the body.

Task Area: History Taking and Performing Examinations
Organ System: Dermatologic

25. a. In the hours following a myocardial infarction, several different enzymes are elevated; however, in order to make an accurate diagnosis, it is important to know which enzymes will be elevated at which time periods. Troponin (choice **a**) is one of the most commonly used cardiac markers because elevated levels can be detected as early as two to four hours after the attack, peak at around seven hours, and remain elevated for a few days. Aspartate transaminase (choice **b**) and lactate dehydrogenase (choice **e**) are other markers of myocardial damage, but they are both fairly nonspecific tests and would not be significantly elevated within four hours after the event. Creatine kinase (choice **c**) is also released from myocardial cells, but its levels usually increase a few hours after troponin; also, while the creatine kinase isoenzyme CK-MB is fairly specific to myocardial tissue, overall creatine kinase levels are not as heavily affected. Creatinine (choice **d**) is a breakdown product of creatine phosphate and is usually elevated when the kidneys are unable to eliminate it effectively, but is not a good cardiac marker.

Task Area: Using Laboratory and Diagnostic Studies

Organ System: Cardiovascular

26. a. Normally, hypertension should provoke a compensatory decrease in heart rate in order to decrease the blood pressure. This patient's combination of hypertension and tachycardia suggests either congestive heart failure or an iatrogenic effect. Drugs that cause hypertension will usually still spark a compensatory decrease in heart rate, but drugs that cause tachycardia will avert this mechanism. The only drug on this list that is known to cause tachycardia is albuterol (choice **a**); while albuterol is fairly selective for β_2 receptors (which cause relaxation of smooth muscle, including bronchi), they also have some cross-reactivity against β_1 receptors (which cause contraction of cardiac muscle). Tachycardia and subsequent hypertension are recognized side effects of inhaled β_2 agonists. Choice **b**, fluticasone, may appear attractive because β-agonists are known to cause hypertension, but this hypertension normally causes a compensatory bradycardia; additionally, inhaled corticosteroids have very little systemic effect. HMG-CoA reductase inhibitors, or statins (choice **c**), occasionally cause muscle pain and rhabdomyolysis but have not been associated with tachycardia or hypertension. Hydrochlorothiazide (choice **d**) and ramipril (choice **e**) are antihypertensive drugs and, consequently, would not contribute to hypertension.

Task Area: Pharmaceutical Therapeutics

Organ System: Pulmonary

27. c. This patient wears contact lenses, which is a common cause of corneal abrasion (choice **c**). Eye pain and foreign body sensation are typical complaints. Choices **a**, chalazion; **b**, blepharitis; and **d**, hordeolum, are incorrect because the patient's eyelids are without lesions. Choice **e**, retinal detachment, is incorrect because this patient's visual acuity is intact.

Task Area: Formulating Most Likely Diagnosis
Organ System: EENT (Eye, Ear, Nose, and Throat)

28. a. When used correctly, proton pump inhibitors (PPIs) are almost universally effective for relief of symptoms related to gastroesophageal reflux disease (GERD). However, in order to inhibit enough proton pumps to provide significant symptom relief, the drug must be used every day. Because this patient is only using them occasionally when he has heartburn (choice **a**), the proton pumps in gastric parietal cells are likely regenerating in between episodes. PPIs are not useful for relieving acute heartburn; antacids and H2-receptor antagonists are more useful for this purpose. Choice **b**, inadequate dosage, is incorrect because even an inadequate dose should provide some relief; while some patients do require larger doses than others, this is not the cause of his poor symptom relief. Insensitivity (choice **c**) and malabsorption (choice **d**) are also possible, but are less likely than misuse. Drug interactions (choice **e**) are fairly common with omeprazole, but these interactions are usually the result of omeprazole's tendency to inhibit some isoforms of cytochrome P450; this may cause increased effects of other drugs or of omeprazole itself, but would not cause this patient's presentation.

Task Area: Pharmaceutical Therapeutics
Organ System: Gastrointestinal/Nutritional

29. a. Because of this patient's family history of osteoporosis, it is important to identify her modifiable risk factors and address as many of them as possible. There is a wide range of known risk factors for osteoporosis, but weight-bearing exercise (choice **a**) is a well-established method of improving a patient's outlook. Resistance training mobilizes osteoblasts to form newer bone tissue and, therefore, stronger bones over time. Other forms of exercise, such as swimming, are more beneficial for joint diseases such as osteoarthritis. Other factors may also influence osteoporosis risk; diet, for instance, is a key modifiable risk factor. While diets high in calcium and vitamin D are likely to reduce a patient's risk, high-protein diets (choice **b**) and low-fat diets (choice **c**) lead to a somewhat increased risk of osteoporosis. Estrogen levels are also important; hormone replacement therapy after menopause (choice **d**) has been shown to reduce the risk of osteoporosis, while the oral contraceptive pill (choice **e**) may have a similar effect.

Task Area: Health Maintenance
Organ System: Musculoskeletal

30. a. While redness and irritation in the eye with a recent history of an upper respiratory tract infection are usually suggestive of conjunctivitis (choice **b**), this is unlikely to present with visual disturbance. However, if a conjunctival infection spreads to the cornea and causes keratitis (choice **a**), a temporary deterioration in visual acuity may be found. Furthermore, glare is a visual feature that is very specific to corneal pathology. Uveitis (choice **c**) is a serious inflammatory process that is common in patients with a history of autoimmune conditions, but it is unlikely in this clinical setting. A corneal abrasion (choice **d**) may present with these visual features, but the redness in the eye is more suggestive of keratoconjunctivitis. Acute angle closure (choice **e**) typically presents with acute onset of severe pain.

Task Area: Formulating Most Likely Diagnosis
Organ System: EENT (Eye, Ear, Nose, and Throat)

31. c. The correct answer is choice **c**, echocardiogram to rule out cardiac valve abnormalities. Disease of the heart valves can cause all of the symptoms the patient is exhibiting: chest pressure, dizziness, shortness of breath, and heart palpitations. Choice **a**, cardiac catheterization, is an excellent choice for ruling out cardiac ischemia, but it is an invasive procedure that is not required in this patient because of a normal EKG. Choice **b**, myocardial perfusion imaging, is also useful, but a normal EKG in the presence of these symptoms makes cardiac ischemia unlikely. Choice **d**, CT scan to rule out pulmonary embolism, is incorrect because the normal D-dimer level makes pulmonary embolism unlikely. Choice **e**, lung ventilation and perfusion imaging to rule out pulmonary embolism, like the CT scan, would be inappropriate because the D-dimer level is normal.

Task Area: Using Laboratory and Diagnostic Studies
Organ System: Cardiovascular

32. e. The tetrad of tremor (resting), rigidity, akinesia (or bradykinesia), and postural instability (TRAP is a good mnemonic) is typical of Parkinson's Disease. Parkinson's Disease is caused by the loss of dopamine-producing neurons in the substantia nigra (choice **e**). There is no significant change in the caudate (choice **a**), the putamen (choice **b**), the thalamus (choice **c**), or the hippocampus (choice **d**).

Task Area: Applying Basic Science Concepts
Organ System: Neurologic

33. e. Dilated cardiomyopathy is associated with a wide range of risk factors, but high blood pressure is one of the most important. Persistently high afterload will add additional stress to the myocardium, thereby progressively worsening the patient's condition. Consequently, lowering this patient's blood pressure can have a positive impact on the prognosis of his dilated cardiomyopathy. This is often achieved with diuretics, but dietary salt restriction (choice **e**) can also contribute significantly to management of hypertension. Increasing dietary protein (choice **a**) may be beneficial for patients who are hoping to build muscle, but there is little evidence to suggest that it has an effect on chronic disease. Increasing fruit and vegetable intake (choice **b**) may have general benefits, but it is not as useful as salt restriction for the management of dilated cardiomyopathy. Decreasing dietary carbohydrates (choice **c**) is likely to help the patient lose weight, but this patient's hypertension is a more pressing concern, and while he is mildly overweight, he is not obese. Decreasing cholesterol intake (choice **d**) is not a high priority for this patient because his plasma cholesterol levels are normal.

Task Area: Health Maintenance
Organ System: Cardiovascular

34. b. Benign prostatic hypertrophy (BPH) is a very common cause of lower urinary tract symptoms, including increased frequency and urgency, urge incontinence, hesitancy, incomplete bladder emptying, straining, decreased force of stream, and dribbling. It is important to monitor patients with BPH because of the potential for malignancy. Prostate-specific antigen (choice **b**) is a fairly sensitive indicator of BPH; although it is not highly specific, it is a good screening tool. A digital rectal examination should also be conducted. Urine culture (choice **a**) may help to identify a urinary tract infection, which would be unlikely to persist for such a long period with no constitutional symptoms. Urine electrolytes (choice **c**) may be affected in a wide range of conditions, none of which would cause this patient's presentation. Plasma creatinine (choice **d**) and blood urea nitrogen (choice **e**) would be raised in the case of renal failure, which is much less likely than prostatic hypertrophy and would not cause lower urinary tract symptoms.

Task Area: Using Laboratory and Diagnostic Studies
Organ System: Genitourinary

35. d. Yellow fever (choice **d**), a mosquito-borne viral illness, is characterized by an initial illness featuring general constitutional symptoms, occasionally followed by a resurgence of symptoms two to three days after resolution of the first bout. The second phase of the illness often includes damage to the myocardium, kidneys, and/or liver (which likely accounts for this patient's jaundice). Yellow fever is generally found in parts of South America and Africa, so this patient's recent history of travel is a critical aspect of this diagnosis. Patients who travel to developing countries should generally consult their clinician at least ten days prior to travel. Hepatitis B (choice **b**) may also present with similar symptoms, but the remission period is unique to yellow fever. Hepatitis A (choice **a**) generally features a somewhat delayed onset of symptoms, while hepatitis C (choice **c**) and hepatocellular carcinoma (choice **e**) are more likely to cause a chronic disease process.

Task Area: Formulating Most Likely Diagnosis
Organ System: Infectious Diseases

36. d. This is a classic presentation of gout, an arthritis caused by the deposition of uric acid crystals in the synovial fluid. Physical examination usually yields a hard nodule known as a tophus; while the tophus usually appears in a big toe, it may also appear in the knee. The most significant risk factor for gout is hyperuricemia, which is an important side effect of therapy with hydrochlorothiazide (choice **d**). A good mnemonic for remembering the side effects of thiazide diuretics is HyperGLUC (hyperglycemia, hyperlipidemia/hypertriglyceridemia, hyperuricemia, and hypercalcemia). While sedentary lifestyle (choice **a**) and smoking (choice **b**) are risk factors for a wide variety of conditions, they are not directly implicated in hyperuricemia or gout; diet, however, may be involved if it contains a high level of protein. Ramipril (choice **c**) has been known to cause some renal toxicity and an intense cough, but again, is not related to hyperuricemia. Patients with hypertension (choice **e**) may be at higher risk for hyperuricemia, but this is usually due to diuretic therapy rather than an effect of the hypertension itself.

Task Area: Pharmaceutical Therapeutics
Organ System: Musculoskeletal

37. c. Graves' Disease and thyroid cancer can both cause hyperthyroidism, which often leads to fever, night sweats (choice **a**), tachycardia, palpitations, resting tremor, and weight loss (choice **b**). Plasma levels of T4 will usually be high (choice **e**) due to a TSH receptor-stimulating antibody in Graves' disease or a T4-secreting tumor in thyroid cancer, while TSH will be low (choice **d**) due to feedback inhibition of TSH production in the presence of high levels of thyroid hormone. However, exophthalmos (choice **c**) is a symptom that is unique to Graves' disease. While the sign has relatively low sensitivity, it is highly specific and is often considered to be pathognomonic. The presence of exophthalmos has no bearing on the seriousness of a patient's condition, and it is unclear whether the eye complications arise directly from Graves' disease or from a closely linked disorder.

Task Area: History Taking and Performing Physical Examinations

Organ System: Endocrine

38. b. The correct answer is choice **b**, electrical cardioversion, which is not immediately indicated in this patient. Treatment for new onset atrial fibrillation that has lasted for more than three days is anticoagulation for four weeks (choices **a**, **d**, and **e**), followed by an attempted cardioversion. The patient is also tachycardic, so treatment with a beta blocker (choice **c**) is also indicated.

Task Area: Clinical Intervention

Organ System: Cardiovascular

39. d. Albuterol is an adrenergic agonist and can therefore cause an increased heart rate (choice **d**). Oral thrush (choice **a**) is caused by inhaled corticosteroids. Hearing loss (choice **c**) can be caused by ototoxic drugs such as aminoglycosides. Many drugs can cause lupus (choice **b**); however, albuterol is not one of them. Drugs such as ACE inhibitors can cause a dry cough (choice **e**).

Task Area: Pharmaceutical Therapeutics

Organ System: Pulmonary

40. c. The correct answer is choice **c**, appendicitis, which has a typical history and physical findings such as a positive psoas sign as described in this case. Choice **a**, gastrointestinal bleed, is incorrect because there is no mention of dizziness, melena, or other typical presentations. Choice **b**, colon cancer, is incorrect because that is usually a diagnosis made on colonoscopy by biopsy. Choice **d**, cholecystitis, is incorrect because this condition typically presents with RUQ pain with positive Murphy's on exam. Choice **e**, pancreatitis, is incorrect because pain is typically in epigastric and/or lower upper quadrant (LUQ) without positive psoas sign.

Task Area: Formulating Most Likely Diagnosis

Organ System: Gastrointestinal/Nutritional

41. b. *Klebsiella pneumoniae* (choice **b**) is a Gram-negative, non-motile, rod-shaped bacterium that is an uncommon cause of pneumonia. However, prolonged abuse of alcohol will suppress the immune system, and *Klebsiella pneumoniae* will be able to colonize and cause pneumonia. Choice **a**, *Legionella pneumophila*, which causes Legionella pneumonia, is most likely to invade the body when aerosols containing the bacterium are inhaled. The most common sources of these aerosols are cooling systems, swimming pools, hot water systems, and fountains. Choice **c**, *Myocplasma pneumoniae*, is a very small bacterium that is the cause of walking pneumonia. Choice **d**, *Chlamydia pneumoniae*, affects otherwise healthy individuals and is the primary cause of community-acquired pneumonia. Choice **e**, *Diplococcus pneumoniae*, is a bacterium that can cause many other conditions other than pneumonia such as sepsis, osteomyelitis, and meningitis.

Task Area: Applying Basic Science Concepts
Organ System: Pulmonary

42. a. Hypercholesterolemia is associated with a wide range of conditions, the most prominent of which are atherosclerosis and coronary artery disease. However, the importance of abdominal aortic aneurysm (choice **a**) as a potential consequence of hypercholesterolemia is often understated. Abdominal aortic aneurysm is the tenth leading cause of death in men over 55 in the United States and is far more likely to occur in patients with atherosclerosis, which is more common in patients with a history of smoking, hypercholesterolemia, and a wide range of other risk factors. Giant cell arteritis (choice **b**) is primarily an immune phenomenon and is not strongly linked to cholesterol. Prinzmetal's angina (choice **c**), unlike other forms of angina, is caused by coronary vasospasm rather than by coronary atherosclerosis. Deep vein thrombosis (choice **d**) and pulmonary embolism (choice **e**) are particularly common in patients with prolonged immobility and often occur in patients who are otherwise healthy.

Task Area: Health Maintenance
Organ System: Cardiovascular

43. a. A Mallory-Weiss tear is a linear mucosal tear in the esophagus, generally at the gastroesophageal junction, and is often associated with alcoholism (choice **a**). Choices **b**, **c**, and **e** are incorrect as this disorder is commonly caused by prolonged vomiting or coughing, which these answer choices do not provoke. Choice **d**, bulimia nervosa, could possibly be the cause of a Mallory-Weiss tear as repeated forced vomiting promotes this condition; however, this condition primarily occurs secondary to repeated vomiting from prolonged alcohol abuse.

Task Area: Using Laboratory and Diagnostic Studies

Organ System: Gastrointestinal/Nutritional

44. a. Septic arthritis (choice **a**) is caused by a systemic spread of bacteria and tends to affect a single joint such as the hip, shoulder, ankle, or wrist. Patients usually present with swelling, fever, joint warmth, effusion, tenderness to palpation, and increased pain with minimal range of motion. Evaluation of the synovial fluid will be positive for bacteria. Choice **b**, reactive arthritis, should be ruled out based on the lack of urinary symptoms, conjunctivitis, and skin rashes. Choice **c**, calcium pyrophosphate dihydrate disease, should be ruled out since the synovial fluid was positive for *Staphylococcus aureus* bacteria and not for calcium pyrophosphate dihydrate crystals. Choice **d**, gout, should be ruled out since the synovial fluid was positive for *Staphylococcus aureus* bacteria and not for uric acid crystals. Choice **e**, osteomyelitis, might be a consideration, but the presence of *Staphylococcus aureus* bacteria in the synovial fluid should rule this out.

Task Area: History Taking and Performing Physical Examinations

Organ System: Musculoskeletal

45. d. Barotrauma (choice **d**) is defined as the inability to equalize barometric stress on the inner ear, resulting in pain. This disorder is caused by auditory tube dysfunction as a result of congenital narrowing or acquired mucosal edema, and is commonly the result of airplane descent, rapid altitude changes, or underwater diving. Choice **a**, otitis externa, should be excluded because there is no drainage, and itching and pain in the ear do not become worse when the ear is touched or pulled. Choice **b**, central vertigo, should be excluded because there is no dizziness or sensation of motion when standing still. Choice **c**, labyrinthitis, should be excluded because there is no vertigo, dizziness, nausea, vomiting, or involuntary eye movement. Choice **e**, tympanic membrane rupture, should be excluded because there is no vertigo, tinnitus, nausea, vomiting, or drainage from the affected ear.

Task Area: Formulating Most Likely Diagnosis

Organ System: EENT (Eye, Ear, Nose, and Throat)

46. a. Osteomalacia (choice **a**) is a disease of defective bone mineralization that occurs in adults and is similar to rickets. Patients may present with muscle weakness in the pelvic girdle and generalized bone pain, and have a history of several fractures. X-rays will reveal a generalized decrease in bone density and Looser's lines that are characteristic of pseudofractures. Blood work will reveal vitamin D deficiency. Choice **b**, rickets might be a consideration because the presentation is identical to osteomalacia; however, rickets only affects children. Choice **c**, Paget's disease, should not be a consideration because the X-rays would show bone enlargements as well as bowing of the long bones. Paget's disease is also associated with an elevated alkaline phosphatase blood level. Choice **d**, osteoporosis, should definitely be considered; however, the presence of Looser's lines indicates osteomalacia. Choice **e**, osteomyelitis, should be ruled out because this disorder is associated with fever, redness, and swelling over the painful area.

Task Area: History Taking and Performing Physical Examinations
Organ System: Endocrine

47. c. A nonseminomatous testicular tumor (choice **c**) is radio-resistant. Treatment for this type of tumor, depending on the stage of the disease, includes retroperitoneal lymph node dissection, chemotherapy, and surgery. Choice **a**, Wilms' tumor; choice **b**, renal cell carcinoma; choice **d**, seminomatous testicular tumor; and choice **e**, pheochromocytoma, will all respond to radiation therapy treatments.

Task Area: Applying Basic Science Concepts
Organ System: Genitourinary

48. b. A Wood's light examination is not useful to evaluate the presence of warts (choice **b**). A Wood's light examination is extremely useful for accentuating hyperpigmented macules (choice **a**), which are associated with the disorder of melasma, or to fluoresce urine for ethylene glycol poisoning (choice **c**). A Wood's light examination is also useful to evaluate fungal and bacterial infections (choices **d** and **e**).

Task Area: Using Laboratory and Diagnostic Studies
Organ System: Dermatologic

49. a. Multiple myeloma (choice **a**) is a malignancy of plasma cells, possibly caused by exposure to a herpes virus. This disorder primarily occurs in individuals around 65 years of age. Patients with multiple myeloma can present with anemia, pain in the back or ribs, and recurrent infections. Choice **b**, chronic lymphocytic leukemia, is a malignancy of the white blood cells, particularly B-lymphocytes. Choice **c**, Hodgkin's lymphoma, is a malignancy of the white blood cells, particularly multinucleated Reed-Sternberg cells. Choice **d**, acute myelogenous leukemia, is a cancer that begins in the bone marrow and attacks immature cells that would develop into white blood cells. Choice **e**, polycythemia vera, is an abnormal increase in the number of red blood cells.

Task Area: Applying Basic Science Concepts
Organ System: Hematologic

50. c. This patient is most likely suffering from Wegener's granulomatosis, a form of vasculitis that primarily affects the lungs and kidneys. Patients typically present with hemoptysis and dyspnea, but hematuria is also a common feature. The presence of circulating antineutrophil cytoplasmic antibodies (c-ANCA) is relatively specific for this condition. Like other autoimmune diseases, Wegener's granulomatosis responds well to cytotoxic agents such as cyclophosphamide (choice **c**). Depending on the location and severity of symptoms, methotrexate and corticosteroids may also be involved in a treatment regimen. Antineoplastic chemotherapy (choice **a**) may also help to control the patient's symptoms, but is not warranted in a patient without cancer because of its narrow therapeutic index. Radiotherapy (choice **b**) is of no clear benefit. Thrombolytic therapy (choice **d**) would be used if this patient's hemoptysis and dyspnea were caused by a pulmonary embolism, but the presence of c-ANCA is highly suggestive of vasculitis. Antimicrobial therapy (choice **e**) would be useful if there were evidence of pneumonia.

Task Area: Clinical Intervention
Organ System: Cardiovascular

51. d. This patient appears to have Ewing's sarcoma, a malignant tumor of the bone that is most common in teenagers. The most common sites are the pelvis and the diaphyses of long bones such as the femur, humerus, and tibia. A radiograph will usually demonstrate a lytic lesion with possible invasion to adjacent soft tissue. The typical cause of Ewing's sarcoma is a chromosomal translocation at (11,22) (choice **d**), and the diagnosis can usually be confirmed with a karyotype. This question can also be answered via process of elimination, since the other four choices are much more well-known mutations. Trisomy 21 (choice **a**), or Down syndrome, may cause a variety of consequences, but bone cancer is not a recognized feature. 47, XXY karyotype (choice **b**), or Klinefelter's syndrome, is characterized by changes related to the sex hormones. (9,22) translocation (choice **c**) is known as the Philadelphia chromosome, which predisposes to chronic myelogenous leukemia. (8,14) translocation (choice **e**) usually leads to Burkitt's lymphoma.

Task Area: Applying Basic Science Concepts
Organ System: Musculoskeletal

52. **c.** Otitis media is a very common illness in children and, in most cases, is self-limiting. However, in the case of bacterial etiology (as would be expected by the presence of a purulent exudate), it is often necessary to institute antibiotic therapy. A wide variety of complications can arise if the infection is allowed to spread, but mastoiditis (choice **c**) is one of the most common of these potential complications. Otitis interna, otitis externa, and chronic suppurative otitis media are also commonly seen. Sepsis (choice **a**) and conjunctivitis (choice **b**) are not typically seen as consequences of otitis media. Meningitis (choice **d**) and facial paralysis (choice **e**) may occasionally appear, but these complications are rare.

Task Area: Health Maintenance

Organ System: EENT (Eye, Ear, Nose, and Throat)

53. **a.** Invasive ductal carcinoma is the most common form of malignant breast cancer and is one of the more aggressive subtypes. Its receptor profile will often dictate the optimal management. HER2-positive breast cancers are more aggressive in nature and carried a relatively poor prognosis until the discovery of trastuzumab, a monoclonal antibody that specifically targets the HER2 receptor and was approved by the FDA for breast cancer therapy in 1998. Meanwhile, estrogen and progesterone receptor positivity in a breast tumor is indicative that it will also respond well to hormone therapy. While the prognosis of a stage 1 breast cancer is relatively good regardless of its hormone profile, the presence of all three receptors (choice **a**) is especially beneficial. Choices **b**, **c**, **d**, and **e** are incorrect because a cancer that is negative for any of these three types of receptors will be less responsive to targeted therapy.

Task Area: Pharmaceutical Therapeutics

Organ System: Reproductive

54. **c.** In the presence of severe headache and neck stiffness, it is important to consider the possibilities of intracranial hemorrhage and meningitis. While meningitis usually presents with a fever, either provisional diagnosis would warrant a CT scan of the head first and then a lumbar puncture. If bloody cerebrospinal fluid (choice **c**) is obtained from the lumbar puncture, it is likely that a bleed in the cranial cavity is responsible for the patient's symptoms. If the cerebrospinal fluid is turbid (choice **a**) or cloudy (choice **b**), the culprit is more likely to be infectious. An increase in cerebrospinal fluid pressure (choice **d**) may be found in either intracranial hemorrhage or meningitis. Low cerebrospinal fluid pressure (choice **e**) is a sign of a cerebrospinal fluid leak, which is unlikely in either of the two conditions in question.

Task Area: History Taking and Performing Physical Examinations

Organ System: Neurologic

55. e. A unilateral lower eyelid spasm, or eyelid myokymia, is a fairly common presentation in general practice. It is most commonly caused by stress and sleep deprivation (choice **e**) and usually resolves with improved sleep habits and reduced stress levels. This patient should be counseled about sleep hygiene and the importance of managing stress and sleep habits. It may also be beneficial for him to reduce his caffeine intake because caffeine has a tendency to act as a CNS stimulant. Neuropathy (choice **a**) may also cause similar symptoms, but this is far rarer than stress-related myokymia. Vaso-spasm (choice **b**) may be felt by a patient but is unlikely to appear as a twitch. Caffeine use may commonly cause eyelid spasms, but caffeine withdrawal (choice **c**) is more likely to cause depressive and sedative symptoms. Blepharospasm (choice **d**), a rare neuro-pathic dystonia that manifests as an eyelid spasm, usually presents with gradual onset and progressive increases in the length of episodes; in some cases, eyelid myokymia can act as a precursor to blepharospasm.

Task Area: Formulating Most Likely Diagnosis
Organ System: Psychiatry/Behavioral Science

56. d. For individuals who have been diagnosed with thrombocytopenia and have undergone a prednisone therapy regimen that has failed, splenectomy (choice **d**) is the indi-cated treatment. Splenectomy offers a defini-tive resolution for this disorder. Choice **a**, continued higher dose of prednisone treat-ment, is incorrect as this condition has already proven resistant to prednisone, so continuing this course of treatment or increasing his dose of prednisone would have no effect. Choice **b**, immunosuppres-sive therapy, is incorrect, as this form of treatment is commonly used to treat auto-immune disorders and is used to prevent rejection after an organ transplant. Choice **c**, stem cell transplantation, may be used as treatment for aplastic anemia or leukemia; however, this course of treatment is not indicated for thrombocytopenia. Choice **e**, blood transfusion, may be a treatment option for this condition; however, for symptomatic, steroid-resistant thrombocy-topenia, splenectomy is the only definitive resolution.

Task Area: Clinical Intervention
Organ System: Hematologic

57. e. While it is important to maintain tight glycemic control in patients with type 2 diabetes, it is generally appropriate to attempt lifestyle changes before initiating pharmaceutical therapy. When a patient's sugar levels are near normal, they can often be controlled using diet and exercise (choice **e**). If the patient is unable to control his sugar with lifestyle changes alone, further measures should be considered. Metformin (choice **a**), a member of the biguanide class of drugs, is generally the first-line drug used for management of type 2 diabetes if lifestyle changes fail. Glyburide (choice **b**), a sulfonylurea, can be used as an alternative if biguanides are contraindicated or as an adjuvant if biguanides alone are ineffective. Insulin (choice **c**) is usually not necessary in type 2 diabetes (hence the term *noninsulin-dependent*) unless sugar levels are uncontrollable with other measures. Because of their renal protective effect in diabetes, ACE inhibitors (choice **d**) are generally used to manage hypertension in diabetic patients, but this patient does not have any clear indication for antihypertensive medications.

Task Area: Health Maintenance
Organ System: Endocrine

58. b. The correct answer is choice **b**, hydrochlorothiazide (HCTZ), which is a diuretic to reduce circulatory volume. Choice **a**, esomeprazole (Nexium), is incorrect because it is a proton-pump-inhibitor used in refractory acid reflux disease. Choice **c**, aspirin, is incorrect because it does not directly improve hypertension, although it is used for cardio-protection. Choice **d**, clopidogrel (Plavix), is incorrect because it is an antiplatelet not used for treating hypertension. Choice **e**, zolpidem (Ambien), is incorrect because it is used for treatment of insomnia.

Task Area: Pharmaceutical Therapeutics
Organ System: Cardiovascular

59. e. The patient's skin lesion is most consistent with a premalignant SCC, which is an actinic keratosis (choice **e**) and can be treated with cryotherapy. Melanoma (choice **a**) usually presents as a pigmented asymmetric lesion. Discoid lupus (choice **c**) presents as moderate scaling plaques. Acne (choice **d**) and warts (choice **b**) are usually present as visually observable lesions.

Task Area: Formulating Most Likely Diagnosis
Organ System: Dermatologic

60. b. 80-90% of kidney stones are composed of calcium oxalate, which generally crystallizes in acidic urine. Alkalinization of the urine choice **b**, consequently, often helps to dissolve these stones over time. Calcium salts tend to be radiopaque (which is why we also often use X-rays to look for calcification in the lungs, the bowels, and several other organs), so the opacity on this patient's X-ray further increases the likelihood of calcium oxalate stones rather than uric acid stones, which are the second most common type. Acute therapy for this patient is more likely to comprise pain relief and referral to a specialist for basket retrieval or lithotripsy of the stone. Long-term therapy will generally be instituted after the diagnosis is confirmed based on the sample that is retrieved; although uric acid stones are highly unlikely based on the radiological findings, it is still necessary to eliminate rarer causes of kidney stones. Because calcium oxalate stones crystallize in acidic urine, acidification (choice **a**) would only accelerate their growth. Allopurinol (choice **c**) might be a useful therapeutic agent for uric acid stones, but it has no benefit for this patient. Antibiotics (choices **d** and **e**) may also be helpful in some cases, but only 10–15% of kidney stones present with infection.

Task Area: Pharmaceutical Therapeutics
Organ System: Genitourinary

Section 2

61. c. This patient has progressive loss of vision and decreasing quality of life as a result. The correct answer is choice **c**, cataract surgery, which is the treatment of choice. Choice **a**, prescription glasses, is incorrect because glasses will not improve the opacity of lenses. Choice **b**, no intervention is indicated at this time, is incorrect because this patient's condition is affecting his quality of life. Choice **d**, vitamin C and E supplementation, is incorrect because, in controlled studies, vitamins have not been shown to treat or even prevent cataracts. Choice **e**, eye drops with artificial tears, is incorrect because it is not the standard of care.

Task Area: Clinical Intervention

Organ System: EENT (Eye, Ear, Nose, and Throat)

62. a. Tachypnea and peripheral cyanosis are fairly nonspecific symptoms, but in a young infant they are fairly suggestive of a congenital heart abnormality. The location of a murmur can often help to localize this sort of abnormality; in this case, it is in the region overlying the great vessels. The continuous machine-like murmur is a classic sign of patency in the ductus arteriosus (choice **a**), a duct that connects the embryonic pulmonary artery to the aortic arch at the origin of the left subclavian artery in order to shunt blood away from the pulmonary vasculature, since fetal oxygen comes from the maternal circulation. Normally, the ductus arteriosus closes soon after birth; however, if this does not happen, it can cause significant circulatory impairment and left ventricular hypertrophy. Usually, a patent ductus arteriosus can be closed pharmaceutically with intravenous indomethacin or ibuprofen, both of which are nonsteroidal anti-inflammatory drugs (NSAIDs) that facilitate vasoconstriction by inhibiting the production of prostaglandins (particularly prostaglandin E_2). A patent foramen ovale (choice **b**) and a patent interventricular foramen (choice **c**) may also cause cyanosis by other mechanisms, but the characteristic murmurs are generally different. The aortic valve (choice **d**) and the pulmonary valve (choice **e**) are affected in the Tetralogy of Fallot, but this would also cause a different murmur.

Task Area: Formulating Most Likely Diagnosis

Organ System: Cardiovascular

63. e. While it is impossible to vaccinate against the presence of a cancer, it is possible to reduce the incidence of risk factors. The so-called "cervical cancer vaccine" (Gardasil®) is an excellent example of this strategy: by vaccinating against the oncovirus that usually causes cervical cancer, the human papillomavirus (HPV), it has the potential to significantly reduce the rates of cervical cancer in future generations. Most commercial vaccines protect against HPV subtypes 16 and 18 (choice **e**) because these are the two most common causes of cervical cancer in the community. HPV is highly prevalent in sexually active patients, so it is important to vaccinate boys and girls before they become sexually active. It is also necessary to educate these patients about the nature of the vaccine; while it covers the two most common causes of cervical cancer, there are several other subtypes of HPV that can still act as oncoviruses. Consequently, it is still important for the patient to return for regular pap smears after she becomes sexually active, while boys should be educated on how to examine themselves for genital warts.

Choices **a**, **b**, **c**, and **d** are incorrect because HPV subtypes 6 and 11 are generally associated with genital warts, but not with cervical cancer.

Task Area: Applying Basic Science Concepts
Organ System: Reproductive

64. d. Patients with a history of systemic lupus erythematosus are at particularly high risk of Goodpasture's Syndrome, a nephritic syndrome characterized by antibodies against the glomerular basement membrane. As with other nephritic syndromes, the chief characteristic symptom is hematuria (choice **d**) in addition to nonspecific symptoms such as dysuria. Meanwhile, it is important to consider the other differential diagnoses associated with dysuria, the most common of which in a young female is urinary tract infection. Urinary incontinence (choice **a**) is another nonspecific symptom that may be associated with caffeine consumption, diabetes, and a range of other disorders. Hypertension (choice **b**) may be a consequence of renal failure but is also very nonspecific. Vaginal bleeding (choice **c**) is not associated with nephritic syndrome; blood is usually found in the urine. Fever (choice **e**) may be associated with Goodpasture's Syndrome, but it is more likely to indicate a urinary tract infection.

Task Area: History Taking and Performing Physical Examinations
Organ System: Genitourinary

65. c. Parathyroid hormone functions to increase calcium and phosphate levels by increasing bone turnover and activation of vitamin D. In pseudohypoparathyroidism (choice **c**), the kidney becomes unresponsive to PTH, thereby causing a decrease in calcium and phosphate levels. This causes a feedback increase in PTH levels as the body attempts to correct the deficiency. Primary hyperparathyroidism (choice **a**) causes an increase in calcium and phosphate levels rather than a decrease. Primary hypoparathyroidism (choice **b**) might explain the patient's symptoms, but it would cause a decrease in plasma PTH levels. Choices **d** and **e** are incorrect because parathyroid hormone levels are not influenced by the pituitary gland.

Task Area: Formulating Most Likely Diagnosis
Organ System: Endocrine

66. d. Barrel chest (choice **d**) is seen in emphysema. Productive cough (choice **a**), dyspnea (choice **b**), clubbing (choice **c**), and orthopnea (choice **e**) can be seen in chronic bronchitis.

Task Area: History Taking and Performing Physical Examinations
Organ System: Pulmonary

67. a. Ultrasound examinations (choice **a**) are now the gold standard for evaluating disorders pertaining to the testicles. Ultrasound exams are the most effective diagnostic procedures for diagnosis of testicular disorders such as torsion and epididymitis. Choice **b**, nuclear medicine testicular scan, might be considered and can be used to rule out testicular torsion; however, this study has been replaced with ultrasound as the gold standard for diagnosis of this condition. Choices **c** and **d**, CT angiogram of the testicles and MRI angiogram of the testicles, may have potential as imaging tools for testicular torsion, but there is no scientific evidence confirming the sensitivity of these modalities for diagnosis of this condition. Choice **e**, X-ray of the pelvis, should not be considered, as this will offer no assistance for diagnosis of testicular abnormalities.

Task Area: Using Laboratory and Diagnostic Studies
Organ System: Genitourinary

68. b. Given this patient's increased risk for strokes, warfarin (Coumadin) (choice **b**) should be used to prevent blood clots as a result of atrial fibrillation. Choice **a**, aspirin, is incorrect because of this patient's increased risk for peptic ulcer complications and for stroke. Choice **c**, hydrochlorothiazide (HCTZ), is incorrect because it is typically used to treat hypertension. Choice **d**, β-blockers, is incorrect because β-blockers do not reduce this patient's risk for stroke, although they are beneficial for rate control. Choice **e**, none of the above, is incorrect for reasons given for choice **b**.

Task Area: Pharmaceutical Therapeutics
Organ System: Cardiovascular

69. a. The correct answer is choice **a**, short-acting bronchodilator: inhaled beta2-agonist, such as albuterol. These agents offer quick relief of symptoms and reverse acute airflow obstruction by relaxing the bronchial smooth muscle. Choice **e** is therefore incorrect. Choice **b**, inhaled corticosteroids, is incorrect because they are preferred for long-term control of asthma, not for immediate rescue. Choice **c**, long-acting bronchodilator: inhaled beta2-agonist, is incorrect because it has delayed onset of action and is not suitable for acute treatment. Choice **d**, oxygen via nasal cannula, is incorrect because it does not relieve the underlying bronchospasm that causes airway obstruction.

Task Area: Clinical Intervention
Organ System: Pulmonary

70. a. The correct answer is choice **a**, ciprofloxacin and metronidazole. This question tests your knowledge of management of diverticulitis (inflammation or infection of a colonic diverticulum). When this condition is suspected and no peritoneal signs are present, reasonable regimens include broad-spectrum oral antibiotics with anaerobic activity. Choice **b**, amoxicillin, is incorrect because additional antibiotics with anaerobic activity are necessary for complete coverage. Choice **c**, acetaminophen (Tylenol), is incorrect because it does not address the underlying inflammatory process. Choice **d**, oxycodone, is incorrect because pain management alone does not address the main pathology. Choice **e**, metronidazole, is incorrect because it does not have activity against aerobic organisms.

Task Area: Pharmaceutical Therapeutics
Organ System: Gastrointestinal/Nutritional

71. c. The patient has temporal arteritis, which is usually associated with elevated erythrocyte sedimentation rate (ESR) (choice **c**), not a reduced ESR (choice **d**). The platelet count is usually not affected (choices **a** and **b**). IL-6 (choice **e**) is usually increased in giant cell arteritis.

Task Area: Using Laboratory and Diagnostic Studies
Organ System: Cardiovascular

72. d. Surgical repair with internal fixation (choice **d**) is the standard of treatment, given that this patient does not have contraindications to surgery. All other choices are incorrect in this case because surgery is the definitive treatment given the high rate of complications with a nonsurgical treatment such as non-union.

Task Area: Clinical Intervention
Organ System: Musculoskeletal

73. a. This patient is most likely immunocompromised, given his uncontrolled diabetes. His inhaled corticosteroid use also predisposes him to infections. The white plaques are consistent with thrush (oral candidiasis), which makes choice **a**, thrush, the correct answer. Choice **b**, tonsillitis, is incorrect because there is no mention of tonsillar exudates. Choice **c**, gastroesophageal reflux disease (GERD), is incorrect because it is inconsistent with the white plaques. Choice **d**, aphthous ulcers, is incorrect because there is no mention of any mucosal ulcers. Choice **e**, cheilitis, is incorrect because there is no mention of lip lesions.

Task Area: Formulating Most Likely Diagnosis
Organ System: EENT (Eye, Ear, Nose, and Throat)

74. d. The correct answer is choice **d**, fibrocystic change, which is the most common benign breast condition. Choice **a**, fibroadenoma, is incorrect because it is typically a non-painful lesion. This condition affects 60% of women between the ages of 30 and 50 and tends to become less of a problem after menopause. Choice **b**, carcinoma, is incorrect because it is a much less likely diagnosis given this patient's age. Choice **c**, hematoma, and choice **e**, fat necrosis, are incorrect, although possible, because they are much less likely than fibrocystic changes.

Task Area: History Taking and Performing Physical Examinations
Organ System: Reproductive

75. d. The correct answer is choice **d**, tamsulosin, which relaxes smooth muscle and improves urine flow. Choice **a**, ciprofloxicin, is incorrect because BPH is not an infectious condition. Choice **b**, NSAIDs, is incorrect because BPH is not an inflammatory condition. Choice **c**, allopurinol, is incorrect because it is indicated in treatment of gout. Choice **e**, fluticasone propionate, is incorrect because it is a nasal spray used for seasonal allergies.

Task Area: Pharmaceutical Therapeutics
Organ System: Genitourinary

76. b. This patient's clinical presentation and chest X-ray result is typical of active TB, which is then confirmed by positive acid-fast bacilli on the sputum smear. Sputum culture is the gold standard. The correct answer, therefore, is choice **b**, pulmonary tuberculosis. All the other options are incorrect because they are inconsistent with the positive acid-fast bacilli finding on the sputum smear.

Task Area: Formulating Most Likely Diagnosis
Organ System: Infectious Diseases

77. d. The most effective treatment option for a localized renal cell carcinoma is a radical nephrectomy (choice **d**). Choices **a** and **b**, radiation therapy and chemotherapy, should be considered; however, neither of these treatment choices has proven effective to prolong survival in early stage, localized renal cell carcinoma. Choice **c**, hormonal therapy, is incorrect as this would have no therapeutic benefit for this condition. Choice **e**, cryosurgery, should not be a consideration as this treatment option is useful for skin lesions and tumors but is not a viable treatment option for localized renal cell carcinoma.

Task Area: Clinical Intervention
Organ System: Genitourinary

78. d. Retinopathy is often the first sign of micro-vascular changes in diabetes; this can often act as an early indicator of the potential of further microvascular disease such as nephropathy and neuropathy. Consequently, it is important for patients with diabetes mellitus to have regular opthalmoscopic examinations, and, when available, retinal photography. In the presence of a chronic hyperglycemic state, retinal capillaries become structurally incompetent. This vascular wall compromise (choice **d**) eventually leads to retinopathy. Papilledema (choice **a**) is a swelling of the optic disc that is usually caused by an increase in intracranial pressure. Optic neuropathy (choice **b**) is most commonly caused by glaucoma and is generally unrelated to the peripheral neuropathy that is commonly seen in diabetes. Vascular occlusion (choice **c**) would be suggestive of a transient ischemic attack or a stroke, which may happen as a result of macrovascular changes in diabetes but is not a feature of diabetic retinopathy. Macular degeneration (choice **e**) is a common age-related cause of blindness.

Task Area: Applying Basic Science Concepts
Organ System: Endocrine

79. b. The patient's abnormal electrocardiogram with ST segment elevation should tell you that this patient is experiencing an acute myocardial infarction. Coronary angiography to evaluate for myocardial infarction (choice **b**) is the appropriate choice because the performing cardiologist can place a stent during the coronary angiography procedure to prevent permanent coronary damage. Choice **a**, ruling out pulmonary embolism with a CT scan of the chest, is incorrect because a normal D-dimer of 0.24 should rule out pulmonary embolism on its own without any radiologic procedure. Choice **c**, myocardial perfusion scan to evaluate for myocardial infarction, is incorrect because the time factor would be an issue in this situation, and no cardiac intervention would take place to prevent permanent cardiac damage. Choice **d**, echocardiogram to evaluate cardiac function, would not be the appropriate choice in this situation because this is an emergent situation, and the patient's vital signs and electrocardiogram indicate an acute myocardial infarction. Choice **e**, CT scan to rule out aortic dissection, would be inappropriate because the ST segment elevation on the electrocardiogram is a classic indication for myocardial infarction.

Task Area: Using Laboratory and Diagnostic Studies
Organ System: Cardiovascular

80. d. The correct answer is choice **d**, chronic obstructive pulmonary disease (COPD). COPD is characterized by progressive shortness of breath and excessive cough with sputum production. Auscultation of the chest should reveal decreased breath sounds, early inspiratory crackles, and prolonged expiration. Chest X-rays should reveal hyperinflation and flat diaphragm. Choice **a**, pneumonia, should definitely be a consideration, but the lack of fever and pain with inspiration should rule out this condition. The presence of excessive cough with sputum production should rule out choice **b**, asthma. Choice **c**, bronchiectasis, is incorrect due to lack of foul-smelling sputum and hemoptysis. Choice **e**, cystic fibrosis, should not be a consideration because of the age of the patient, as cystic fibrosis is diagnosed in childhood or adolescence.

Task Area: Formulating Most Likely Diagnosis
Organ System: Pulmonary

81. e. The correct answer is choice **e**, all of the above. Choice **a**, low-salt diet, is correct because a high-salt diet has been shown to worsen hypertension, which can cause CHF. Choice **b**, moderate physical activity, is correct because this patient has remained asymptomatic and stable on his medications, at which time physical activity is recommended as tolerated. Choice **c**, tobacco cessation, is correct given this patient's long pack-year and tobacco's numerous health risks. Choice **d**, diet low in fat and high in fruits and vegetables, is correct because this plan can help to reduce BMI, which is beneficial to heart health.

Task Area: Health Maintenance
Organ System: Cardiovascular

82. c. The correct answer is choice **c**, bronchiolitis. Ribavirin is indicated for use as treatment for bronchiolitis with the presence of respiratory syncytial virus (RSV). A three- to seven-day regimen of ribavirin has been proven to reduce mortality, length of hospitalization, and duration of mechanical ventilation for patients with RSV-induced bronchiolitis. Choice **a**, Tetralogy of Fallot, is only effectively treated via open heart surgery. Choice **b**, epiglottitis, is treated with intubation, humidified oxygen, antibiotics, and corticosteroids. Choice **d**, hyaline membrane disease, is most effectively treated with intubation and surfactant replacement. Choice **e**, respiratory distress syndrome, is commonly treated with warm, moist oxygen.

Task Area: Pharmaceutical Therapeutics
Organ System: Pulmonary

83. c. The correct answer is choice **c**, fever of greater than 100.4°F, tender anterior cervical adenopathy, lack of cough, and pharyngotonsillar exudates. Presence of three of the four criteria is highly suggestive of streptococcal pharyngitis. Presence of two of the four criteria indicates a need for a culture. Presence of one of the four criteria makes streptococcal pharyngitis highly unlikely. None of the other choices accurately describe the Centor Criteria.

Task Area: Applying Basic Scientific Concepts
Organ System: EENT (Eyes, Ears, Nose, and Throat)

84. c. A lack of thyroid hormone decreases the metabolic rate, which causes weight gain (choice **c**). Tachycardia (choice **a**), diarrhea (choice **b**), and profuse sweating (choice **d**) are consistent with hyperthroidism. Bulging of the eyes (choice **e**) can be seen in Graves' opthalmolopathy, which occurs in about half of all patients with Graves' disease. None of the other choices accurately describe the Centor Criteria.

Task Area: History Taking and Performing Physical Examinations
Organ System: Endocrine

85. b. The correct answer is choice **b**, infertility. Clomiphene citrate is commonly prescribed for anovulatory women to promote ovulation. A five-day regimen of 50 to 100 mg is administered beginning on day 3, 4, or 5 of the menstrual cycle. Choice **a**, ectopic pregnancy, is most effectively treated with methotrexate. Choice **c**, oral contraception, is achieved by several medications containing estrogen or progesterone. Choice **d**, transdermal contraception, is achieved by using the Ortho-Evra patch. Choice **e**, emergency contraception, is achieved by using high-dose progestin-only pills.

Task Area: Pharmaceutical Therapeutics
Organ System: Reproductive

86. b. The correct answer is choice **b**, stroke involving posterior circulation. The basilar and vertebral arteries are responsible for perfusion of the posterior aspect of the brain. These arteries supply the brain stem, cerebellum, thalamus, and portions of the occipital and temporal lobes. Strokes occurring in these vessels are commonly associated with evidence of brain stem dysfunction such as coma, drop attacks, vertigo, nausea, vomiting, and ataxia. Choice **a**, stroke involving anterior circulation, is incorrect because strokes involving the anterior circulation generally produce unilateral symptoms such as one-sided weakness and difficulty with speech. Choice **c**, transient ischemic attack (TIA), can produce dizziness, tingling, and numbness to one side of the body, but individuals generally do not lose consciousness. Choice **d**, hemorrhagic stroke, is caused by an aneurysm or blowout of a blood vessel; strokes of this type primarily cause sudden death. Choice **e**, thrombotic stroke, is much like strokes involving anterior circulation in that they cause unilateral symptoms such as one-sided weakness and difficulty with speech.

Task Area: Applying Basic Scientific Concepts
Organ System: Neurologic

87. c. The correct answer is choice **c**, seasonal affective disorder (SAD). Light therapy, otherwise known as phototherapy or heliotherapy, has been proven successful for patients who suffer from SAD. Light therapy consists of exposure to daylight or to specific wavelengths of light using lasers, light-emitting diodes, or fluorescent lamps. Light therapy treatments are administered for a prescribed amount of time and/or at a certain time of day. Choice **a**, obsessive-compulsive disorder (OCD), would most commonly be treated with cognitive behavioral therapy. Choice **b**, melancholia, or clinical depression, is commonly treated with cognitive behavioral therapy and the administration of antidepressants. Choice **d**, atypical depression, is also treated with cognitive behavioral therapy and the administration of antidepressants. Choice **e**, catatonic depression, is most effectively treatment with the administration of benzodiazepines such as lorazepam.

Task Area: Clinical Intervention
Organ System: Psychiatry/Behavioral Science

88. d. The correct answer is choice **d**, vasodilation. Minoxidil's ability to slow or stop hair growth and promote regrowth is due to its antihypertensive and vasodilatory properties. This medication is the safest, most effective treatment for male pattern baldness. Choices **a**, **b**, **c**, and **e** are all incorrect because minoxidil does not use any of these mechanisms to promote hair growth.

Task Area: Pharmaceutical Therapeutics
Organ System: Dermatologic

89. e. In a small child, exertional dyspnea and cyanosis (i.e., a "blue baby") should always raise concerns about congenital defects. The most common congenital cyanotic heart defect is the Tetralogy of Fallot, a network of abnormalities that includes pulmonary valve stenosis (choice **a**), right ventricular myocardial hypertrophy (choice **b**), the aorta overlying part of the pulmonary valve (choice **c**), and ventricular septal defects (choice **d**). Choice **e** is correct because the pulmonary artery is unaffected. It is important to remember that the pulmonary valve (part of the heart's endocardial tissue) and the pulmonary artery (vascular tissue) are two separate entities and that *pulmonary stenosis* refers to the valve rather than to the artery. Symptoms are not related to heart failure; they generally arise in response to systemic vasodilation (most commonly caused by exertion), which lowers afterload and left-ventricular resistance, thereby increasing the amount of right-to-left shunting.

Task Area: Applying Basic Science Concepts
Organ System: Cardiovascular

90. d. Tuberculosis (choice **d**) is one of the most common causes of lung disease worldwide, and while rates in Japan have dropped in recent years, older Japanese patients are still at high risk. Only about 10% of people infected with *Mycobacterium tuberculosis* will ever develop tuberculosis, so many patients have been unknowingly exposed to the infection. Tuberculosis presents with many of the same symptoms and test results as lung cancer and sarcoidosis: productive cough, weight loss, night sweats, and bilateral hilar lymphadenopathy on a chest X-ray. However, pulmonary fibrosis (choice **a**) is more likely to present with dyspnea and diffuse opacity in the lung fields. Choices **b** and **c**, small-cell carcinoma of the lung and sarcoidosis, are incorrect simply because tuberculosis is far more common, especially in Japanese populations. Additionally, tuberculosis nodules are more likely to appear in the apical lung fields. COPD (choice **e**) usually presents with an FEV_1/FVC below 70% and a very different radiologic appearance (no nodules, enlarged lung fields).

Task Area: Formulating Most Likely Diagnosis
Organ System: Pulmonary

91. d. This is a classic presentation of acute pancreatitis, an inflammatory condition in which patients usually complain of severe epigastric pain often accompanied by vomiting. The most common risk factor of acute pancreatitis is a history of excessive alcohol consumption, but it can also be caused by a wide range of other risk factors. A good mnemonic is *GET SMASHED*, which stands for *Gallstones, Ethanol, Trauma, Steroids, Mumps, Autoimmune, Scorpion stings, Hypercalcemia/Hyperlipidemia/Hypothermia, ERCP (endoscopic retrograde cholangiopancreatography), Drugs*. Acute pancreatitis typically causes a significant increase in the pancreatic enzymes, including lipase (choice **d**) and amylase. Aspartate transaminase, alanine transaminase, and gamma glutamyl transpeptidase (choices **a**, **b**, and **c**) are more likely to be elevated in liver disease; while this patient's chronic alcohol use may also have caused liver damage, pancreatitis is much more likely based on the clinical scenario. Gastrin (choice **e**) is a hormone that induces the release of gastric acid, but is not an enzyme and it is not related to pancreatitis.

Task Area: Using Laboratory and Diagnostic Studies
Organ System: Gastrointestinal/Nutritional

92. d. Ankylosing spondylitis (choice **d**) is a form of inflammatory arthritis that first manifests in the sacroiliac joints and progressively moves to other joints, especially in the back. As with rheumatoid arthritis, symptoms are usually most significant in the morning and improve over the course of the day as the joint is used. The specific cause is not known, but the most important risk factor is the HLA-B27 gene, which also predisposes to reactive arthritis, psoriatic arthritis, anterior uveitis, and inflammatory bowel disease; this patient's family history of Crohn's disease suggests that he is at a higher risk of other diseases related to HLA-B27. The gene is fairly common in the general population, although the prevalence varies between 1% in and 25% in different ethnic groups. Patients with ankylosing spondylitis almost always have HLA-B27, but the majority of patients with HLA-B27 do not develop any autoimmune disease. Trauma (choice **a**) is always an important differential diagnosis to consider for a young patient with pain, but trauma is unlikely to cause occasional pain that does not resolve over time. Gonococcal arthritis (choice **b**) is also particularly common in younger patients, but it is less likely to be confined to the sacroiliac joints and usually also causes dysuria due to urethritis. Reactive arthritis (choice **e**) also causes urethritis and typically presents within one to two months of a significant infection. Psoriatic arthritis (choice **c**) is not limited to the sacroiliac joints and is usually associated with psoriatic rashes.

Task Area: Formulating Most Likely Diagnosis
Organ System: Musculoskeletal

93. b. Diazepam is the indicated course of treatment for individuals who suffer from acute episodes of vertigo (choice **b**). Diazepam should be administered intravenously or rectally for the most effective treatment. Bed rest may also be required with acute episodes of vertigo. Diazepam is contraindicated for elderly patients because the sedative effect may make their situations worse. Choice **a**, barotrauma, is commonly treated medically with antihistamines, steroids, or decongestants. Choice **c**, motion sickness, is most commonly treated with scopolamine or meclizine (Antivert). Choice **d**, labyrinthitis, will commonly resolve on its own after a few days; however, meclizine is often prescribed for treatment of this disorder. Choice **e**, presbycusis, is not treatable, but hearing loss is often treated with hearing aids.

Task Area: Pharmaceutical Therapeutics
Organ System: EENT (Eye, Ear, Nose, and Throat)

94. c. This patient's knees appear to be affected by osteoarthritis, a degenerative condition caused by years of wear on the joints. Osteoarthritis is usually managed with NSAIDs for pain relief and, if necessary, joint replacement. However, before recommending surgical intervention, it is advisable to suggest lifestyle changes for the patient. Features of osteoarthritis have been shown to be alleviated by a regimen of non-weight-bearing exercise such as swimming (choice **c**). Weight loss (choice **a**) is beneficial for managing lower limb osteoarthritis in patients who are overweight, but it is unlikely to provide relief for this patient because her weight is already in the acceptable range. Weight-bearing exercise (choice **b**) is useful for patients with osteoporosis, but it generally exacerbates symptoms of osteoarthritis. Increasing intake of calcium (choice **d**) and vitamin D (choice **e**) is also beneficial for osteoporosis and some other bone disorders but is unlikely to improve symptoms of joint degeneration.

Task Area: Health Maintenance
Organ System: Musculoskeletal

95. b. This patient has a classic presentation of Cushing's syndrome, a disorder caused by excess glucocorticoid concentrations. Cushing's syndrome usually causes amenorrhea, central obesity, hypertension, hyperglycemia, and a variety of other signs and symptoms that are fairly nonspecific on their own, but may be diagnostic when present together. There are several possible causes of Cushing's syndrome, but the most common is the use of corticosteroid therapy (choice **b**); less common causes include Cushing's disease (ACTH-producing pituitary tumor), a cortisol-producing tumor in the adrenal glands, or ectopic production of ACTH or cortisol. Hydrochlorothiazide (choice **a**) can also cause hyperglycemia but is not associated with most of this patient's other symptoms. Methotrexate (choice **c**) often causes bone marrow suppression but does not account for any of the symptoms here. Naproxen (choice **d**) may cause peripheral edema, but it is a fairly safe NSAID that is unlikely to cause significant complications. The oral contraceptive pill (choice **e**) may affect levels of estrogen and progesterone but is less likely to affect glucocorticoids.

Task Area: Pharmaceutical Therapeutics
Organ System: Endocrine

96. b. This patient has a spinal cord hemisection, also known as Brown-Sequard syndrome. In Brown-Sequard syndrome, all motor and sensory function is lost in the areas supplied by upper motor neurons of the corticospinal tract as well as the sensory neurons in the dorsal column and the spinothalamic tract below the level of the lesion. However, because reflexes are mediated by the spinal cord via lower motor neurons, and the upper motor neuron connection to the brain will only inhibit reflexes, an upper motor neuron deficit causes reflexes to become hyperactive. Therefore, choice **b** is correct. Choices **a** and **c** are incorrect because there is no mechanical lesion that can cause hyperactive sensation. Choice **d** describes a situation that may be consistent with a lower motor neuron lesion, but an upper motor neuron lesion will not cause hyporeflexia or areflexia. Choice **e** might occur if the patient's paralysis is not because of a nerve lesion, but this is unlikely because of the unilateral nature of the symptoms, the history of major trauma, and the severe back pain.

Task Area: History Taking and Performing Physical Examinations

Organ System: Neurologic

97. e. The patient has a pneumoperitoneum that was caused by perforation during the colonoscopy. The treatment for this condition is immediate surgery (choice **e**). Triple therapy (choice **a**) is used to treat H. pylori. Infliximab (choice **b**) and corticosteroids (choice **c**) are used to treat Crohn's disease. This is not the primary concern. A second colonoscopy (choice **d**) would cause more harm.

Task Area: Clinical Intervention

Organ System: Gastrointestinal/Nutritional

98. e. Polycystic ovarian syndrome is not associated with hypotension (choice **e**). It is associated with hyperandrogenism, which causes hirsutism (choice **c**) and baldness (choice **d**). It is also associated with metabolic syndromes which cause obesity (choice **a**) and acanthosis nigricans (choice **b**).

Task Area: History Taking and Performing Physical Examinations

Organ System: Reproductive

99. b. This patient seems to have chronic obstructive pulmonary disease (COPD), a very common smoking-related syndrome that includes emphysema and chronic bronchitis. The effect of the chronic bronchitis is known to be exacerbated by beta-blockers, especially nonselective beta-blockers like propranolol, because of their tendency to cause bronchoconstriction. Cessation of propranolol (choice **b**) is likely to cause a significant reduction in bronchoconstriction and, consequently, should improve this patient's symptoms considerably. It is also important to recommend smoking cessation (choice **a**) in order to prevent further deterioration in patients with COPD, but this does not generally cause an improvement in the patient's current pulmonary function. Hydrochlorothiazide (choice **c**) does not have any significant effect on this process. Albuterol (choice **d**) is a short-acting bronchodilator, so while it may help to alleviate acute symptoms, daily therapy is not useful. Fluticasone (choice **e**) and other inhaled corticosteroids are often used in patients with COPD, but their effect is generally minor, and their efficacy has only been proven in patients with severe pulmonary disease.

Task Area: Pharmaceutical Therapeutics

Organ System: Pulmonary

100. **d.** Malignant hypertension, which occurs in approximately 1% of patients with essential hypertension, is a medical emergency that should be treated quickly in order to address the patient's symptoms and to prevent the development of hypertrophic cardiomyopathy and renal failure. A hypertensive emergency consists of substantial effects on the cardiovascular, nervous, and renal systems; however, the presence of papilledema (choice **d**) must be established in order to make a diagnosis. Irregular heartbeat (choice **a**) generally signifies a cardiac arrhythmia, which is not related to malignant hypertension. Hepatomegaly (choice **b**) is a nonspecific sign that may be associated with portal hypertension, but it is unlikely to be caused by arterial hypertension. Crackles in the lung fields (choice **c**) are usually caused by pulmonary edema, which may be related to pulmonary hypertension but is less sensitive and specific for systemic hypertension. Carotid bruits (choice **e**) are likely to be found in carotid artery stenosis.

Task Area: History Taking and Performing Physical Examinations
Organ System: Cardiovascular

101. **b.** Although the pathophysiology of this disease has not been completely elucidated, it is understood that dopamine (choice **b**) is involved in the disease and is therefore a good target for therapy. Acetylcholine (choice **a**) levels are depleted in Alzheimer's disease. Norepinephrine (choice **c**) and serotonin (choice **d**) levels are altered in depression and anxiety. Histamine (choice **e**) depletion causes sedation.

Task Area: Applying Basic Science Concepts
Organ System: Psychiatry/Behavioral Science

102. **d.** The depth of the lesion (choice **d**) is the most important prognostic factor for melanoma. Inflammatory markers such as erythrocyte sedimentation rate (ESR) (choice **a**) and C-reactive protein (CRP) (choice **b**) are not affected by melanoma. Prostate-specific antigen (PSA) (choice **c**) is a nonspecific marker for prostate cancer. Vascularity (choice **e**) is not used for grading or staging melanoma.

Task Area: Using Laboratory and Diagnostic Studies
Organ System: Dermatologic

103. **c.** A CD4 count below 200/mm^3 puts the patient at risk of *Pneumocystis jirovecii* infection. *Pneumocystis jirovecii* is a fungus and would be unresponsive to ceftriaxone (choice **a**), penicillin (choice **b**), vancomycin (choice **d**), and doxycycline (choice **e**).

Task Area: Clinical Intervention
Organ System: Infectious Diseases

104. **a.** A Hampton's hump (choice **a**) is denoted by a shallow, wedge-shaped opacity along the periphery of the lung. This sign results from a pulmonary embolism causing an infarct at the site of the embolism. Choice **b**, apple core lesion, is incorrect as this is the classic sign for annular carcinomas of the colon. Choice **c**, Codman's triangle, is incorrect as this is the classic sign for osteosarcoma. Choice **d**, cookie cutter lesion, is incorrect as this is a classic sign for bone metastases or Paget's disease. Choice **e**, crescent sign, is incorrect as this is the classic sign for avascular necrosis of the femoral head.

Task Area: Using Laboratory and Diagnostic Studies
Organ System: Pulmonary

105. c. Chronic pancreatitis (choice **c**) is predominantly caused by alcohol abuse. Chronic pancreatitis will present as epigastric pain that radiates to the back and may be relieved when the patient leans forward or lies in the fetal position. This disorder differs from acute pancreatitis by the presence of fat malabsorption and steatorrhea. Serum amylase and lipase levels will be elevated. Choice **a**, esophageal varices, should be considered due to the patient's history of alcoholism; however, the absence of bleeding and endoscopic confirmation should rule this out. The lack of fever, nausea, vomiting, and diaphoresis should exclude choice **b**, acute pancreatitis. Choice **d**, pancreatic neoplasm, might be considered and a work-up performed; however, from the patient's presentation, the lack of nausea, vomiting, weight loss, and loss of appetite should exclude this diagnosis. The fact that the pain is relieved when lying in the fetal position and the lack of fever, nausea, jaundice, and vomiting should rule out choice **e,** cholelithiasis.

Task Area: Formulating Most Likely Diagnosis
Organ System: Gastrointestinal/Nutritional

106. d. Polymyositis (choice **d**) is an inflammatory disease of striated muscles affecting the proximal limbs, neck, and pharynx. Patients may present with proximal muscle weakness, dysphagia, malar or heliotrope skin rash, muscle aches, or muscle atrophy. Serum creatinine phosphokinase and aldolase will be elevated. Choice **a**, septic arthritis, should be ruled out because of the lack of pain and swelling in a joint area. Lack of urinary symptoms and conjunctivitis should rule out choice **b**, reactive arthritis. Choice **c**, calcium pyrophosphate dihydrate disease, should be ruled out because of the lack of pain and swelling in joint spaces. Choice **e**, multiple myeloma, should be ruled out because of the lack of bleeding problems and bone pain.

Task Area: History Taking and Performing Physical Examinations
Organ System: Musculoskeletal

107. d. For individuals who suffer from acute episodes of vertigo, intravenous or rectal administration of diazepam (choice **d**) is the preferred treatment. Bed rest may also be required with acute episodes of vertigo. Choice **a**, scopolamine, is primarily used to treat nausea and motion sickness. Choice **b**, meclizine, is also used to treat nausea, vomiting, and motion sickness. Choice **c**, dimenhydrinate, is an antihistamine used to treat nausea, vomiting, and motion sickness. Choice **e**, adenosine, should not even be considered as it is used to treat cardiac conditions such as supraventricular tachycardia.

Task Area: Pharmaceutical Therapeutics
Organ System: EENT (Eye, Ear, Nose, and Throat)

108. **c.** Menopause (choice **c**) is clinically confirmed when the level of follicle-stimulating hormone (FSH) exceeds 30 IU/mL. The rise in FSH levels is directly proportional to the ovaries slowing down production of estrogen. FSH levels are not associated with choices **a**, **b**, **d**, and **e**.

Task Area: Using Laboratory and Diagnostic Studies

Organ System: Reproductive

109. **b.** Mitral valve prolapse (choice **b**), an upward displacement of at least one of the two cusps of the mitral valve, is the most common valvular heart disease in the general population. It is associated with a variety of causes, and genetic inheritance is a major contributing factor. Patients are usually asymptomatic until they develop mild intermittent palpitations, and although some complications are possible, the prognosis is generally benign. Physical examination usually reveals a systolic click, which is produced by the sudden tensing of the valve apparatus as its leaflets prolapse into the left atrium, followed by a systolic murmur that is best heard at the apex. Mitral valve stenosis (choice **a**) produces a similar murmur, but it is not associated with a click. Pulmonary valve stenosis (choice **c**) leads to a systolic murmur that is best heard at the superior aspect of the left sternal border. Pulmonary valve prolapse (choice **d**) is uncommon and, if present, would also be loudest at the superior left sternal border. Multiple valvular defects (choice **e**) are possible, but there is no evidence to suggest their presence in this case.

Task Area: Formulating Most Likely Diagnosis

Organ System: Cardiovascular

110. **c.** Diverticulitis is caused by an infection of a diverticulum, an abnormal outpouching in the intestinal wall. One of the strongest risk factors for diverticulitis is an established history of diverticulosis, which is supported by a past history of an intestinal bleed (choice **c**). Intestinal bleeds are a common complication of diverticulosis; if this is elicited in a history, diverticulitis should be considered as a provisional diagnosis. Usually, an intestinal bleed would manifest as either melena or blood on the patient's toilet paper. The diagnosis can be further supported by an elevated white blood cell count as well as bowel wall thickening on an abdominal X-ray. Recent travel to certain countries, including much of South America (choice **a**), is a risk factor for bloody diarrhea. If other members of his household have experienced a similar illness (choice **b**), gastroenteritis is a more likely culprit. If he has recently undergone an antibiotic regimen, particularly one that included clindamycin (choice **d**), pseudomembranous colitis should be considered. Recent abdominal surgery (choice **e**) may raise the possibility of a bleed or an incisional hernia.

Task Area: History Taking and Performing Physical Examinations

Organ System: Gastrointestinal/Nutritional

111. b. The most common cause of knee pain in adolescents is Osgood-Schlatter disease, a rupture of the growth plate on the superior end of the tibia (choice **b**). Osgood-Schlatter disease is far more common in patients who engage in regular athletic activity and typically appears during a growth spurt. The diagnosis can be confirmed with a knee X-ray, which will demonstrate a lesion at the tibial tuberosity near the site of the soft tissue swelling. Usually, rest and supportive therapy will allow the condition to heal. Lesions at the patella (choice **a**), fibula (choice **c**), or tibialis anterior tendon (choice **d**) should also be considered, but these are less common in this population and are usually associated with clear trauma. A rupture of the patellar tendon (choice **e**), also known as Sinding-Larsen and Johansson syndrome, may also present in this sort of patient but is less common than Osgood-Schlatter disease.

Task Area: Applying Basic Science Concepts
Organ System: Musculoskeletal

112. a. Even in the absence of bereavement, the *DSM-IV* criteria for diagnosis of major depressive disorder require the presence of symptoms for at least two months. After the death of a loved one, it is normal for a patient to experience grief-related depressive symptoms for several months. This is particularly likely if the patient's loved one was young and the death was sudden and unexpected. Consequently, it is inappropriate to start addictive or invasive therapy at this stage; instead, most patients will benefit from grief counseling or psychotherapy (choice **a**). Fluoxetine (choice **b**) may become necessary if the patient's symptoms persist, but is not indicated at this stage because of its addictive nature. Electroconvulsive therapy (choice **c**) is also not indicated at this stage because of its invasiveness and the potential for significant complications. Temazepam (choice **d**) may help with the patient's insomnia, but it should also be avoided if possible because of its tendency to cause addiction. Phototherapy (choice **e**) is useful for patients with seasonal affective disorder but has not been shown to provide benefits to other forms of depression.

Task Area: Clinical Intervention
Organ System: Psychiatry/Behavioral Science

113. **d.** Actinic keratosis is a common cause of skin lesions in areas that are openly exposed to the sun. They generally appear many years after the causative sun exposure and can be treated with cryotherapy, immunomodulatory cream, radiotherapy, or surgical excision. While the lesion itself is unlikely to spread beyond the skin, it has a 20% chance of conversion to squamous cell carcinoma (choice **d**), a skin cancer that carries a small chance of local invasion or metastasis. Local tissue invasion (choice **a**) is not an established consequence of actinic keratosis, although it is possible in some cases if the lesion develops into a squamous cell carcinoma. Malignant melanoma (choice **b**), lentigo maligna (choice **c**), and basal cell carcinoma (choice **e**) are not associated with actinic keratosis in any situation.

Task Area: Health Maintenance

Organ System: Dermatologic

114. **a.** HIPAA (choice **a**) is the legislation designed to insure the privacy and security of personal health information. Choice **b**, MIPPA, is incorrect as this legislation is used to adjust Medicare reimbursement to certain facilities. Choice **c**, Patient Bill of Rights, is incorrect as this legislation requires healthcare providers to inform all patients of their rights as patients receiving medical treatment. Choice **d**, EMTALA, is incorrect as this legislation legally obligates healthcare facilities to provide emergent care regardless of citizenship, legal status, or ability to pay. Choice **e**, SMDA, is incorrect as this piece of legislation requires users of medical devices to report any incidents that could in any way suggest that the device caused death, serious injury, or illness to a patient.

Task Area: Clinical Intervention

Organ System: Cardiovascular

115. **d.** Aortic stenosis (choice **d**) is characterized by chest pain, shortness of breath and even sudden death. Fluid in the lungs may accompany aortic stenosis if the condition is severe enough to cause heart failure. Classic echocardiogram of aortic stenosis is a calcified, poorly functioning aortic valve. Choice **a**, carotid stenosis, is a viable option; however, without a Doppler study of the carotid arteries, a proper diagnosis cannot be made. Choice **b**, pericarditis, would be an incorrect diagnosis in this case because the echocardiogram did not reveal any fluid surrounding the heart. Choice **c**, mitral valve prolapse, is also incorrect because the echocardiogram revealed a poorly functioning aortic valve. Choice **e**, congestive heart failure, might be a consideration; however, this condition is usually accompanied by fluid collection in the abdomen, feet, and ankles, as well as weight gain, which the patient does not present.

Task Area: Formulating Most Likely Diagnosis

Organ System: Cardiovascular

116. **c.** This patient experiences situational panic attacks, so the correct answer is choice **c**, panic disorder. Choice **a**, generalized anxiety disorder, is incorrect because this disorder is excessive anxiety for most days for more than six months. Choice **b**, delusional disorder, is incorrect as patients with this disorder have isolated and implausible beliefs. Choice **d**, schizoid disorder, is incorrect because patients with this disorder have difficulty in social situations, are fascinated by unusual ideas, and appear to others as odd or eccentric. Choice **e**, attention-deficit disorder, is incorrect because patients with this disorder have difficulty focusing to perform normal daily activities.

Task Area: History Taking and Performing Physical Examinations

Organ System: Psychiatry/Behavioral Science

117. **c.** Pilocarpine, commonly referred to as Salagen, is used to increase salivary flow for patients who experience dry mouth as a result of Sjögren's syndrome (choice **c**). This medication is used when other therapies such as artificial saliva and increasing oral fluid intake fail to provide adequate treatment. Choice **a**, Parkinson's disease, is commonly treated with levodopa, amantadine, and benztropine. Choice **b**, Meniere's disease, is commonly treated with antivert, hydrochlorothiazide, and valium. Choice **d**, Hashimoto's disease, is commonly treated by replacing the deficient thyroid hormone with levoxyl or synthroid. Choice **e**, Wilson's disease, is treated with penicillamine and trientine, which will lower the levels of copper in the body.

Task Area: Pharmaceutical Therapeutics
Organ System: Musculoskeletal

118. **e.** Macrocytic anemias are characterized by mean corpuscular volumes greater than 100 fL (choice **e**). These forms of anemia can be caused by conditions such as acute hemorrhage and hemolysis. These forms of anemia also include deficiencies that ultimately lead to megaloblastic states. Choices **a**, **b**, **c**, and **d** are all incorrect as macrocytic anemia are characterized by mean corpuscular volumes greater than 100 fL.

Task Area: Using Laboratory and Diagnostic Studies
Organ System: Hematologic

119. **b.** Proton pump inhibitors (choice **b**) are a group of medications that are very effective and offer long-lasting reduction of gastric acid production. This group is the most powerful medication for treatment of GERD. Proton pump inhibitors are the first line of defense in the treatment of moderate to severe GERD, patients who are unresponsive to histamine blockers, and patients with evidence of erosive gastritis. Choice **a**, antacids, is incorrect. Even though antacids are a mainstay treatment for GERD, the extent of this patient's condition indicates the use of proton pump inhibitors. Nitrates (choice **c**) would not be effective for this disorder as these medications may only make the condition worse. Calcium channel blockers (choice **d**), would not be effective for this disorder as these medications may only make the condition worse. Choice **e**, ACE inhibitors, is also incorrect as they may worsen the condition.

Task Area: Health Maintenance
Organ System: Gastrointestinal/Nutritional

120. d. A migraine headache (choice **d**) often presents unilaterally with throbbing or pulsing discomfort. Migraine headaches occur more in women than in men and often follow the menstrual cycle pattern. Patients who suffer from migraines can also present with aura involving visual changes, nausea, vomiting, photophobia, phonophobia, and anorexia. Choice **a**, cerebral aneurysm, is incorrect because this condition can be associated with double vision, loss of vision, neck pain, and mental status changes. Choice **b**, subarachnoid hemorrhage, is incorrect because this condition is associated with mental status changes, dilated pupils, intraocular hemorrhaging and a quick, sudden, "thunderclap" headache. Choice **c**, cluster headache, can be similar to a migraine headache; however, the pain usually occurs in the eye regions, and lying down will not alleviate the pain of a cluster headache. In contrast to people with migraine, people with cluster headache usually avoid lying down during an attack because this position seems to increase the pain. Choice **e**, tension headache, is not appropriate because this condition is associated with a dull aching pain in the forehead or the back of the head and can include pain in the neck and shoulders.
Task Area: Formulating Most Likely Diagnosis
Organ System: Neurologic

Section 3

121. d. Clomiphene modulates estrogen receptors in the hypothalamus (choice **d**). Mifepristone is a peripheral acting progesterone antagonist (choice **e**) and is used as an abortifacient. Bromocriptine is a central acting dopamine agonist (choice **b**) and can be used to treat hyperprolactinemia. Many synthetic estrogens act as estrogen agonists in the periphery (choice **c**). There is no major drug that is considered to be a peripheral acting estrogen antagonist (choice **a**).
Task Area: Pharmaceutical Therapeutics
Organ System: Reproductive

122. c. This patient most likely has rheumatic heart disease, as evidenced by his symptoms of mitral stenosis as well as his history of a childhood illness that resembles rheumatic fever. Rheumatic heart disease is caused by Antistreptolysin O, an antibody whose primary purpose is to fight the *Streptococcus pyogenes* that caused this patient's childhood infection. Antistreptolysin O often goes on to develop cross-reactivity against endocardial tissue, including the heart valves. Heart symptoms usually appear in the fourth or fifth decade of life and generally manifest as significant exertional dyspnea that appears fairly rapidly. The most common pathological change is mitral valve stenosis, which causes a diastolic murmur that is most prominent over the apex (choice **c**), which is where the sound from the mitral valve is loudest. Choice **a** describes the sound that would be heard from mitral valve regurgitation, which may also be present in rheumatic heart disease, but is far less common than mitral valve stenosis. Choice **b** represents aortic valve stenosis, which is also a less common consequence of rheumatic heart disease and several other conditions. Choice **d** suggests aortic valve regurgitation, which is also less likely. Choice **e** might appear in the presence of a ventricular septal defect, which is usually a congenital abnormality.

Task Area: History Taking and Performing Physical Examinations
Organ System: Cardiovascular

123. e. Both Crohn's disease and ulcerative colitis are associated with presence of the HLA-B27 gene, which is also associated with uveitis (choice **e**), ankylosing spondylitis, reactive arthritis (Reiter's syndrome), and primary sclerosing cholangitis. Patients with one of these syndromes are considered to be at considerably higher risk for any of the others; uveitis is an important potential complication of IBD (inflammatory bowel disease), ankylosing spondylitis, and reactive arthritis, and warrants immediate attention and treatment to prevent blindness. While sulfa-drug allergy (choice **a**) is occasionally seen in response to sulfasalazine, it usually causes skin rashes and systemic symptoms and is unlikely to be confined to the eyes. Choices **b** and **c** are incorrect because although corticosteroids can induce rash or Cushing's syndrome (which can cause increased intraocular pressure), these are both unlikely to cause photophobia. Keratoconjunctivitis (choice **d**) is also unlikely to cause photophobia, and this patient is not at particularly high risk.

Task Area: Pharmaceutical Therapeutics
Organ System: EENT (Eye, Ear, Nose, and Throat)

124. e. Cystic fibrosis (choice **e**) is characterized by cough, excess sputum, sinus pain, nasal discharge, diarrhea, and abdominal pain. Steatorrhea and decreased exercise tolerance may also be presented. A physical exam can reveal clubbing, apical crackles, and increased anteroposterior chest diameter. A CT scan can reveal bronchiectasis. A chest X-ray can reveal hyperinflation, mucous plugging, peribronchial cuffing, focal atelectasis or pneumothorax. Choices **a**, pneumonia; **b**, asthma; and **d**, COPD, are all ruled out because of the presence of excess sputum, sinus pain, nasal discharge, diarrhea and abdominal pain. Choice **c**, bronchiectasis, is a consideration and is often present with cystic fibrosis; however, the presence of nasal discharge, diarrhea, and abdominal pain, as well as the age of the patient should warrant further investigation.

Task Area: Formulating Most Likely Diagnosis
Organ System: Pulmonary

125. a. A volvulus (choice **a**) is a twisting of any part of the bowel on itself. This disorder usually involves the sigmoid or cecal areas of the bowel. Patients with volvulus may present with abdominal pain, distention, nausea, vomiting, fever, or tachycardia. Choice **b**, celiac disease, is incorrect, as this condition is characterized by damage to the small intestine that prevents it from absorbing nutrients from food. Choice **c**, Crohn's disease, is incorrect, as this is a form of inflammatory bowel disease. Choice **d**, bowel obstruction, is incorrect, as this occurs without a twisting of any part of the bowel. Choice **e**, obstipation, is incorrect as this is a form of bowel obstruction that occurs without the bowel being twisted.

Task Area: Applying Basic Science Concepts
Organ System: Gastrointestinal/Nutritional

126. b. This presentation is consistent with aortic stenosis, or a narrowing of the aortic valve that causes an obstruction in the outflow of oxygenated blood from the heart. The characteristic physical examination finding is a systolic ejection murmur that is loudest over the region of the aortic valve and often radiates to the neck. When aortic stenosis becomes symptomatic (with angina, exertional dyspnea, or syncope with effort), the prognosis can be fairly poor. The diagnosis can generally be confirmed with an echocardiogram (choice **b**), which can quantify the extent of stenosis by reporting an ejection fraction. Elevated troponin levels (choice **a**) are indicative of myocardial damage (usually due to infarction), which is not a concern for this patient. A resting electrocardiogram (choice **c**) may be helpful to test for the presence of left ventricular hypertrophy, but an echocardiogram would provide a more specific answer regarding aortic stenosis. An exercise stress electrocardiogram (choice **d**) may demonstrate ischemia, but would be no more beneficial than a resting electrocardiogram for diagnosis and grading of aortic stenosis. A chest X-ray (choice **e**) may demonstrate a dilated cardiomyopathy, but again would not be useful here.

Task Area: Using Laboratory and Diagnostic Studies
Organ System: Cardiovascular

127. c. A gluten-free diet (choice **c**) is imperative for individuals diagnosed with celiac disease. Celiac disease is characterized by small bowel inflammation due to the digestion of gluten-containing products such as wheat, rye, and barley. A gluten-free diet will allow individuals diagnosed with celiac disease avoid flareups. Choices **a**, **b**, **d**, and **e** are all incorrect, as maintaining a lactose-free, sugar-free, fat-free, or fructose-free diet will have no impact on celiac disease flareups.

Task Area: Health Maintenance
Organ System: Gastrointestinal/Nutritional

128. c. This is a classic presentation of oral candidiasis, commonly known as thrush. Thrush is a common fungal infection of the tongue which, if not treated, may spread to the esophagus. It can be treated with a variety of antifungal agents, but the standard treatment is an oral nystatin suspension (choice **c**). The patient swishes the suspension in her mouth in order to maximize contact of the affected area with the drug. Nystatin resistance is uncommon, and the treatment regimen is highly effective. Additionally, it may be beneficial to order an HIV test; while the presence of HIV is unlikely, oral thrush occasionally presents as the first manifestation of a systemic immunocompromised state. Systemic amphotericin B (choices **a** and **b**) is a powerful method for clearing systemic fungal infections, but amphotericin B is a relatively toxic drug, and local nystatin is more useful for thrush. Penicillin (choice **d**) is not useful because a bacterial infection is unlikely. Antiseptic mouthwash (choice **e**) is believed to help prevent thrush but is not as effective as targeted antifungal therapy for resolving an existing infection.

Task Area: Clinical Intervention
Organ System: EENT (Eye, Ear, Nose, and Throat)

129. c. The correct answer is choice **c**, troponin I and T, which are cardiac-specific when elevated. Choice **a**, ESR, is incorrect because it is a nonspecific test that, when increased, may indicate any underlying infection or inflammation. Choice **b**, D-dimer, is used to rule out pulmonary emboli and deep vein thrombosis. Choice **d**, CK-MM, is incorrect because it is an isoenzyme of creatine kinase more specific to muscle injury. Choice **e**, WBC, is incorrect because it is usually elevated due to inflammatory or infectious etiologies and is not specific to ischemic heart injury.

Task Area: Using Laboratory and Diagnostic Studies

Organ System: Cardiovascular

130. d. This patient's unusual tendency to fracture with minimal trauma is suggestive of impaired bone formation. While this would typically suggest calcium deficiency (choice **b**) or hyperparathyroidism (choice **c**), the presence of blue sclerae is a sign that is fairly specific for osteogenesis imperfecta, an inherited disorder that leads to deficiency of type I collagen. Osteogenesis imperfecta is usually inherited in an autosomal dominant pattern (choice **d**), although autosomal recessive forms also exist. Choice **e** is incorrect; even if an X-linked recessive form of osteogenesis imperfecta existed, X-linked recessive traits are exceedingly rare in females. Choice **a** is incorrect because a viral infection plays no role in this process.

Task Area: Applying Basic Science Concepts

Organ System: Musculoskeletal

131. e. The correct answer is choice **e**, percutaneous coronary intervention (PCI), which should be performed within 90 minutes to reduce mortality up to 50%. Choice **a**, continue to observe, is incorrect because in the setting of STEMI, percutaneous coronary intervention (PCI) is the standard of treatment. Choice **b**, electrocardioversion, is incorrect because the patient is conscious. Choice **c**, give a beta-blocker, is incorrect because it is an adjunctive therapy that is initiated after the patient has been stabilized. Choice **d**, perform immediate chest compressions, is incorrect because the patient is conscious with a pulse.

Task Area: Clinical Intervention

Organ System: Cardiovascular

132. b. The correct answer is choice **b**, high-pitched wheezes more pronounced on expiration. Choice **e**, none of the above, is therefore incorrect. Choice **a**, clear bilateral lung sounds, is incorrect because wheezing on bilateral lung fields is usually appreciated on auscultation during acute exacerbation. Choice **c**, body temperature of 102°F, is incorrect because asthma alone typically does not induce fever without secondary bacterial infection. Choice **d**, no symptomatic relief after albuterol use, is incorrect because bronchodilator responsiveness is a strong indicator of asthma.

Task Area: History Taking and Performing Physical Examinations

Organ System: Pulmonary

133. e. The correct answer is choice **e**, all of the above, because several factors may contribute to gastroesophageal reflux disease (GERD). Choice **a**, weight loss, is correct because body weight, especially truncal obesity, can increase abdominal pressure and lead to GERD. Choice **b**, smoking cessation, is correct because nicotine relaxes the lower esophageal sphincter. Choice **c**, avoid overeating, and choice **d**, sitting upright for three hours before lying supine, are both good measures to prevent increasing the lower esophageal sphincter pressure.

Task Area: Health Maintenance
Organ System: Gastrointestinal/Nutritional

134. d. The correct answer is choice **d**, bisphosphonates, which are antiresorptives indicated to reduce risk of fractures. Choice **a**, Omega 3 fish oil, is incorrect because it is indicated in lowering cholesterol. Choice **b**, vitamin E, is incorrect because it is not indicated in treatment of osteoporosis. Choice **c**, tamsulosin (Flomax), is incorrect because it is used to treat benign prostate hypertrophy. Choice **e**, estrogen replacement therapy, is incorrect because it is associated with increased risk of breast cancer, stroke, venous thromboembolism, and perhaps coronary disease.

Task Area: Pharmaceutical Therapeutics
Organ System: Musculoskeletal

135. b. The correct answer is choice **b**, hydatidiform mole (molar pregnancy), given the characteristic "snowstorm" appearance on ultrasound. hCG is typically very high. Choice **a**, normal pregnancy, is incorrect because spotting and high hCG are not normal. Choice **c**, spontaneous abortion, is incorrect because the ultrasound finding is inconsistent with this option. Choice **d**, atopic pregnancy, is incorrect because the ultrasound finding is more consistent with molar pregnancy. Choice **e**, preterm labor, is incorrect because this patient is still in her first trimester.

Task Area: Formulating Most Likely Diagnosis
Organ System: Reproductive

136. d. Pulmonary embolism (choice **d**) presents clinically with pleuritic chest pain, dyspnea, and hemoptysis. Cough and diaphoresis may also be present. A physical examination reveals tachycardia, tachypnea, low-grade fever lasting one to seven days, crackles, and accentuation of the pulmonary component of the second heart sound. Choice **a**, myocardial infarction, should definitely be a consideration, but the lack of ST segment elevation on the electrocardiogram should warrant further evaluation. Choice **b**, bronchiectasis, is not a consideration because of the absence of foul-smelling sputum. The presence of hemoptysis and tachycardia should rule out choice **c**, pulmonary hypertension. Choice **e**, cystic fibrosis, should be ruled out because of the absence of excess sputum, sinus pain, nasal discharge, diarrhea, and abdominal pain.

Task Area: History Taking and Performing Physical Examinations
Organ System: Pulmonary

137. e. This question tests your knowledge of the initial workup for patients with panic attacks. This patient is most likely experiencing panic attacks given her recent distress over her daughter and her clinical presentation. The correct answer is choice **e**, all of the above. It is important to rule out possible medical conditions that may be contributing to this patient's psychological symptoms.

Task Area: Using Laboratory and Diagnostic Studies

Organ System: Psychiatry/Behavioral Science

138. d. The term *dew drops on a rose petal* is frequently used to describe the appearance of impetigo (choice **d**), a bacterial infection of the skin. Choice **e**, none of the above, is therefore incorrect. Choice **a**, vitiligo, is incorrect because there is no mention of depigmentation. Choice **b**, paronychia, is incorrect because this is generally a fingernail condition. Choice **c**, acne vulgaris, is incorrect because of this patient's young age and the appearance of the lesion.

Task Area: History Taking and Performing Physical Examinations

Organ System: Dermatologic

139. b. This question tests your ability to differentiate types of anemia. The lab results and peripheral blood smear showing megalocytes clearly point to a diagnosis of pernicious anemia (choice **b**), which is often caused by vitamin B12 and/or folic acid deficiencies. Choice **a**, iron deficiency anemia, is incorrect because iron deficiency anemia is a microcytic anemia. Choice **c**, aplastic anemia, is incorrect because the reticulocytes in aplastic anemia will typically be elevated because of increased production. Choice **d**, G6PD deficiency, and choice **e**, sickle cell anemia, are incorrect because the blood smear result in this case is inconsistent with these diagnoses.

Task Area: Formulating Most Likely Diagnosis
Organ System: Hematologic

140. d. A Milwaukee brace (choice **d**), also known as a cervico-thoraco-lumbo-sacral orthosis, is a back brace designed specifically to treat curvatures of the spine. Custom made from a mold of the patient's torso, these braces are designed specifically to prevent progression of the curvature. If the curvature worsens despite the brace, surgical intervention may be required. Choice **a**, oral corticosteroids, should not be considered, as they will have no corrective effect on the kyphosis. Choice **b**, oral anti-inflammatories, may be useful for some pain relief, but will not correct the kyphosis. Exercises (choice **c**) are effective when the curvature is less than 45 degrees. Choice **e**, surgical correction, is advised if the curvature is greater than 60 degrees and has not been decreased or corrected with a Milwaukee brace.

Task Area: Clinical Intervention
Organ System: Musculoskeletal

141. c. A Water's view X-ray is routinely ordered for the diagnosis of sinusitis (choice **c**). Positive X-rays for this disorder will reveal opacities in the sinus area. A CT scan may also be required for further evaluation of this disorder. Choice **a**, nasal fracture, would not be appreciated on a Water's view since this view examines only the sinuses and the maxillofacial bones. Choice **b**, blow-out fracture of the orbital floor, can only be evaluated by specific X-rays of the orbits. Choice **d**, mastoiditis, cannot generally be diagnosed with a simple X-ray. A CT scan or MRI scan is often needed for proper diagnosis of this condition. Choice **e**, rhinitis, generally can be diagnosed based on symptoms alone, and imaging procedures are usually not needed for diagnosis of this condition.

Task Area: Using Laboratory and Diagnostic Studies

Organ System: EENT (Eye, Ear, Nose, and Throat)

142. b. The correct answer is choice **b**, inhibits myometrial contractility mediated by calcium. Magnesium sulfate, or $MgSO_4$, is very effective in slowing or stopping pre-term uterine contraction because this medication inhibits myometrial contractility mediated by calcium. Side effects include nausea, fatigue, and muscle weakness. Toxicity from magnesium sulfate can lead to decreased reflexes, respiratory depression, and cardiac collapse. Choices **a, c, d**, and **e** are all incorrect because they are not effective in treating pre-term uterine contractions.

Task Area: Pharmaceutical Therapeutics
Organ System: Reproductive

143. c. In a patient with acute onset of unilateral eye irritation and photophobia, a corneal abrasion (choice **c**) is one of the most likely differential diagnoses. An area of increased fluorescein uptake further affirms this diagnosis. The abrasion will usually heal with rest, but an antibiotic eye ointment is often prescribed in order to provide lubrication and decrease the patient's likelihood of developing a bacterial infection. Keratitis (choice **a**) is usually accompanied by conjunctivitis (which is characterized by redness over the sclerae) and is unlikely to present with a small localized area of increased fluorescein uptake. Uveitis (choice **b**) affects the layer posterior to the cornea and does not respond to fluorescein staining. An entropion (choice **d**), or inward folding of the eyelid, may lead to a corneal abrasion but would not otherwise cause this sort of presentation. Sjögren's syndrome (choice **e**) is an autoimmune condition that features dry eyes and may also lead to a corneal abrasion, but again would not otherwise cause this sort of presentation.

Task Area: Formulating Most Likely Diagnosis
Organ System: EENT (Eye, Ear, Nose, and Throat)

144. b. This patient appears to have hypothyroidism. While thyroid hormone levels are often normal in patients who are clinically hypothyroid, elevated TSH is a much more sensitive and specific marker because it indicates that the thyroid must be overworked in order to achieve normal levels of thyroxine. While the most common cause of hypothyroidism worldwide is iodine deficiency, in the United States, the most common cause is Hashimoto's thyroiditis, an autoimmune disease in which thyroid hormone levels are affected by an antithyroid peroxidase antibody (choice **b**), and TSH must be excessively stimulated in order to maintain adequate levels of thyroid hormone. An anti-TSH receptor antibody (choice **a**) is an antibody that stimulates the thyroid and causes Graves' disease. A pituitary MRI (choice **c**) or pituitary hormone levels (choice **d**) might help identify a pituitary tumor or hypopituitarism; while either of these processes may cause thyroid dysfunction, they are both less likely than thyroiditis. A thyroid ultrasound (choice **e**) may help to identify a goiter but is unlikely to help establish the specific cause of the goiter.

Task Area: Using Laboratory and Diagnostic Studies
Organ System: Endocrine

145. e. Pneumonia (choice **e**) classically presents with a one- to ten-day history of cough, purulent sputum, tachycardia, shortness of breath, chest pain, fever, and sweats. Auscultation of the chest reveals altered breath sounds with crackles, dullness to percussion, and bronchial breath sounds over an area of consolidation. The short history and the presence of fever and sweats should rule out choice **a**, chronic obstructive pulmonary disease. The positive chest X-ray should rule out choice **b**, acute bronchitis. The lack of a sudden fever, sore throat, and muffled voice should eliminate choice **c**, acute epiglottitis, from consideration. The absence of anorexia, weight loss, and hemoptysis should rule out choice **d**, tuberculosis.

Task Area: History Taking and Performing Physical Examinations
Organ System: Infectious Diseases

146. c. A history of dyspnea, hemoptysis, and pleuritic pain is strongly suggestive of a pulmonary embolism. This differential diagnosis is further strengthened by the patient's history of calf swelling and pain after a long flight; this is suggestive of a deep vein thrombosis, a very common source of the clot that causes a pulmonary embolism. To confirm the diagnosis, a clinician may choose to use a CT pulmonary angiogram (choice **c**) or a ventilation/perfusion scan, depending on the resources available. It may also be useful to order an ultrasound of the right calf in order to determine whether any intervention is necessary for her deep vein thrombosis. A full blood count (choice **a**) might show a decreased platelet count, but that is a very nonspecific finding. A chest X-ray (choice **b**) is another useful tool for detecting lung pathology, but there are no chest X-ray findings that are specific for a pulmonary embolism. Spirometry (choice **d**) can help distinguish obstructive lung disease from restrictive lung disease but cannot make any further distinctions. Methacholine challenge test (choice **e**) is one of the best ways to diagnose asthma, but again is of no use for a pulmonary embolism.

Task Area: Using Laboratory and Diagnostic Studies
Organ System: Pulmonary

147. d. ACE inhibitors such as ramipril (choice **d**) slow cardiac remodeling and are indicated in heart failure. Atropine (choice **a**) has no antiarrythmic activity. Thiazide, nifedipine, and prazosin (choices **b**, **c**, and **e**) are antihypertensives but have no effect on cardiac remodeling.

Task Area: Pharmaceutical Therapeutics
Organ System: Cardiovascular

148. **d.** Pancreatic cancer generally carries a poor prognosis but may be treated with a pancreaticoduodenectomy, also known as the Whipple procedure. This involves resection of tissue supplied by the gastroduodenal artery, which includes the gastric antrum (choice **a**), the proximal two-thirds of the duodenum (choice **c**), the gallbladder (choice **b**), the common bile duct (choice **e**), and the head of the pancreas. The distal duodenum and the jejunum (choice **d**) are generally left intact.

Task Area: Applying Basic Science Concepts
Organ System: Gastrointestinal/Nutritional

149. **e.** Valproate is considered to be first-line therapy for epilepsy, but it carries a well-established risk of neural tube defects because of its tendency to act as a folic acid antagonist. However, for the safety of both the mother and the future fetus, it is important to minimize the risk of seizures during the pregnancy. In order to ensure effective management of both of these risks, carbamazepine (choice **e**) can be used for pregnant women; it is almost as effective as valproate (especially for partial epilepsy) and has been shown to be significantly less teratogenic. Folic acid should also be added to the carbamazepine therapy, as it would be for any other pregnant woman. It should also be emphasized that no anti-epileptic drug is completely safe in pregnancy, so the patient should be fastidious in the monitoring of her epilepsy. Choice **a** is incorrect because valproate is not the only option for control of her epilepsy. Folate supplementation (choice **b**) should be recommended to all pregnant women in order to help reduce the chances of neural tube defects, but it has not been shown to mitigate the teratogenicity of valproate; switching to carbamazepine is a better choice. Choices **c** and **d** are incorrect because it is important to ensure adequate control of the patient's epilepsy.

Task Area: Pharmaceutical Therapeutics
Organ System: Neurologic

150. b. Anorexia nervosa (choice **b**) is an eating disorder characterized by an excessive desire to lose weight. Patients usually avoid food wherever possible and often exercise regularly; despite being underweight, patients with anorexia still feel a compulsion to lose more weight. Advanced cases also cause endocrine disorders, which typically manifest as amenorrhea in women and decreased libido in men. Referral to a nutritionist and a mental health professional is usually warranted. Because of the patient's age, family involvement may also be appropriate. Bulimia nervosa (choice **c**) is a similar disorder that involves binging on food followed by purging, but this is less likely in this case because amenorrhea is far less common in bulimia. Pregnancy (choice **a**) initially seems like a viable choice, but after four months of amenorrhea, a physical examination would reveal some level of tenderness. Depression (choice **d**) may cause a decrease in appetite, but it rarely leads to enough weight loss to cause amenorrhea. Iron deficiency (choice **e**) is usually responsible for an anemia that would explain the patient's lethargy, but none of the other symptoms.

Task Area: Formulating Most Likely Diagnosis
Organ System: Psychiatry/Behavioral Science

151. c. This patient most likely has a basal cell carcinoma (BCC), the most common skin cancer worldwide. Key risk factors for a BCC include light skin color and large amounts of sun exposure; however, the lesion generally appears several years after the exposure itself. A BCC will typically present as a painless skin lesion with an approximately circular appearance and a shiny red color. The standard treatment is excision, although certain topical treatments are also effective. The lesion continues to grow if left untreated (choice **c**), but its long-term consequences are mostly cosmetic; the most serious potential consequence arises if it grows to the point of causing a mechanical obstruction. Metastasis (choices **a** and **b**) is seen commonly in melanoma and occasionally in squamous cell carcinoma, but is not a typical consequence of basal cell carcinoma. Choices **d** and **e** might appear attractive if the initial diagnosis is incorrect; infection and sepsis might be seen in a wide range of other dermatological conditions, but they are not generally associated with a BCC.

Task Area: Clinical Intervention
Organ System: Dermatologic

152. a. The patient has signs and symptoms consistent with an aortic dissection (choice **a**). The systolic murmur is indicative of aortic regurgitation, which occurs with a dissection of the proximal aorta. Dissection of the distal aorta (choice **b**) usually does not need surgical intervention. Abdominal aortic aneurism (choice **c**) presents with a palpable abdominal mass. This patient does not have signs or symptoms consistent with STEMI or NSTEMI (choices **d** and **e**).

Task Area: Formulating Most Likely Diagnosis
Organ System: Cardiovascular

153. a. A rise in C-peptide levels indicates that the patient is producing indigenous insulin and therefore rules out type 1 diabetes (choice **a**). Hyperglycemia based on lab results choices **b**, **c**, **d**, and **e** can be used to distingish the severity of type 1 diabetes and type 2 diabetes.
Task Area: Using Laboratory and Diagnostic Studies
Organ System: Endocrine

154. b. Furosemide inhibits reabsorption of sodium and chloride in the ascending loop of Henle (choice **b**). Drugs like acetazolamide work on the proximal convoluted tubule (choice **c**). Thiazides work on the distal convoluted tubule (choice **d**). Potassium sparing diuretics work on the cortical collecting duct (choice **e**). There are drugs that work on the thin descending loop choice **a**.
Task Area: Pharmaceutical Therapeutics
Organ System: Genitourinary

155. b. Pemphigus is caused by antibodies directed against junctions between epidermal cells (choice **b**). Antibodies directed against basal lamina (choice **a**) cause Goodpasture's syndrome. IgE mediated degranulation (choice **c**) causes asthma. Rheumatoid factor (choice **d**) is seen in variety of connective tissue disease. Anti-dsDNA (choice **e**) is seen in lupus.
Task Area: Applying Basic Science Concepts
Organ System: Dermatologic

156. c. Approximately 90% of cases of chronic pancreatitis (choice **c**) in the United States are caused by alcohol abuse. Because alcohol abuse is the cause of this disorder, a high percentage of chronic pancreatitis cases can be resolved by decreasing alcohol consumption. Choice **a**, cirrhosis, is an irreversible liver condition primarily caused by excessive alcohol consumption. Decreasing alcohol consumption may slow the progression of cirrhosis, but will not resolve the condition. Choice **b**, diverticulitis, is incorrect as this disorder is not associated with alcohol consumption. Choice **d**, acute cholecystitis, is generally not associated with alcohol consumption; however, if alcohol consumption causes pancreatitis, acute cholecystitis may develop. Choice **e**, chronic cholecystitis, is generally not associated with alcohol consumption; however, if alcohol consumption causes pancreatitis, chronic cholecystitis may develop.
Task Area: Clinical Intervention
Organ System: Gastrointestinal/Nutritional

157. c. Temporomandibular joint disorder (TMJD or TMJ syndrome) (choice **c**) is the most common cause of facial pain. Facial pain, generally located anterior to the pinna, is aggravated by movement of the jaw, such as eating. In addition, a click or pop may be felt or heard while eating. The jaw may have limited range of motion. Choice **a**, whiplash, should be ruled out because this disorder is associated with pain, swelling, and tenderness of the neck; also, there is no indication that the patient suffered a whiplash-like injury. Choice **b**, extension injury of the cervical spine, might be a consideration; however, this injury would not cause a click or pop to heard or felt during eating. Choice **d**, rheumatoid spondylitis, should not be a consideration, as this disorder primarily affects the spine and pelvis. Choice **e**, jaw osteonecrosis, is associated with high doses of bisphosphonate medications, which this patient does not take, and is indicated by lesions on the mandible and the maxilla.

Task Area: History Taking and Performing Physical Examinations

Organ System: Musculoskeletal

158. b. A lateral soft tissue X-ray of the neck shows a classic thumb sign if epiglottitis is present, choice **b**. A CT scan of the neck, MRI of the neck, and ultrasound of the neck are all viable options in order to diagnose epiglottitis. Choice **a**, croup, might be a consideration based on the patient's presentation; however, the classic thumb sign on the X-ray is a classic finding for epiglottitis. Choices **c** and **d** should be excluded based on presence of fever and sore throat and absence of foreign body on X-ray. Choice **e**, acute parotitis, should be excluded because of the lack of swelling in the neck area and the presence of thumb sign on X-ray.

Task Area: Using Laboratory and Diagnostic Studies

Organ System: EENT (Eye, Ear, Nose, and Throat)

159. d. For patients who are symptomatic and have a confirmed diagnosis of parathyroid adenoma, surgical removal (choice **d**) of the affected parathyroid gland is the recommended treatment. Choices **a**, **b**, and **c** are all incorrect because there is no scientific evidence proving effectiveness of any of these therapeutic options. If, however, the clinician feels the patient has yet to reach the point of having the glands surgically removed, a wait-and-see approach is appropriate; in this case, estrogen replacement may help ameliorate postmenopausal symptoms and prevent bone loss. Choice **e**, oral prednisone, would have no value in the treatment of parathyroid adenoma.

Task Area: Clinical Intervention

Organ System: Endocrine

160. e. Individuals with factitious disorder (choice **e**) intentionally fake signs and symptoms of medical or psychiatric disorders with the primary motivation of being taken care of and assuming the sick role. Patients will attempt to gain hospital admission under several different names with several different illnesses and, when confronted, normally become angry and check themselves out. Patients are unable to provide reliable medical history; however, they are fairly knowledgeable about the disease processes. Choice **a**, hypochondriasis, is incorrect because this condition is actually a disorder in which a patient has an irrational fear of contracting a serious illness. This disorder is commonly associated with anxiety and depression. Choice **b**, somatization disorder, might be a consideration because individuals with this disorder complain of pain in one or more body parts; however, in individuals who have this condition, the pain is real and not feigned. Choice **c**, body dysmorphic disorder, should be ruled out immediately because this condition characterizes an individual who is excessively concerned with his or her body image. Choice **d**, conversion disorder, should be ruled out because it is characterized by an unexplained condition of the nervous system such as blindness, numbness, or paralysis.

Task Area: Formulating Most Likely Diagnosis
Organ System: Psychiatry/Behavioral Science

161. e. Atenolol and timolol are both beta blockers, a class of drugs that act as antagonists at beta adrenergic receptors. Beta blockers have a wide range of indications, but they are most commonly used to treat hypertension, tachycardia, arrhythmia, and glaucoma. The use of two different beta blockers can produce a synergistic effect, even if one of the drugs is only used as an eye drop. One of the most significant of these potential effects is heart block (choice **e**), which can also occur in some cases of therapy with only a single beta blocker. The half-life of atenolol (choices **a** and **b**) is unlikely to be affected as a result of a drug interaction because it is not eliminated by the liver. Hepatotoxicity (choice **c**) is also unlikely because timolol is metabolized only partially by the liver, and atenolol is metabolized entirely by the kidney. Metabolic alkalosis (choice **d**) is not a consequence of beta blocker therapy, although metabolic acidosis is a possibility.

Task Area: Pharmaceutical Therapeutics
Organ System: Cardiovascular

162. d. Pulmonary fibrosis is an umbrella term that encompasses several different types of fibrous deposits in the lungs; these deposits may be composed of asbestos, iodine, silica, carbon, or a variety of other agents. It is a restrictive lung disease that usually presents with exertional dyspnea, a dry cough, fine inspiratory crackles in the lung fields, and an elevated FEV_1/FVC ratio. There is little useful therapy available, and prognosis is generally poor. Risk factors are often related to occupational toxin exposure. Employment in a shipyard (choice **d**), for instance, carried a high risk of asbestos exposure until recent years. Patients with a long history of such exposure will often develop asbestosis years later; exposed occupations include firefighters, construction workers, steel and iron workers, carpenters, and a wide range of other industrial workers. A long smoking history (choice **a**) also contributes to the development of pulmonary fibrosis and exacerbates the symptoms, but only acts as a risk factor if it is combined with occupational toxin exposure. A history of recurrent pneumonia (choice **b**) or COPD (choice **c**) is not associated with an increased risk of developing any type of pulmonary fibrosis. Some autoimmune diseases (choice **e**) may contribute, but a family autoimmune history alone is not sufficient to increase clinical suspicion of pulmonary fibrosis.

Task Area: History Taking and Performing Physical Examinations
Organ System: Pulmonary

163. c. Vitamin D is necessary for the dietary absorption of calcium; its deficiency is a common cause of brittle bones in older patients. Patients with darker skin generally have higher sunlight requirements in order to maintain normal vitamin D levels; however, in some cultures with a high prevalence of people with darker skin, further skin tanning is considered to be cosmetically undesirable. Consequently, these patients are at higher risk of developing osteomalacia (choice **c**), a condition associated with poor bone mineralization due to deficiency of calcium or vitamin D. This leads to a higher incidence of fractures and bone pain. Osteoporosis (choice **a**) is a common bone condition that is exacerbated by low vitamin D levels, but its pathophysiology involves imbalance of osteoblast and osteoclast activity rather than calcium and vitamin D levels. Osteoarthritis (choice **b**) is a degenerative joint disease that is unrelated to calcium and vitamin D. Osteopenia (choice **d**) is simply an early stage of osteoporosis. Rickets (choice **e**) is a growth abnormality caused by vitamin D deficiency in children, but because it is intrinsically related to growth, it is not found in adults.

Task Area: Health Maintenance
Organ System: Gastrointestinal/Nutritional

164. c. Pelvic inflammatory disease (choice **c**) is a fairly common condition in female patients who have a history of multiple sexual partners. The classic presentation features a short history of lower abdominal inflammatory pain associated with fever, cervical discharge, and pelvic tenderness. It is usually caused by infection with *Neisseria gonorrhoeae* or *Chlamydia trachomatis* and can be diagnosed by a culture and/or Gram stain of cervical discharge. Antibiotic treatment should generally be initiated as soon as possible in order to avoid long-term damage to the reproductive system. Ectopic pregnancy (choice **a**) is a rare complication of pregnancy in which the fetus implants in the Fallopian tube or elsewhere outside the uterus; this causes lower abdominal pain but is unlikely to present with acute onset or a fever. Endometriosis (choice **b**) is a growth of endometrium outside the uterine cavity, often causing a gradual onset of dysmenorrhea, dyspareunia, and dysuria in addition to pelvic pain. Vaginal candidiasis (choice **d**) and bacterial vaginosis (choice **e**) cause a white vaginal discharge but are not associated with pain or fever.

Task Area: Formulating Most Likely Diagnosis
Organ System: Reproductive

165. c. Diabetes is a very common condition that often requires a very complex management plan because of the wide range of comorbidities and complications that are generally present in affected patients. This patient appears to have early signs of diabetic nephropathy, as evidenced by the presence of microalbuminuria and impaired creatinine clearance. In order to answer this question, it is important to know which drugs are unsafe in patients with kidney disease and hyperglycemia. Metformin (choices **a** and **b**) is usually first-line therapy for type 2 diabetes, but it is contraindicated in patients with impaired kidney function. Glyburide (choices **c** and **d**), by contrast, is a safe option for glycemic control in these patients. Insulin (choice **e**) is generally only used in type 1 diabetes or very advanced cases of type 2 diabetes. Thiazide diuretics (choices **b** and **d**) are known to cause hyperglycemia, so they should be avoided in diabetic patients. Ramipril (choices **a** and **c**) is normally contraindicated in renal failure, but diabetic nephropathy is an exception; ACE inhibitors are actually known to be protective against diabetic nephropathy, so ramipril therapy should be safe in this patient. Choice **c** is the only correct answer because glyburide and ramipril are likely to be both safe and effective in this patient.

Task Area: Pharmaceutical Therapeutics
Organ System: Endocrine

166. b. When a child suffers an injury that is not consistent with the history, it is important to rule out the possibility of child abuse. A fall onto an outstretched hand, for instance, usually causes a fracture in the distal radius rather than the shaft of the humerus. Additional suspicion may be raised by the fact that the boy's father did not seek medical attention after the injury. In many cases of child abuse, full body X-rays (choice **b**) will demonstrate spiral fractures or old fractures that have not healed properly due to inadequate medical attention. If the full body X-ray increases the suspicion of child abuse, it may be appropriate to contact local authorities (choice **a**); however, it is important to avoid prematurely breaching confidentiality if the suspicion is only mild. A right arm X-ray (choice **c**) would be beneficial for investigating the presenting injury, but is less likely to provide information about child abuse. A genetic screen (choice **d**) for osteogenesis imperfecta may be useful if multiple fractures are found, while von Willebrand's disease need not be suspected in the absence of any bleeding symptoms. It may be helpful to talk to the boy's father (choice **e**), but this will usually yield an unreliable history and may lead the father to take the boy home.

Task Area: Using Laboratory and Diagnostic Studies

Organ System: Psychiatry/Behavioral Science

167. a. The correct answer is choice **a**, a six-month regimen of isoniazid, rifampin, pyrazinamide, and ethambutol. Choices **b** to **e** are all incorrect.

Task Area: Pharmaceutical Therapeutics

Organ System: Pulmonary

168. d. Although gonorrhea is commonly recognized as an infection of the urethra, it is also the most common cause of septic arthritis in the United States. The presentation is often similar to that of reactive arthritis, which also causes urethritis. However, reactive arthritis usually affects the sacroiliac joints and the large joints of the lower limbs, while gonococcal arthritis is more likely to affect the smaller joints of the upper limbs. The presence of wrist arthritis (choice **d**), therefore, is more suggestive of a gonococcal etiology. Uveitis (choice **a**), sacroiliitis (choice **b**), and knee arthritis (choice **c**) are features that are commonly seen in reactive arthritis. Fever choice **e** is a nonspecific sign that can be found in either gonorrhea or reactive arthritis.

Task Area: History Taking and Performing Physical Examinations

Organ System: Genitourinary

169. c. This patient is experiencing an acute hemolytic crisis, a condition in which a large number of red blood cells are destroyed in the circulation. Features of hemolytic crisis include sudden-onset dyspnea, bloody urine, and scleral icterus. This is particularly common in the African-American population because of the high prevalence of sickle cell disease and glucose-6-phosphate dehydrogenase (G6PD) deficiency. Patients with G6PD deficiency will often experience a hemolytic crisis in response to sulfur-containing drugs, so it is important to avoid these drugs whenever possible. On the basis of this patient's acute presentation and recent history, it is likely that he has G6PD deficiency and is currently suffering from a reaction to trimethoprim/sulfamethoxazole (choice **c**). Sickle cell disease (choice **a**) may also present in a similar way, but is likely to be diagnosed at a young age and is not related to sulfa drug allergy. A urinary tract infection may spread to the systemic circulation and cause sepsis (choice **b**), but this is a rare complication, and this patient's symptoms are not consistent with sepsis. Autoimmune hemolytic anemia (choice **d**) also causes a hemolytic crisis similar to this one, but it is far rarer than G6PD deficiency and is not related to sulfa drug allergy. Malaria (choice **e**) may present with similar symptoms, but the onset of symptoms is not as acute and should not be suspected unless there is a recent history of travel to a country where malaria is endemic.

Task Area: Pharmaceutical Therapeutics
Organ System: Hematologic

170. d. Diseases of defective bone mineralization, such as osteomalacia and rickets, are most commonly caused by a vitamin D deficiency (choice **d**). Other causes may include deficiencies in calcium or phosphate. Aluminum toxicity can also cause these disorders. Choices **a**, **b**, **c**, and **e** are all incorrect as the conditions of osteomalacia and rickets are commonly caused by a deficiency of vitamin D, not vitamins B6, B12, C, or E.

Task Area: Applying Basic Science Concepts
Organ System: Musculoskeletal

171. d. Circumcision (choice **d**) is the proper treatment for symptomatic phimosis. If phimosis is asymptomatic, it can be left alone and should resolve as patient gets older. Antibiotics and steroid creams may be useful to relieve symptoms, but the only true way to remedy a symptomatic phimosis is through circumcision. Choice **a** is a viable treatment course; however, when the condition becomes symptomatic, circumcision should be performed. Choices **b**, **c**, and **e** are incorrect as they may be useful to alleviate symptoms associated with phimosis, but have no benefit to resolve the condition.

Task Area: Clinical Intervention
Organ System: Genitourinary

172. a. Vancomycin can trigger histamine release, which would cause flushing (choice **a**) and hypotension commonly referred to as *red man syndrome*. Aplastic anemia (choice **b**) can be caused by drugs such as chloramphenicol. Tetracyclines can cause phototoxicity (choice **c**). Pulmonary fibrosis (choice **d**) can be caused by amiodarone. Phenytoin can cause drug-induced lupus (choice **e**).

Task Area: Pharmaceutical Therapeutics
Organ System: Infectious Diseases

173. b. Uterine leiomyomata (choice **b**), or fibroids, are fairly common benign tumors of the uterus. They are often asymptomatic, but larger leiomyomata can cause severe pelvic pain that is exacerbated by pressure. Ultrasound typically shows a focal mass with a heterogeneous texture. Surgery may be indicated if symptoms are severe, but they can often be safely left with no intervention. Metastatic transformation, which generally manifests as a uterine sarcoma (choice **a**) is an uncommon consequence of uterine leiomyomata. Endometriosis (choice **c**) may fit this clinical presentation, but it is unlikely to present with a painful mass on ultrasound. Endometrial carcinoma (choice **d**) and ectopic pregnancy (choice **e**), which can usually be ruled out with a pregnancy test, are also far less common than leiomyomata.

Task Area: Formulating Most Likely Diagnosis
Organ System: Reproductive

174. b. A cluster headache (choice **b**) is a severe, unilateral, periorbital headache that lasts for 30 to 90 minutes and can occur several times a day over a period of weeks to months. Bouts of frequent attacks, known as cluster periods, may last from weeks to months and are usually followed by remission periods when the headache attacks stop completely. These headaches are often accompanied by ipsilateral lacrimation, conjunctival injection, nasal congestion, myosis, and ptosis. Choice **a**, subarachnoid hemorrhage, is incorrect because this condition is associated with mental status changes, dilated pupils, intraocular hemorrhaging, and a quick, sudden, so-called "thunderclap" headache. Choice **c**, migraine headache, often presents unilaterally with throbbing or pulsing discomfort. Migraine headaches occur more in women than in men and often follow the menstrual cycle pattern. Patients who suffer from migraines can also present with aura involving visual changes, nausea, vomiting, photophobia, phonophobia, and anorexia. Choice **d**, tension headache, is not appropriate because this condition is associated with a dull aching pain in the forehead or the back of the head and can include pain in the neck and shoulders. Choice **e**, cerebral aneurysm, is incorrect because this condition can be associated with double vision, loss of vision, neck pain, and mental status changes.

Task Area: History Taking and Performing Physical Examinations
Organ System: Neurologic

175. **c.** Micturition syncope (choice **c**) is a temporary drop in blood pressure during urination. This condition usually occurs in the elderly. Choice **a**, septicemia, would be a consideration if the patient had an elevated white blood cell count, but the patient's lab values are all within normal limits. Choice **b**, vasovagal reaction, is incorrect because a vasovagal reaction is not associated with the urinary tract. Choice **d**, orthostatic hypotension, is incorrect because the dizziness is not associated with a change in position. Choice **e**, transient ischemic attack, is incorrect because these attacks usually do not occur during urination and are usually accompanied by other symptoms, such as tingling, numbness, and muscle weakness.

Task Area: Formulating Most Likely Diagnosis
Organ System: Cardiovascular

176. **c.** Premature infants have a substantially increased risk of neonatal respiratory distress syndrome (NRDS). At 31 weeks gestation, this risk is approximately 25%. NRDS is a syndrome that includes atelectasis and interstitial edema. Due to an inadequate amount of surfactant, the lung is unable to expand fully. Administration of surfactant via the endotracheal tube (choice **c**) is essentially curative; symptoms are fully resolved until the lungs mature. Thoracentesis (choice **a**) is a useful treatment option for a pneumothorax (or similar condition), but this is unlikely in a neonate. Intravenous indomethacin (choice **b**) is curative for a patent ductus arteriosus, which is a common congenital cause of dyspnea but is less likely than NRDS in a premature infant. Inhaled albuterol (choice **d**) is used for acute asthma exacerbations but will not be useful in the presence of atelectasis. Intravenous antibiotic therapy (choice **e**) may be helpful if the patient has pneumonia, but pneumonia generally presents with fever and coughing.

Task Area: Clinical Intervention
Organ System: Pulmonary

177. a. Pulmonary atresia (choice **a**) is a congenital heart defect in which the pulmonary valve fails to develop properly, preventing blood flow from the right ventricle to the pulmonary artery. Patients are born with severe cyanosis and tachypnea. Auscultation of the chest should reveal a hyperdynamic apical impulse and a single S1 and S2 sound. An echocardiogram may reveal tricuspid regurgitation. Choice **b**, Tetralogy of Fallot, is a combination of four congenital heart defects including pulmonary stenosis, over-riding aorta, ventricular septal defect, and right ventricular hypertrophy. Infants with this disorder present with extreme cyanosis, polycythemia, hyperpnea, and agitation. Auscultation of the chest reveals right ventricle impulse at left lower sternal border and a loud S2. Choice **c**, hypoplastic left heart syndrome, is associated with lethargy, poor pulse, liver enlargement, and tachycardia. Choice **d**, transposition of the great vessels, is associated with blue skin, clubbing of fingers and toes, poor feeding, and shortness of breath. Auscultation of the chest will reveal a single loud S2 and a systolic murmur. Choice **e**, hyaline membrane disease, is associated with rapid, labored grunting respirations, retractions above and below the breast bone, and flaring of the nostrils, occurring shortly after delivery.
Task Area: History Taking and Performing Examinations
Organ System: Cardiovascular

178. b. Computerized tomography, commonly known as a CT scan (choice **b**), is the recommended imaging modality to use during the acute phase in order to differentiate between ischemic and hemorrhagic strokes. Choice **a**, PET scan, is generally used for dementia and is generally not useful for stroke evaluation. Choice **c**, angiogram, can be useful to indicate blood flow to the brain and evaluate exactly which blood vessel is occluded; however, the invasive nature of this procedure would not make this a viable option for this situation. Choice **d**, ultrasound, is not of any value for differentiation of stroke types. Choice **e**, MRI, could be useful; however, the time warranted to obtain MRI images could mean the difference between life or death for a stroke patient and therefore is not the preferred imaging modality.
Task Area: Using Laboratory and Diagnostic Studies
Organ System: Neurologic

179. e. Understanding how to reduce the risk of falls is a very important aspect of aged care. Because this patient's recent history of a fall significantly increases her falls risk, it is necessary to identify and address all other risk factors. A patient's pharmaceutical regimen is a key aspect of a falls risk assessment; psychotropic drugs, including selective serotonin reuptake inhibitors such as fluoxetine (choice **e**), are among the most potent of these risk factors. Diuretics such as furosemide (choice **a**) can also significantly increase a patient's falls risk if they are causing postural hypotension, but this would be detected as part of a thorough physical examination. Atorvastatin (choice **b**) is a relatively safe drug that is not associated with an increase in falls risk. Warfarin (choice **c**) may increase the risk of bleeding after a fall but does not increase the risk of a fall itself unless it is caused by a drug interaction. Alendronate (choice **d**) is effective for preventing fractures and does not contribute to falls risk.

Task Area: Pharmaceutical Therapeutics
Organ System: Musculoskeletal

180. a. In a patient with a long history of smoking, an FEV_1/FVC ratio below 70% is almost always indicative of chronic obstructive pulmonary disease (COPD). Continued smoking generally leads to further deterioration in lung function, which manifests as a progressive increase in the patient's dyspnea and cough. If the patient quits smoking, however, the deterioration in her lung function will revert to that of the general population. While the current damage to her lungs is mostly irreversible, smoking cessation may still provide her with a reasonable chance of avoiding long-term respiratory failure. While an aerobic exercise program (choice **b**) is nearly always a good recommendation, it is unlikely to be sustainable in a patient with irreversible exertional dyspnea. Bronchodilator therapy (choice **c**) and inhaled corticosteroid therapy (choice **d**) have been shown to be mildly beneficial to COPD patients, but their effect is relatively mild, and they will not prevent long-term deterioration if the patient is still smoking. Chemotherapy (choice **e**) may be effective if the patient develops a lung cancer, but this patient's presentation is much more likely to be associated with COPD. For this patient, it is still valuable to recommend inhaled therapy as well as aerobic exercise. If these actions are combined with smoking cessation, they are likely to provide considerable long-term benefit. However, smoking cessation is most powerful as a single independent recommendation to maximize prognosis.

Task Area: Health Maintenance
Organ System: Pulmonary

Section 4

181. **e.** Drug-induced lupus is highly associated with the presence of anti-histone antibodies (choice **e**). Anti-dsDNA antibodies (choice **a**) are seen in systemic lupus erythematosus (SLE). Anti-centromere antibodies (choice **b**) occur in autoimmune disorders such as limited systemic scleroderma. Anti-streptolysin O antibodies (choice **c**) are seen in rheumatic fever and post-streptococcal glomerulonephritis. Anti-IgM antibodies (choice **d**) are seen in rheumatoid arthritis.

Task Area: Using Laboratory and Diagnostic Studies

Organ System: Musculoskeletal

182. **a.** Ursodiol is a bile acid. It acts to decrease the production of cholesterol and to dissolve the cholesterol already present in the bile so that it cannot form gallstones (choice **a**). Ursodiol is prescribed for patients who either do not want or cannot have surgery to remove gallstones. Choices **b**, **c**, **d**, and **e** are all incorrect as ursodiol is designed specifically to be used to dissolve gallstones and prevent gallstones from forming, particularly in obese individuals who are losing weight rapidly.

Task Area: Clinical Intervention

Organ System: Gastrointestinal/Nutritional

183. **b.** While short stature alone does not necessarily suggest any pathological process, the presence of a bitemporal hemianopia is very specific for a lesion pressing on the optic chiasm. This is usually caused by a pituitary tumor, the presence of which can be confirmed with an MRI (choice **b**). A pituitary tumor may cause excess hormone secretion, as in the case of an adenoma, or may cause decreased hormone secretion, as in the case of a craniopharyngioma. Because of this patient's stunted growth, it is likely that he suffers from impaired secretion of growth hormone (somatotropin), probably due to a craniopharyngioma. Slit lamp examination (choice **a**) is an excellent test for many ophthalmic conditions, but is unlikely to provide an answer regarding a lesion in the brain. Pituitary hormone levels (choice **c**) would probably reveal decreased levels of somatotropin, but would not identify the cause. A nutritional assessment (choice **d**) may help to explain poor growth if it is related to malnutrition, but the patient's bitemporal hemianopia suggests a brain lesion. Inflammatory markers (choice **e**) are not indicated for any reason.

Task Area: Using Laboratory and Diagnostic Studies

Organ System: Neurologic

184. e. A neonate's viability, or the probability that the neonate will survive, is generally around 30% at 23 weeks gestation. In many cases, neonatal intensive care is not recommended for these patients because even if their life is maintained, their lifetime disability will be severe. The viability reaches 50% at 24 weeks gestation and 90% at 27 weeks gestation, so intensive care may be advisable at 24 weeks and beyond. At 23 weeks gestation, it is unlikely that the neonate will even survive long enough to be discharged from the hospital; consequently, the most likely prognosis is a life expectancy of less than one year (choice **e**). The chance of normal growth with little to no disability (choices **a** and **b**) becomes greater than 50% around 25 to 26 weeks gestation. Severe disability (choice **c**) is more likely at 24 weeks gestation. Death between ages one and six (choice **d**) is unlikely at any stage of gestation; preterm neonates who survive the initial hospital stay are likely to live into adulthood.

Task Area: Health Maintenance
Organ System: Reproductive

185. c. With a prevalence of 1 in 100, von Willebrand's disease (choice **c**) is the most common coagulopathy in the general population. It is caused by a deficiency in von Willebrand factor (vWF), a protein that acts in several parts of the coagulation cascade. The disease often goes unnoticed, but in some cases patients will present with excessive bruising or bleeding. The diagnosis can usually be confirmed by checking the levels of vWF. Hemophilia A (choice **a**) and B (choice **b**) can cause a similar presentation but are much less common than von Willebrand's disease, with a prevalence of 1 per 10,000 and 1 per 100,000, respectively. Vitamin K deficiency (choice **d**) is common in neonates who have not yet been able to produce their own vitamin K but is not usually found in other children. Child abuse (choice **e**) should always be considered in a patient with excessive bruising, but when laboratory investigations are suggestive of a coagulopathy, child abuse should not be the primary differential diagnosis.

Task Area: Formulating Most Likely Diagnosis
Organ System: Hematologic

186. **c.** This patient appears to have tuberculosis, a pulmonary infection caused by the bacterium *Mycobacterium tuberculosis. M. tuberculosis* is highly prevalent in most of the developing world (as well as much of the developed world), and should be considered as the most likely diagnosis in any patient from a high-prevalence country who presents with a chronic productive cough along with night sweats and weight loss. The pulmonary nodule on chest X-ray further increases the likelihood of tuberculosis, but in order to exclude some less-common diagnoses like lung cancer and sarcoidosis, a sputum sample should be taken. *M. tuberculosis* generally grows slowly in culture and does not appear on a Gram stain (choice **a**), but an acid-fast stain (choice **c**) can effectively detect the presence of the bacteria. The presence of acid-fast bacteria is strongly suggestive of the presence of *Mycobacterium* species. A sputum coagulase test (choice **b**) is used to distinguish *Staphylococcus aureus* from other *Staphylococcus* species. A blood culture (choice **d**) may grow some *M. tuberculosis* but is far less sensitive than a sputum culture or acid-fast stain. A hilar lymph node biopsy (choice **e**) is highly sensitive and specific, but it is very invasive and is unnecessary at this stage.

Task Area: Using Laboratory and Diagnostic Studies
Organ System: Infectious Diseases

187. **b.** This patient has experienced an asthma attack, which characteristically includes acute onset of dyspnea and wheeze. While acute episodes are effectively resolved by short-acting β-agonists like albuterol, these are ineffective for long-term prevention. The best drugs for long-term prevention are inhaled corticosteroids like fluticasone along with long-acting β-agonists like salmeterol (choice **b**). Choice **a** is incorrect because it is a short-acting β-agonist, so it is only useful for reversal of acute symptoms, or as a rescue inhaler. Choice **c** is incorrect because systemic corticosteroids are less effective for asthma and also cause Cushing's syndrome when used regularly. Choice **d** is incorrect because while antihistamines may be useful for prevention of general atopic symptoms, they are not as effective as directed inhaled therapy for asthma prevention. Choice **e** is incorrect because weight is not strongly linked to asthma. However, it is probably reasonable to recommend management of the child's weight, possibly with the help of a pediatrician who specializes in weight management.

Task Area: Health Maintenance
Organ System: Pulmonary

188. d. Amiodarone is an effective antiarrhythmic agent that can often be used when other drugs have been unsuccessful, but it is generally avoided because of its tendency to cause significant long-term consequences. Because it contains iodine (hence the *iod* in *amiodarone*), it is very difficult for the body to eliminate. This causes it to form deposits in the lungs, the thyroid, and the liver, eventually leading to pulmonary fibrosis, thyroid dysfunction, and hepatotoxicity. Among other investigations, liver enzymes (choice **d**) should be monitored in patients on amiodarone in order to ensure early diagnosis of any possible liver dysfunction. A full blood count (choice **a**) is more useful for drugs that are known to cause bone marrow dysfunction, which leads to pancytopenia, or autoimmunity, which leads to leukocytosis. Blood urea nitrogen and creatinine levels (choice **b**) should be monitored in drugs that cause nephrotoxicity. Plasma electrolyte levels (choice **c**) are affected by a variety of drugs, the most common of which are diuretics. Pancreatic enzyme levels (choice **e**) are affected by some drugs, the most common of which is alcohol.

Task Area: Pharmaceutical Therapeutics
Organ System: Cardiovascular

189. c. Rickets (choice **c**) is classically noted on a plain chest radiograph with a rachitic rosary, or string-of-beads, appearance. This appearance is due to the thickening of costochondral margins. Choice **a**, cardiomyopathy, may be an initial diagnosis because of the widened mediastinum on the X-ray; however, the presence of thickened costochondral margins is classic indication for rickets. Choice **b**, hyaline membrane disease, is incorrect as this disorder is classified by a "ground glass" appearance on X-ray. Choice **d**, croup, is incorrect as this disorder is characterized by a steeple sign on X-ray. Choice **e**, epiglottitis, is incorrect as this disorder is characterized by a classic thumb sign on lateral neck X-ray.

Task Area: Using Laboratory and Diagnostic Studies
Organ System: Musculoskeletal

190. d. Pelvic inflammatory disease (PID) is caused by an infectious agent, which in developed countries is usually *Chlamydia trachomatis* (choice **d**). HPV (choice **c**) can cause cervical cancer. None of the other choices have any relationship to PID.

Task Area: Applying Basic Science Concepts
Organ System: Genitourinary

191. a. While a wide variety of fractures can occur as a result of a fall onto the outstretched hand (also known as a FOOSH injury), the most common is known as Colles' Fracture, which happens at the distal radius (choice **a**). These fractures may present in a variety of ways, but an X-ray is generally required for confirmation. None of the other choices are as likely to fracture under these circumstances.

Task Area: Formulating Most Likely Diagnosis
Organ System: Musculoskeletal

192. c. Vitamin D aids calcium absorption from the gut, which is required for bone deposition (choice **c**). Vitamin K helps synthesize certain clotting factors (choice **a**). Vitamin A is required to detect light (choice **b**). Many vitamins are required to metabolize fat (choice **d**) and sugars (choice **e**), but vitamin D is not one of them.

Task Area: Applying Basic Science Concepts
Organ System: Gastrointestinal/Nutritional

193. c. The characteristics of this lesion are consistent with a melanoma (choice **c**). A good mnemonic for the diagnosis of melanoma is *ABCD*: asymmetry, border irregularity, color variation, and diameter (>6mm is suggestive of malignancy and most lesions are >10mm). These features are a very sensitive way to distinguish a melanoma from other pigmented skin lesions. Basal cell carcinoma (choice **a**) is the most common skin cancer worldwide, but generally appears as a uniform pearly nodule. Squamous cell carcinoma (choice **b**) is also more common than melanoma, but presents as a red, scaly, or crusted bump that is often accompanied by pain. Seborrheic keratoses (choice **d**) usually have regular, clearly-defined borders and are generally seen in older patients. Melanocytic nevi (choice **e**) are benign neoplasms composed of melanocytes; they usually have a relatively uniform color and are unlikely to grow over time.

Task Area: Formulating Most Likely Diagnosis
Organ System: Dermatologic

194. c. Glaucoma is a progressive optic neuropathy that is caused by a buildup of intraocular pressure. 90% of glaucoma cases can be described as "open-angle," a painless hindrance in the outflow of aqueous humor due to an obstruction of the Canal of Schlemm (choice **c**). In closed-angle glaucoma, flow is obstructed between the iris and the lens; this process is more likely to cause pain. Both types of glaucoma eventually lead to optic neuropathy and visual field deficit, but the primary pathology is usually the obstruction. The anterior capsule (choice **a**) is normally involved in closed-angle glaucoma but will not be the site of a primary abnormality in an open-angle glaucoma. The macula (choice **b**) is affected in age-related macular degeneration, a common cause of central vision loss. Retinal abnormalities (choice **d**) in glaucoma are limited to optic neuropathy (choice **e**), which is secondary to the abnormality in the Canal of Schlemm.

Task Area: Applying Basic Science Concepts
Organ System: EENT (Eye, Ear, Nose, and Throat)

195. **c.** Vitamin B3 (niacin) deficiency, also known as pellagra, is fairly common in alcoholics and otherwise malnourished populations. It is accompanied by a characteristic syndrome that can be summarized by the mnemonic *diarrhea, dermatitis, dementia, and death.* This patient seems to be experiencing dementia; the presence of dermatitis, which may manifest as a peripheral rash (choice **c**), would further increase the likelihood of this diagnosis. Dysphasia (choice **a**) is a feature of vitamin B6 (thiamine) deficiency, which is also common in alcoholics. Confusion (choice **b**) may accompany any sort of dementia, which may be caused by either B3 or B6 deficiency. Peripheral neuropathy (choice **d**) is more common in vitamin B12 deficiency, which is usually caused by pernicious anemia or dietary deficiency. Pallor (choice **e**) may also be seen in B12 deficiency or other forms of anemia.

Task Area: History Taking and Performing Physical Examinations
Organ System: Gastrointestinal/Nutritional

196. **a.** The correct answer is choice **a**, pseudodementia. Patients with pseudodementia appear to be demented without actually having a psychiatric illness. They will present with the appearance of being distressed or upset and will complain of memory problems. Examination will reveal concentration and attention span to be intact. Choice **b**, frontotemporal dementia, is incorrect because this disorder is associated with degeneration of the frontal lobe of the brain and may include the temporal lobe. Patients with this disorder may present with memory loss, abrupt mood swings, inability to function in social situations, lack of personal hygiene, and obsessive compulsive behavior. Choice **c**, vascular dementia, is incorrect because this disorder is caused by prolonged decrease of blood flow to the brain, normally as a result of multiple strokes. Choice **d**, Alzheimer's disease, is incorrect as it presents much like frontotemporal dementia with memory loss and mood swings; this disorder is also associated with diminished vocabulary and word fluency. Choice **e**, Huntington's disease, is associated with hallucinations, paranoia, psychoses, and abnormal involuntary muscle movements.

Task Area: Formulating Most Likely Diagnosis
Organ System: Neurologic

197. d. The correct answer is choice **d**, acute pericarditis, which is associated with characteristic pericardial friction rub. Choice **a**, mitral regurgitation, is incorrect because this patient's disease duration is acute, and no typical heart murmur is found. Choice **b**, gastroesophageal reflux disease (GERD), is incorrect because GERD is not typically associated with pleuritic chest pain or pericardial friction rub. Choice **c**, aortic stenosis, is incorrect because of the lack of heart murmurs. Choice **e**, cor pulmonale, is incorrect because this patient has no prior pulmonary history such as chronic obstructive pulmonary disease (COPD).

Task Area: History Taking and Performing Physical Examinations
Organ System: Cardiovascular

198. e. This question tests your knowledge of health maintenance measures to prevent cardiovascular diseases. This patient has a family history and a personal history of conditions that increase his risk for cardiovascular diseases. The correct answer is choice **e**, all of the above. All of these options are appropriate for promoting good health in this patient.

Task Area: Health Maintenance
Organ System: Endocrine

199. e. The correct answer is choice **e**, myocardial infarction, because of the EKG finding of ST elevation, which indicates myocardial injury. Choice **a**, GERD, and choice **b**, anxiety attack, are both good differentials; however they are incorrect because neither of them results in ST changes in the EKG. Choice **c**, aortic stenosis, is incorrect because the onset of symptoms is usually more gradual, and there should not be ST elevation on the EKG. Choice **d**, pulmonary embolism, is incorrect because of the EKG finding.

Task Area: Formulating Most Likely Diagnosis
Organ System: Cardiovascular

200. b. Knee injuries caused by lateral clipping are fairly common among football players and other athletes. A severe injury is most commonly associated with the so-called unhappy triad, often known as a *blown knee*, which features damage to the anterior cruciate ligament (choice **a**), the medial collateral ligament, and either meniscus (choices **c** and **d**). This typically leads to persistent pain, reduced weight bearing, and impaired range of motion (choice **e**). The posterior cruciate ligament, however, is generally intact, so the posterior drawer test is likely to be normal (choice **b**).

Task Area: History Taking and Performing Physical Examinations
Organ System: Musculoskeletal

201. **c.** This patient has signs and symptoms consistent with rheumatic fever (choice **c**), which occurs after an infection with a group A streptococcus, not a group B streptococcus (choice **e**). Dressler's syndrome (choice **a**) is an autoimmune pericardial inflammation that occurs weeks after a myocardial infarction. SLE (choice **b**) patients have anti double-stranded DNA antibodies. Sarcoidosis (choice **d**) is a pathological gathering of granulomas in multiple organ systems.

Task Area: Formulating Most Likely Diagnosis
Organ System: Cardiovascular

202. **c.** The correct answer is choice **c**, an increase in FEV_1/FVC after treatment. Spirometry measures the extent of airflow obstruction. A short-acting bronchodilator typically improves FEV_1 and therefore FEV_1/FVC (ratio of forced expiratory volume in one second to forced vital capacity) by relaxing the bronchial smooth muscle so that air trapping is reduced. Choice **a**, no change in FEV_1/FVC after treatment, is incorrect because the patient shows improvement after treatment. Choice **b**, a decrease in FEV_1/FVC after treatment, is incorrect because FEV_1/FVC should be increased with improvement after bronchodilator treatment. Choice **d**, a decrease in FEV_1 after treatment, and choice **e**, no change in FEV_1 after treatment, are incorrect because FEV_1 should increase with reduced air trapping.

Task Area: Applying Basic Science Concepts
Organ System: Pulmonary

203. **e.** The correct answer is choice **e**, all of the above, because all of the choices given are beneficial as health maintenance measures for patients with osteoporosis to prevent further bone loss.

Task Area: Health Maintenance
Organ System: Musculoskeletal

204. **c.** Pulmonary hypertension (choice **c**) presents clinically with shortness of breath, retrosternal chest pain, weakness, fatigue, cyanosis, and syncope. Edema and ascites may also be present. Auscultation of the chest can reveal narrow splitting and accentuation of the second heart sound and a systolic ejection click. A chest X-ray will reveal enlarged pulmonary arteries. A lack of infiltrates on the chest X-ray and lack of edema accumulation in the lower extremities should rule out choice **a**, congestive heart failure. Choice **b**, bronchiectasis, is not a consideration because of the lack of foul-smelling sputum and hemoptysis. Lack of pleuritic chest pain, hemoptysis, and diaphoresis should rule out choice **d**, pulmonary embolism. Choice **e**, cystic fibrosis, should be ruled out because there is no excess sputum, sinus pain, nasal discharge, diarrhea, or abdominal pain.

Task Area: History Taking and Performing Physical Examinations
Organ System: Pulmonary

205. d. This question tests your knowledge of how to determine when surgery is indicated in gallstone pancreatitis in pregnancy, which complicates more than 3% of pregnancies. The correct answer is choice **d**, laparoscopy cholecystectomy. The development of pancreatitis from cholelithiasis is usually indication for surgery, and the laparoscopic approach is the gold standard. Choice **a**, avoidance of fatty foods, is incorrect because it does not address the presence of gallstones and the ongoing inflammation of the pancreas. Choice **b**, ciprofloxacin, is incorrect because it does not address the presence of gallstones. Choice **c**, open cholecystectomy, is incorrect because it is associated with increased maternal and fetal mortality rate compared to the laparoscopic approach. Choice **e**, appendectomy, is incorrect because this patient does not have appendicitis.

Task Area: Formulating Most Likely Diagnosis
Organ System: Reproductive

206. d. This question tests your knowledge of managing malignant thyroid disease. The FNA biopsy confirms the malignant nature of this nodule. The correct answer is choice **d**, subtotal thyroidectomy. Choice **a**, levothyroxin, is incorrect because it is indicated in treatment of hypothyroidism. Choice **b**, propylthiouracil, is incorrect because it is indicated in treatment of hyperthyroidism. Choice **c**, radioactive iodine therapy, is incorrect because it is used in treating hyperthyroidism. Choice **e**, observation for now, is incorrect because surgery is the definitive treatment in this case.

Task Area: Clinical Intervention
Organ System: Endocrine

207. d. The positive blood acetylcholine antibody establishes the diagnosis of myasthenia gravis (choice **d**). Choice **a**, hypothyroidism; choice **b**, hyperthyroidism; choice **c**, Guillain-Barré syndrome (GBS); and choice **e**, asthma, are all incorrect because they are inconsistent with the lab finding.

Task Area: Using Laboratory and Diagnostic Studies
Organ System: Neurologic

208. b. The correct answer is choice **b**, GABA (gamma-amino butyric acid) receptors agonist. Alprazolam (Xanax) belongs to the class of benzodiazepines. They are widely used to treat a variety of anxiety disorders. The other choices are incorrect.

Task Area: Applying Basic Science Concepts
Organ System: Psychiatry/Behavioral Science

209. b. Blepharitis (choice **b**) is characterized by itching eyelids, burning eyes, and light sensitivity. It is also characterized by red eyelid margins, swollen eyelids, frothy tears, and crusting of the eyelashes. Choice **a**, chalazion, is incorrect because this disorder is characterized not by itching and redness, but by a lump on the eyelid caused by a blocked oil gland. Choice **c**, glaucoma, is caused by a blockage of the outflow of aqueous humor. The intraocular pressure then builds, and the increased intraocular pressure can then damage the optic nerve. Choice **d**, cataracts, is incorrect because this disorder is a clouding of the lens of the eye, and vision is adversely affected. Choice **e**, orbital cellulitis, might be a possibility; however, this condition is accompanied by a fever, a bulging eye, eye pain with movement of the affected eye, and decreased vision, which this patient is not experiencing.

Task Area: History Taking and Performing Physical Examinations
Organ System: EENT (Eye, Ear, Nose, and Throat)

210. a. This patient's lesion is highly suspicious for basal cell carcinoma (BCC), given the pearly appearance. This is the most common form of malignant lesion affecting sun-exposed areas in fair-skinned individuals. The correct answer is choice **a**, a biopsy with complete excision, which is the treatment of choice for BCC. Choice **b**, electrodesiccation, is incorrect because it is not recommended for head and neck lesions. Choice **c**, continue observation, is incorrect because this lesion needs immediate biopsy for a diagnosis to prevent metastasis. Choice **d**, topical antibiotic ointment, and choice **e**, topical corticosteroid ointment, are incorrect because a biopsy is needed first to characterize the lesion.

Task Area: Clinical Intervention
Organ System: Dermatologic

211. b. A rapid irregular pulse is strongly suggestive of an arrhythmia, the most common of which is atrial fibrillation. Atrial fibrillation causes stasis in the blood of the left atrium, which leads to thrombus formation over time. Eventually, this thrombus falls into the left ventricle and is ejected into the aorta. Often, this leads to a thromboembolism in the cerebral circulation, thereby causing a cerebrovascular attack (choice **b**). In order to prevent this possibility, patients with atrial fibrillation are usually treated with prophylactic anticoagulants such as warfarin. A pulmonary embolism (choice **a**) is also a possible consequence if a thrombus comes from the right atrium or from a systemic vein, but the vast majority of thrombi in atrial fibrillation are formed in the left atrium. A myocardial infarction (choice **c**) may happen if a thrombus becomes lodged in a coronary artery, but the cerebral circulation is a much more common site of embolization. Heart block (choice **d**) is a common consequence of a myocardial infarction. Aortic stenosis (choice **e**) is unlikely, although mitral stenosis has been shown to have an association with atrial fibrillation.

Task Area: Health Maintenance
Organ System: Cardiovascular

212. c. This question tests your knowledge of treatment for microcytic anemia. The most common cause of microcytic anemia is iron deficiency; in young female patients, menstrual blood loss plays a major role in this deficiency. The correct answer is choice **c**, iron supplement. Choice **a**, vitamin B12 injections, and choice **b**, folic acid supplement, are incorrect because deficiencies in these two elements will result in macrocytic anemia. Choice **d**, vegetarian diet, is incorrect because this diet is often the cause of vitamin B12 deficiency and will not alleviate iron deficiency anemia. Choice **e**, no treatment is necessary, is incorrect because this patient may become symptomatic if the anemia worsens.

Task Area: Pharmaceutical Therapeutics
Organ System: Hematologic

213. c. Chemotherapy is the treatment of choice for small cell lung carcinoma, or oat cell carcinoma (choice **c**). Oat cell carcinoma is more likely to spread early, and surgery is rarely successful. Chemotherapy has proven to increase survival, although patients rarely live five years after diagnosis. Chemotherapy should not be considered for choice **a**, chondroadenoma, as it is a benign tumor. Choice **b**, solitary pulmonary nodule, is most appropriately treated with surgical removal. Choice **d**, non-small cell carcinoma, is most appropriately treated with surgical removal. Choice **e**, carcinoid tumor, is also most successfully treated with surgical removal.

Task Area: Clinical Intervention
Organ System: Pulmonary

214. a. A form of orthostatic hypotension (choice **a**) occurs in young people when they are active or standing for long periods of time. The body responds with a drop in heart rate and blood pressure causing dizziness, nausea, and sometimes fainting. Choice **b**, adrenal insufficiency, can cause dizziness; however, the absence of fatigue and muscle weakness makes this diagnosis unlikely. Choice **c**, vasovagal reaction, is incorrect because there is no stimulus such as vomiting or an intravenous injection. Choice **d**, micturition syncope, occurs in elderly people during urination, so the patient's age alone rules this out. Choice **e**, septicemia, would be an inappropriate diagnosis because the white blood cell count is not elevated.

Task Area: Formulating Most Likely Diagnosis
Organ System: Cardiovascular

215. c. Ceftriaxone is the treatment of choice for men and women infected with gonorrhea (choice **c**). Gonorrhea is resistant to several other common medications, such as penicillin, tetracyclines, and fluoroquinolones, making ceftriaxone the drug of choice. Choice **a**, chlamydia, is most frequently treated with the antibiotics Zithromax or doxycycline. Choice **b**, syphilis, is normally treated with an intramuscular injection of penicillin. Genital warts (choice **d**) are commonly treated with substances that are applied directly to the skin, such as Imiquimod, podophyllin, and tricholoracetic acid. Choice **e**, HIV, is commonly treated with zidovudine (AZT).

Task Area: Pharmaceutical Therapeutics
Organ System: Infectious Diseases

216. d. The correct answer is choice **d**, yawn or swallow when he feels pressure begin to increase. The physical act of yawning or swallowing can autoinflate the auditory tube to equalize pressure to rapid change in altitude. Equalizing pressure in the inner ear is critical because increased pressure in the inner ear can lead to rupture of the tympanic membrane. Chewing gum during ascent and descent may also be helpful, as may pseudoephedrine (Sudafed). Choice **a**, taking scopolamine prior to take off, and choice **b**, placing his head between his legs prior to takeoff, are both effective remedies for treatment of motion sickness that may result from an airplane flight, but neither is an effective remedy to prevent barotrauma. Choice **c**, reclining his seat prior to takeoff, may make the airplane flight more comfortable, but it will have no bearing on the prevention of barotrauma. Choice **e**, taking diuretics the day prior to eliminate mucosal edema, may ward off any shortness of breath or hyperventilation that may be associated with anxiety of airplane travel, but will not prevent barotrauma.

Task Area: Health Maintenance
Organ System: EENT (Eye, Ear, Nose, and Throat)

217. c. Alteplase (choice **c**) is a form of thrombolytic therapy known as recombinant tissue plasminogen activator. Recombinant tissue plasminogen activator is a protein that is involved in the breakdown of blood clots. Types of recombinant tissue plasminogen activators include alteplase, reteplase, and tenecteplase. Alteplase is the indicated form for treatment of acute ischemic strokes, whereas reteplase is indicated for acute myocardial infarction. Choice **a**, heparin, and choice **b**, warfarin, are anticoagulants and can be used to dissolve blood clots; however, these medications are generally used to prevent blood clots and should not be chosen for stroke therapy. Choice **d**, reteplase, is a form of recombinant tissue plasminogen activator that is primarily used for treatment of myocardial infarction and not for treatmentment of strokes. Choice **e**, tenecteplase, is a form of recombinant tissue plasminogen activator primarily used for treating and reducing mortality in the acute phase of myocardial infarction.

Task Area: Pharmaceutical Therapeutics
Organ System: Neurologic

218. b. A weak or delayed femoral pulse in an infant is almost pathognomonic for a coarctation of the aorta, a condition in which the aorta (usually in its descending phase) is significantly narrowed, thereby hindering adequate blood delivery to the lower limbs. The narrowing leads to a significantly increased systemic vascular resistance, thereby accelerating the rate of left ventricular hypertrophy (choice **b**). Early-onset left ventricular hypertrophy is a common problem for patients with an aortic coarctation. Turner syndrome (choice **a**) is also associated with aortic coarctations, but this is a chromosomal abnormality and the coarctation is a consequence of Turner syndrome; however, the converse is not true. Dilated cardiomyopathy (choice **c**) may also arise when the heart is unable to pump blood adequately through the circulatory system, but this usually occurs in cases where ventricular pump function is impaired and hypertrophy is not possible. Peripheral neuropathy (choice **d**) may occur if there is inadequate blood supply to the peripheral nerves, but this is not a common consequence of a coarctation. Pulmonary embolism (choice **e**) might a possibility if the patient's symptoms were caused by a venous thrombosis, but this is unlikely to cause a diminished arterial pulse.

Task Area: Health Maintenance
Organ System: Cardiovascular

219. d. Pulmonary edema is a fluid accumulation in the lungs that leads to impaired gas exchange, often causing dyspnea and hemoptysis. The dyspnea also may manifest as orthopnea, which can be elicited in a history by asking about the number of pillows that a patient uses at night. There are a variety of causes, but hypertension (along with congestive heart failure) is a key risk factor. On physical examination, pulmonary edema is almost always associated with end-inspiratory crackles on auscultation (choice **d**). Dullness to percussion (choice **a**) is a sign of pulmonary congestion, which is usually a consequence of pneumonia. Hyperresonance to percussion (choice **b**), on the other hand, is more likely to be caused by lung hyperinflation, a feature of emphysema. Inspiratory wheezes (choice **c**) may be associated with asthma or bronchitis. Reduced air entry (choice **e**) is a nonspecific sign that may be caused by a wide range of pulmonary conditions.

Task Area: History Taking and Performing Physical Examinations
Organ System: Pulmonary

220. e. Amoxicillin (choice **e**) should only be used in bacterial infections. Pseudoephedrine (choice **a**) and oxymetazoline hydrochloride (choice **c**) vasoconstrict nasal vessels and reduce mucus production. Saline nasal spray (choice **b**) and guaifenesin (choice **d**) are thought to reduce the viscosity of mucus, which would aid in its secretions.

Task Area: Pharmaceutical Therapeutics
Organ System: EENT (Eye, Ear, Nose, and Throat)

221. e. The T-score is a measure of a patient's bone mineral density, measured as the number of standard deviations from the mean; for example, a T-score of –2.0 suggests that the patient's bone mineral density is 2.0 standard deviations below the mean. In the absence of a fracture, a T-score of –2.5 is labeled *osteoporosis*, and a T-score between –1.0 and –2.5 is labeled *osteopenia* (therefore, choice **a** is incorrect). However, a diagnosis of osteoporosis can also be established if a patient with an osteopenic T-score experiences a fracture caused by minor trauma (trauma no more severe than that of a fall from standing height) (choice **e**). Choices **b**, **c**, and **d** are incorrect because they only cause calcium deficiency. While this may exacerbate osteoporosis, it can only directly lead to osteomalacia (poor bone mineralization).

Task Area: Using Laboratory and Diagnostic Studies

Organ System: Musculoskeletal

222. d. Genital warts are a common consequence of infection with human papillomavirus, a pathogen that is very highly prevalent in the sexually active population. While many reference materials show advanced cases, most patients present with small, soft, painless white warts. There is no specific antiviral therapy, but because the consequences of HPV in males are fairly benign, this is not usually necessary; cryotherapy (choice **d**), however, is an effective way to treat the warts. It is also important to counsel the patient regarding the effect of sexually transmitted infections, including the potential of HPV to lead to cervical cancer in his partner and the importance of using a condom while having sexual intercourse. Antibiotic therapy (choices **a** and **b**) is not useful because the symptoms are not related to a bacterial infection, and chemotherapy (choice **c**) is not useful because there is no reason to suspect cancer. Steroid therapy (choice **e**) is not likely to be beneficial because inflammatory issues are not involved.

Task Area: Clinical Intervention

Organ System: Reproductive

223. d. This patient is suffering from alcohol withdrawal syndrome, a condition that often occurs when a chronic alcoholic wakes up after several hours with no alcohol consumption. Ethanol binds to postsynaptic gamma amino butyric acid (GABA) receptors, which open chloride channels to activate inhibitory neurons; this causes the sedative effect of ethanol. In chronic alcoholics, the brain begins to attempt to compensate by downregulating GABA receptors, thereby preventing this excess sedation by removing much of the inhibitory signal. When such patients withdraw from alcohol, the inadequate inhibition (and excess excitation) often manifests as seizures. Patients may also present with delirium, tachycardia, tremor, GI upset, headache, nausea or vomiting, palpitations, and a variety of other symptoms related to neural overexcitation. This condition is usually treated with diazepam (choice **d**), which mimics the effects of alcohol by acting as agonists at GABA receptors. The dose is gradually decreased in order to allow the brain to rebuild its GABA receptors without causing any further seizures. The other answer choices are psychiatric drugs that may be used for a variety of conditions, but are not beneficial in alcohol withdrawal. Lithium (choice **a**) is a mood stabilizer with a mechanism that is not fully understood, but it has no use for this patient. Clozapine (choice **b**) is an antipsychotic that acts at serotonin and dopamine receptors but is not related to GABA. Carbamazepine (choice **c**) is an anticonvulsant that is useful for prevention of epileptic seizures and has some GABA-potentiating activity, but its activity is mostly related to sodium channels, and it is not particularly useful for alcohol withdrawal, which involves chloride channels. Phenytoin (choice **e**) is also a sodium channel modulator, so while it is useful for epilepsy, it has no role in the management of alcohol withdrawal.

Task Area: Pharmaceutical Therapeutics
Organ System: Psychiatry/Behavioral Science

224. b. Diabetes insipidus is a condition in which a reduction in the effect of antidiuretic hormone (ADH) leads to polyuria. This can be either nephrogenic (impaired sensitivity to ADH in the collecting duct) or neurogenic (impaired production of ADH in the pituitary). Nephrogenic diabetes insipidus (choice **b**) is particularly common in patients undergoing therapy with lithium or doxycycline; because this patient is taking lithium, he is at particularly high risk. Choice **a** is incorrect because benign prostatic hyperplasia is generally accompanied by dysuria and urge incontinence. Choice **c**, neurogenic diabetes insipidus, is incorrect because this patient has no risk factors for this disorder, so the nephrogenic variant is much more likely. Choice **d** is possible because hydrochlorothiazide often causes hyperglycemia, but this is unlikely to present with no symptoms other than poluyria. Choice **e**, hypernatremia, could cause polyuria in isolation, but there is no reason to suspect that in this patient.

Task Area: Formulating Most Likely Diagnosis
Organ System: Genitourinary

225. e. There is no evidence linking malignant hyperthermia (choice **e**) to smoking. However, patients who stop smoking eight weeks prior to surgery should have quicker wound healing (choice **a**), lower risk of infection (choice **b**), lower CO concentrations (choice **c**), and better peripheral oxygenation (choice **d**).

Task Area: Health Maintenance
Organ System: Pulmonary

226. **a.** Lactulose sequesters nitrogenous waste products in the gut and aids in their excretion (choice **a**). Its laxative properties (choice **c**) are not beneficial in hepatic encephalopathy. It does not affect hepatic blood flow (choice **b**) or urine pH (choice **d**), nor does it restore thiamine levels (choice **e**).

Task Area: Pharmaceutical Therapeutics
Organ System: Gastrointestinal/Nutritional

227. **e.** In menopause, there is a rise in follicle-stimulating hormone (FSH) (choice **e**) and a rise (not a drop) in lutenizing hormone (LH) (choice **d**). Menopause also results in a decline (not a rise) of ovarian function such as progesterone production (choice **b**). Estriol (choice **a**) is raised in pregnancy.

Task Area: Applying Basic Science Concepts
Organ System: Reproductive

228. **a.** Obstructive shock (choice **a**) is a type of shock that can arise from tension pneumothorax, pericardial tamponade, and massive pulmonary embolism. Shock can cause low blood pressure, tachycardia, orthostatic changes, and altered mental status. Choice **b**, cardiogenic shock, is incorrect as this condition is caused by the heart being damaged to the point where it cannot adequately supply the organs with blood. Choice **c**, hypovolemic shock, is incorrect as this condition results from decreased blood volume. Choice **d**, septic shock, is incorrect as this condition is caused by severe infection that leads to vasodilatation. Choice **e**, neurogenic shock, is incorrect as this condition is caused by trauma to the spinal cord.

Task Area: Formulating Most Likely Diagnosis
Organ System: Cardiovascular

229. **c.** The patient is in diabetic ketoacidosis (DKA), most likely precipitated by the pneumonia. He is clinically dehydrated and should not be given a diuretic (choice **c**). Treatment involves insulin (choice **a**) and glucose infusion (choice **b**). Potassium imbalance (choice **d**) often occurs but must be monitored. The triggering event of DKA (pneumonia) should also be treated (choice **e**).

Task Area: Clinical Intervention
Organ System: Endocrine

230. **c.** Perioral dermatitis (choice **c**) is primarily found in young women. This disorder is characterized by redness, inflammation, burning, and eruptions of the skin around the mouth. Choice **a**, seborrheic keratosis, should be excluded because this condition is associated with wartlike growths on the face, chest, and back, which are usually painless and without redness. Choice **b**, seborrheic dermatitis, should be excluded because this condition causes flaky white or yellow scales to form on the scalp or in the ears. The small eruptions associated with the condition in question should rule out choice **d**, cellulitis. Choice **e**, erythema muliforme, should be excluded because other symptoms, such as fever or joint aches, are not present in this patient. In addition, the eruptions associated with this disorder are surrounded by rings, which give them a target or bull's-eye appearance.

Task Area: Formulating Most Likely Diagnosis
Organ System: Dermatologic

231. e. The left anterior descending artery (choice **e**) is the most common coronary artery to become occluded in a myocardial infarction. In cases of instant death following myocardial infarction, the proximal left anterior descending artery is the most likely culprit; for this reason, it is often colloquially called *the widowmaker*. It supplies the anterior myocardium, the apex, and the interventricular septum. In most patients, it is singlehandedly responsible for supplying half of the left ventricle. Consequently, a proximal embolus can lead to an infarction of a large portion of the left ventricle, thereby making it very difficult for the heart to supply the systemic circulation. The right main coronary artery (choice **a**) supplies about one-third of the left ventricle, so an infarct is usually less severe than left anterior descending infarct; furthermore, it is relatively short, so infarcts are less common. The right marginal artery (choice **b**) and the posterior interventricular artery (choice **c**) are usually branches of the right coronary artery, so infarcts here are likely to be less severe than infarcts in the right coronary artery. The left circumflex artery (choice **d**) supplies about 20% of the left ventricle, so an infarct here will usually have a smaller impact on the systemic circulation than an infarct in the right coronary artery or the left anterior descending artery.

Task Area: Applying Basic Science Concepts
Organ System: Cardiovascular

232. d. Proton pump inhibitors are among the most widely-prescribed drugs in the United States because of their relative safety and excellent efficacy in patients with gastroesophageal reflux disease (GERD), a very common cause of chronic heartburn. However, most proton pump inhibitors are known to inhibit various cytochrome P450 isoforms, many of which are also responsible for the metabolism of warfarin. This leads to reduced elimination of warfarin, thereby causing increased bleeding. Pantoprazole (choice **d**), however, has been shown to have fewer such interactions, and is generally considered to be the safest choice in patients undergoing warfarin therapy. Omeprazole, esomeprazole, and lansoprazole (choices **a**, **b**, and **c**) are other proton pump inhibitors that are commonly used, but all three are known to inhibit cytochrome P450 isoform 2C19, which is partially responsible for the metabolism of warfarin. Cimetidine (choice **e**) is a histamine receptor antagonist that is also often used for acid suppression, but it is also known to inhibit isoform 2C19.

Task Area: Pharmaceutical Therapeutics
Organ System: Gastrointestinal/Nutritional

233. d. This patient's presentation is typical of Kawasaki disease, an autoimmune or infectious necrotizing vasculitis of smaller vessels throughout the systemic circulation. Kawasaki disease is often seen in children and is particularly common in patients of East Asian descent. The diagnosis is mostly clinical, and most patients present with at least five days of fever along with peripheral erythema and edema, polymorphous rash starting in the groin, swelling and erythema in the lips and tongue, bulbar conjunctivitis (choice **d**), and in some cases, cervical lymphadenopathy. Reduced visual acuity (choice **a**) in a small child is usually suggestive of myopia, and it is important to recognize that conjunctivitis does not affect visual acuity. Diminished visual fields (choice **b**) are also not present in conjunctivitis. Eye pain (choice **c**) is uncommon unless the cornea is also involved, although some eye irritation is often noted. Diplopia (choice **e**) is generally suggestive of pathology in the ocular muscles.

Task Area: History Taking and Performing Physical Examinations

Organ System: EENT (Eye, Ear, Nose, and Throat)

234. a. This patient is experiencing primary amenorrhea, a complete absence of menstruation by age 16; secondary amenorrhea, by contrast, refers to six months of amenorrhea after the onset of menarche. The most common cause of primary amenorrhea in the United States is Turner syndrome, a form of gonadal dysgenesis that is related to the presence of a single X chromosome. Patients with Turner syndrome are phenotypically female and possess a small uterus and ovaries, but require hormone replacement therapy in order to undergo normal female development. Additional features include short stature and a webbed neck. The diagnosis can usually be confirmed with a chromosomal karyotype (choice **a**), which will demonstrate the presence of a single X chromosome. Inflammatory markers (choice **b**) are usually used to diagnose an autoimmune disease, which is unlikely to be contributing to this patient's presentation. A pituitary MRI (choice **c**) may help to diagnose hypogonadism due to a pituitary tumor, which may cause this patient's symptoms, but this is less common than Turner syndrome and is unlikely to produce a webbed neck. A blood glucose test (choice **d**) may help to diagnose amenorrhea due to an eating disorder, but this is more likely to present as a secondary amenorrhea. An IQ test (choice **e**) is unlikely to be useful because patients with Turner syndrome do not usually exhibit cognitive impairment.

Task Area: Using Laboratory and Diagnostic Studies

Organ System: Reproductive

235. b. This patient appears to be suffering from schizophrenia, a common psychotic condition caused by an excess of dopamine and serotonin. This leads to a constellation of positive and negative symptoms. Positive symptoms include cognitive disorder, delusions, hallucinations, and exceptionally irrational belief systems. Negative symptoms include dull affect, social withdrawal, and reduced ability to perform goal-oriented activities. The presence of these symptoms for over six months suggests a diagnosis of schizophrenia; by contrast, if the symptoms had been present for more than two weeks but less than six months, the most likely diagnosis would be schizophreniform disorder, an early-stage psychosis that usually develops into schizophrenia if left untreated. Patients with schizophrenia are generally treated with an antipsychotic medication like risperidone (choice **b**), along with cognitive behavioral therapy as necessary. Other antipsychotic medications may also be useful, but risperidone is often used as first-line therapy. This treatment regimen has been shown to provide a significant improvement in symptoms, although cessation of therapy usually leads to recurrence. Cognitive behavioral therapy alone (choice **a**) may also be beneficial, especially in a patient with contraindications to antipsychotic drugs, but it is unlikely to be as effective as antipsychotic therapy. Fluoxetine (choice **c**) is a selective serotonin reuptake inhibitor that is generally used for depressive disorders. Methylphenidate (choice **d**) is a stimulant that is usually used to treat attention-deficit disorders. Lithium (choice **e**) is approved for treatment of manic episodes in bipolar disorder.
Task Area: Clinical Intervention
Organ System: Psychiatry/Behavioral Science

236. e. Hypernatremia is a fairly common condition that is associated with a wide range of differential diagnoses. It often leads to lethargy and weakness, but because these signs are relatively nonspecific, a fluid state examination should be conducted. Because of this patient's low blood pressure with a postural drop and a reflex tachycardia, it is important to suspect hypovolemia (choice **e**), which is the most common cause of hypernatremia in the general population. Hypovolemia is particularly common in the elderly due to inadequate intake of water. Diabetes insipidus (choice **a**), diabetes mellitus (choice **b**), and Cushing's syndrome (choice **d**) should also be investigated as possible causes of this patient's hypovolemia, but dehydration is the most likely cause. Kidney failure (choice **c**) is unlikely in the presence of normal creatinine levels.
Task Area: Formulating Most Likely Diagnosis
Organ System: Genitourinary

237. b. Tetralogy of Fallot (choice **b**) is actually a combination of four congenital heart defects: pulmonary stenosis, overriding aorta, ventricular septal defect, and right ventricular hypertropy. Infants with this disorder present with extreme cyanosis and with polycythemia (hematocrit may be more than 60%) if the cyanosis is severe and long-standing, predisposing the patient to thrombosis. Hyperpnea and agitation are also symptoms associated with this disorder. Auscultation of the chest reveals right ventricle impulse at left lower sternal border and a loud S2. Choice **a**, pulmonary atresia, is associated with severe cyanosis and tachypnea without dyspnea. Auscultation of the chest should reveal a hyperdynamic apical impulse and a single S1 and S2 sound. An echocardiogram may reveal tricuspid regurgitation. Choice **c**, hypoplastic left heart syndrome, is associated with lethargy, poor pulse, liver enlargement, and tachycardia. Choice **d**, transposition of the great vessels, is associated with blue skin, clubbing of fingers and toes, poor feeding, and shortness of breath. Auscultation of the chest will reveal a single loud S2 and a systolic murmur. Choice **e**, hyaline membrane disease, is associated with rapid, labored grunting respirations, retractions above and below the breast bone, and flaring of the nostrils that occur shortly after delivery.

Task Area: History Taking and Performing Physical Examinations
Organ System: Cardiovascular

238. c. Maintenance therapy for chronic asthma consists of daily use of inhaled corticosteroids (choice **c**), which provides the greatest anti-inflammatory results and allows for the best management of this disorder. Choice **a**, antibiotics, is incorrect as these medications are used to treat infections. Choice **b**, anticholinergics, is incorrect as this type of medication is commonly used to treat acute attacks of asthma as well as chronic conditions such as emphysema and chronic bronchitis. Choice **d**, β-adrenergic agonists, is incorrect as this type of medication is commonly used to treat acute attacks of asthma. Choice **e**, diuretics, is incorrect as these medications are used to rid the body of excess fluids. Diuretics have no bronchodilatory effects.

Task Area: Health Maintenance
Organ System: Pulmonary

239. a. Esophageal adenocarcinoma (choice **a**) generally presents with dysphagia in patients with a long history of GERD. This is a rare consequence of Barrett's esophagus, which is a metaplasia in which squamous cells in the lower esophagus are replaced by intestinal goblet cells; metaplastic cells exhibit a considerably darker color on endoscopy. While the majority of Barrett's esophagus cases are benign, a small portion will become dysplastic and form a mass in the esophagus. Most patients with Barrett's esophagus (choice **c**) will not develop esophageal adenocarcinoma, so the presence of a clinically significant mass is not a feature of a precancerous metaplasia. Squamous cell carcinoma (choice **b**) is somewhat common in the general population but is far less likely than adenocarcinoma in a patient with a history of GERD and demonstrated endoscopic evidence of Barrett's esophagus. Infectious esophagitis (choice **d**) is not typically seen in immunocompetent individuals, and autoimmune esophagitis (choice **e**) generally presents as diffuse swelling with no color change.

Task Area: Formulating Most Likely Diagnosis
Organ System: Gastrointestinal/Nutritional

240. b. Individuals with seasonal affective disorder (choice **b**) usually experience lethargy, depression, and loss of interest with onset of symptoms primarily occurring in the fall and winter months. This disorder is most commonly found in the northern latitudes, where the nights are longer, and usually goes into remission in the spring. Choice **a**, melancholia, is also characterized by depression and social withdrawal; however, time of year is not a factor for this disorder. Choice **c**, atypical depression, is also possible, but once again, time of year is not a factor for this disorder. Choice **d**, catatonic depression, is incorrect, as this type of depression renders individuals motionless for long periods of time. Choice **e**, malingering, is incorrect as this disorder is characterized by exaggerating illness for secondary gain.

Task Area: History Taking and Performing Physical Examinations
Organ System: Psychiatry/Behavioral Science

Section 5

241. b. Mesothelioma (choice **b**) is a malignant tumor of mesothelial tissue, which forms the lung's pleura. While the disease is fairly rare in the general population, it is especially common in patients with a history of asbestos exposure (which was particularly common in shipyard workers), and the risk is further increased in patients with a history of smoking. The signs and symptoms are related to the diffuse growth of the pleura, which leads to pleuritic pain and decreased air space in the lung. This also leads to a restrictive pattern in the lungs, thereby increasing the FEV_1/FVC ratio. Squamous cell carcinoma (choice **a**) is a much more common form of lung cancer, but it generally presents with hemoptysis and a very different radiological appearance. Asbestosis (choice **c**) may also be present in this patient, but the pleural wall thickening and rapidly worsening chest pain suggest that his symptoms are caused by the mesothelioma. Interstitial pneumonia (choice **d**) is another restrictive lung disease, but it would also present with a more diffuse pattern on imaging and on physical examination. Emphysema (choice **e**) is an obstructive lung disease, so its features are very different; it would include lung hyperexpansion and a decreased FEV_1/FVC ratio.

Task Area: Formulating Most Likely Diagnosis
Organ System: Pulmonary

242. b. ACE inhibitors such as ramipril (choice **b**) are considered to be the best antihypertensive therapy for diabetic patients, primarily because of their renal protective effect. This may seem counterintuitive since ACE inhibitors are slightly nephrotoxic to nondiabetic patients, but their positive effect is well established. Lifestyle changes (choice **a**) are always a good option, but this patient has already implemented considerable lifestyle changes without significant success; at this point, pharmaceutical intervention is easily justifiable. β-blockers (choice **c**) are not recommended for diabetic patients because their negative inotropic effect can mask the symptoms of hypoglycemic shock, which include tachycardia and palpitations. Thiazide diuretics (choice **d**) are known to cause hyperglycemia, which makes them particularly unfavorable in diabetes. Angiotensin receptor blockers (choice **e**) are a reasonable choice if ACE inhibitors are not well tolerated, but ACE inhibitors are still considered to be first-line therapy due to their greater efficacy and renal protective effects.

Task Area: Pharmaceutical Therapeutics
Organ System: Cardiovascular

243. b. Hypochromic microcytic anemia, otherwise known as iron deficiency anemia, can easily be treated and maintained by oral administration of ferrous sulfate (choice **b**). An oral dose of 325mg of ferrous sulfate taken three times a day prior to mealtimes should be sufficient to bring the patient's serum iron level back to normal. Choice **a**, folic acid, is incorrect as this is an effective maintenance therapy for folic acid deficient anemia. Choice **c**, erythropoietin, may be useful for maintenance therapy for many forms of anemia; however, in order to treat hypochromic microcytic anemia, ferrous sulfate is the only therapeutic option. Choice **d**, vitamin B12, is incorrect as this is used for treatment of pernicious anemia. Choice **e**, vitamin E, should not be a consideration as this will have no therapeutic benefit for any form of anemia.
Task Area: Health Maintenance
Organ System: Hematologic

244. b. Spontaneous abortion (choice **b**) is defined as the termination of pregnancy, by any means, before 20 weeks of gestation. Vaginal bleeding is a classic sign for spontaneous abortion. An open cervix does not permit the female to maintain the pregnancy, so termination of the pregnancy is inevitable. Choice **a**, placenta previa, should be immediately excluded by a gynecological exam because the placenta obstructing the cervix should be appreciated on physical exam. That being said, any pregnant patient beyond the first trimester who presents with vaginal bleeding requires a speculum examination followed by diagnostic ultrasound, unless previous documentation confirms no placenta previa. This does not apply here because the patient presents with an open cervix: if the cervix is *not* open, a digital examination is absolutely contraindicated because of the risk of provoking a life-threatening hemorrhage. Choice **c**, ectopic pregnancy, might be a consideration; however, this condition is associated with abdominal or pelvic pain, dizziness, nausea, and fatigue. Choice **d**, gestational trophoblastic disease, also known as hydatidiform mole (or molar pregnancy), might also be a consideration; however, this condition is associated with increased uterine size, nausea, vomiting, and hypertension. Lack of intestinal changes, urinary changes, pelvic pain, and abdominal swelling should rule out choice **e**, uterine cancer.
Task Area: Formulating Most Likely Diagnosis
Organ System: Reproductive

245. b. A barium swallow (choice **b**) is the most appropriate diagnostic procedure for the diagnosis of hiatal hernia. A barium swallow is used to examine the upper gastrointestinal tract and the stomach. To obtain this evaluation, the patient must ingest a mouthful of barium solution, which will line the esophagus and stomach to enable the evaluation. Choices **a**, chest X-ray, and **c**, CT scan of the chest, are incorrect; these exams may offer diagnostic capability for hiatal hernia, but a barium swallow is the diagnostic procedure of choice for this condition. Choice **d**, endoscopy, is incorrect because although this diagnostic procedure will definitely diagnose a hiatal hernia, it is an invasive procedure that may not be tolerated well by patients. Choice **e**, esophageal transit study, is incorrect because although this procedure is used to determine the function of the esophagus in the presence of a hiatal hernia, it is not useful for diagnosing hiatal hernia.

Task Area: Using Laboratory and Diagnostic Studies

Organ System: Gastrointestinal/Nutritional

246. b. A varicocele (choice **b**) is the formation of a varicose vein in the spermatic vein. This disorder will present with a chronic, nontender mass generally on the left side of the scrotum. The lesion will have the consistency of a "bag of worms," will increase in size when the Valsalva maneuver is performed, and will decrease in size with elevation of the testicles or when the patient is supine. Choice **a**, epididymitis, is associated with fever, chills, and a heavy sensation in the scrotum that gets worse with pressure. Choice **c**, hydrocele, should be ruled out because this disorder is characterized by a swollen testicle that feels like a water balloon. Choice **d**, spermatocele, is associated with a swollen scrotum and possible infertility. Choice **e**, testicular torsion, should be immediately ruled out because this condition is associated with sudden, excruciating pain in a testicle, swelling on one side of the scrotum, nausea, and lightheadedness. *Torsion* means *twisting* (of the testicle), which cuts off blood supply. Immediate surgery is needed to unwind the testicle and anchor it to the inner scrotum to prevent the loss of the testicle.

Task Area: Formulating Most Likely Diagnosis

Organ System: Genitourinary

247. c. Ototoxicity, which often manifests as tinnitus, is a recognized side effect of many antibiotics. Some of these antibiotics are also more likely to cause vestibular dysfunction, although this additional symptom is often not present. The antibiotics best known for their ototoxicity are the aminoglycosides (streptomycin, gentamicin, neomycin, amikacin, tobramycin, and the like), but other drugs, including vancomycin and the macrolides, are also somewhat ototoxic. In patients who are undergoing the standard tuberculosis treatment regimen, it is important to monitor for ototoxicity due to streptomycin (choice **c**) as well as for conjunctivitis due to rifampicin and optic neuritis due to ethambutol. The rest of the antibiotics used in tuberculosis treatment also have certain characteristic adverse effects in addition to the side effects that are common to many different antibiotics. Isoniazid (choice **a**) is known for causing hepatotoxicity, peripheral neuropathy, and drug interactions. Rifampin (choice **b**) is more likely to cause conjunctivitis, redness in the mucus membranes, and drug interactions. Ethambutol (choice **d**) may cause optic neuritis, peripheral neuropathy, arthralgia, and some chronic effects. Pyrazinamide (choice **e**) is known to cause arthralgia and hepatotoxicity.

Task Area: Pharmaceutical Therapeutics

Organ System: EENT (Eye, Ear, Nose, and Throat)

248. c. This patient appears to have deep vein thrombosis (DVT), a condition in which a clot becomes trapped in the deep veins of her leg. DVT is particularly common in young women with a history of oral contraceptive use; additionally, it is far more likely after an intercontinental flight or other extended period of immobility. It often presents with several hours of calf tenderness followed by a few hours of severe pain. The diagnosis can be confirmed with a venogram or an ultrasound, and it is often also useful to measure the plasma levels of D-dimers (which are usually elevated in a patient with a DVT). If no treatment is initiated, the clot often follows the venous system into the right atrium of the heart, after which it is ejected from the right atrium into the pulmonary circulation to cause a pulmonary embolism. In most cases, anticoagulant therapy (choice **c**) and close monitoring are necessary to prevent a pulmonary embolism. Compression stockings (choice **a**) are often used in the hospital to prevent a DVT in patients who are at risk, but are not as useful in the case of an existing thrombus. Thrombolytic therapy (choice **b**) may be as beneficial as anticoagulant therapy, but it usually leads to more adverse effects. An IVC filter (choice **d**) can also be as beneficial as anticoagulant therapy, but is not first-line therapy because it is more likely to cause recurrent DVT. Massage (choice **e**) is contraindicated because it may cause a piece of the thrombus to break off and shoot into circulation.

Task Area: Clinical Intervention

Organ System: Cardiovascular

249. b. Guillain-Barré syndrome (choice **b**) is a rapidly progressive peripheral neuropathy caused by autoimmune destruction of myelin in the peripheral nervous system. Symptoms usually start in the lower limbs and gradually move upward over the course of hours to days. The autoimmunity is believed to be a response to a recent infection; the most common pathogen is *Campylobacter jejuni*, which is a common cause of bloody diarrhea. Because the lesion is in peripheral nerves, reflexes will be absent or reduced. Myasthenia gravis (choice **a**) is another autoimmune destruction of nerves, but it usually starts in the eyes and progressively moves downward; also, reflexes are usually preserved. A stroke (choice **c**) in a young healthy patient is unlikely, and if it were to occur (usually as a result of vasculitis), the symptoms would occur instantaneously rather than progressively. Upper motor neuron lesions (choice **d**) always present with hyperreflexia rather than areflexia. A conversion disorder (choice **e**) would not present with areflexia, and there is no particular reason to suspect it.
Task Area: Formulating Most Likely Diagnosis
Organ System: Neurologic

250. a. This patient appears to have adrenocortical insufficiency, also known as Addison's disease. This is a syndrome characterized by dysfunction of the adrenal glands, which causes a decrease in cortisol levels and a constellation of signs and symptoms that includes myalgia and weakness (due to hypokalemia), hypotension, hypernatremia, and nausea/vomiting. In primary adrenal insufficiency, decreased cortisol levels cause feedback stimulation of the pituitary, which also leads to tanned skin due to increased production of melanocyte-stimulating hormone. The presence of adrenal insufficiency can be tested by an ACTH stimulation test (choice **a**); this will stimulate cortisol production in secondary adrenal insufficiency, but not in primary adrenal insufficiency. A dexamethasone suppression test (choice **b**) achieves the opposite goal; it is used to diagnose Cushing's syndrome, a state of excess cortisol production, by suppressing cortisol release. Plasma glucose levels (choice **c**) may help to diagnose diabetes mellitus or hyperglycemia. A urine dipstick (choice **d**) or serum creatinine levels (choice **e**) may be useful if there is a clinical suspicion of genitourinary pathology as a cause of hyponatremia and hyperkalemia, but this patient's presentation is more consistent with Addison's disease.
Task Area: Using Laboratory and Diagnostic Studies
Organ System: Endocrine

251. b. Alcoholics are at especially high risk of aspiration pneumonia, a form of pneumonia that is caused by inhalation of a foreign body. In aspiration pneumonia, the foreign body is most likely to travel down the right main bronchus because it is more vertical than the left main bronchus. Generally, gravity carries the body in the direction of the middle and lower lobes. The right middle and lower lobes are the most common site of aspiration pneumonia in patients who aspirate a foreign body while standing upright. Because alcoholics are usually in the prone position at the time of aspiration, they have a somewhat higher chance of aspirating into the right middle lobe (choice **b**) than does the general population. Right upper lobe aspiration pneumonia (choice **a**) is also more likely in alcoholic patients, but right middle or lower lobe pneumonia is still the most likely possibility. Choices **c**, **d**, and **e** are incorrect because aspiration to the left lung is generally less common than aspiration to the right lung.

Task Area: Applying Basic Science Concepts
Organ System: Pulmonary

252. a. Polyarteritis nodosa and giant cell arteritis (GCA) are two of the most common vasculitides in the general population and can often present with similar symptoms. While there are some differences in signs and symptoms, this patient's presentation is fairly nonspecific. The key distinguishing factor here is the patient's age (choice **a**). While polyarteritis nodosa usually occurs in patients between 30 and 50 years of age, giant cell arteritis is almost exclusively limited to patients over 50; it is most commonly seen in patients around 70 years of age. Choices **b**, **c**, **d**, and **e** are incorrect because they are features that are common to both polyarteritis nodosa and giant cell arteritis.

Task Area: History Taking and Performing Physical Examinations
Organ System: Cardiovascular

253. e. This question tests your knowledge of management of subarachnoid hemorrhage due to intracranial aneurysms. The correct answer is choice **e**, all of the above, because all of the choices are required to stabilize the patient. Surgical clipping of the aneurysm base is the definitive treatment to prevent further hemorrhages.

Task Area: Clinical Intervention
Organ System: Neurologic

254. d. This question tests your knowledge of initial treatment for diabetes mellitus. Given this patient's HgA1c level, medication therapy is indicated. The correct answer is choice **d**, metformin. Choice **a**, continue diet and exercise, is incorrect because the worsening HgA1c has been refractory to diet and exercise. Choice **b**, furosemide, is incorrect because it does not provide blood glucose control. Choice **c**, metoprolol, is incorrect because it is a beta blocker not indicated in initial treatment of diabetes. Choice **e**, levothyroxin, is incorrect because it is used in hypothyroidism.

Task Area: Pharmaceutical Therapeutics
Organ System: Endocrine

255. a. Appendicitis is a medical emergency that usually requires surgical removal of the appendix. Its clinical presentation is often similar to gastroenteritis, which is a far more common cause of fever, nausea, vomiting, and in some cases, lower abdominal pain. Rebound tenderness in the right lower quadrant (choice **a**), however, is a clinical sign that is fairly specific for appendicitis. If this clinical suspicion is present, it is important to obtain an ultrasound or CT image of the appendix. Inguinal lymphadenopathy (choice **b**) is more suggestive of pathology in the lower limbs or the pelvis. Digital rectal examination (choice **c**) has not been shown to be of any diagnostic benefit for appendicitis. Abdominal distention (choice **d**) and hypotension (choice **e**) are more likely to be found in a patient with gastroenteritis.

Task Area: History Taking and Performing Physical Examinations
Organ System: Gastrointestinal/Nutritional

256. e. The correct answer is choice **e**, surgery. For individuals diagnosed with non-small cell carcinoma, surgery is a viable treatment option. Non-small cell lung carcinomas such as squamous cell carcinoma, adenocarcinoma, and large cell carcinoma grow slowly and have a greater chance of treatment via surgery than small cell carcinoma. The five-year survival rate after resection is 35% to 40%. Choice **a**, cryotherapy, is used to treat skin lesions such as warts, moles, and skin tags. Choice **b**, chemotherapy, is a viable option but is usually not used until the disease has spread. Because this disease progresses slowly, surgical intervention gives the patient the greatest chance of survival. Choice **c**, radiation therapy, is not used as a first-line treatment for this disease, but is often used in conjunction with chemotherapy when surgery is not possible. Choice **d**, hormonal therapy, is useful to alleviate gastrointestinal issues secondary to non-small cell carcinoma, but it has no benefit for curing this disorder.

Task Area: Clinical Intervention
Organ System: Pulmonary

257. b. The physical exam and diagnostic finding are consistent with acute angle-closure glaucoma (choice **b**), which is a medical emergency. All other choices are incorrect, although they are good differentials.

Task Area: Laboratory and Diagnostic Studies
Organ System: EENT (Eye, Ear, Nose, and Throat)

258. c. The correct answer is choice **c**, thiazide diuretics, which are the most effective in relieving symptoms in patients with congestive heart failure (CHF). Choice **a**, antitussives, is incorrect because antitussives do not address the underlying cause of the patient's symptoms, which is CHF. Choice **b**, esomeprazole, is incorrect because it is used in acid reflux diseases. Choices **d**, aspirin, and **e**, clopidogrel, are incorrect because they are antiplatelets that are generally not indicated in CHF patients without the presence of atrial fibrillation or previous stroke.

Task Area: Pharmaceutical Therapeutics
Organ System: Cardiovascular

259. e. The correct answer is choice **e**, quantitative pilocarpine iontophoreses sweat test, which should be performed on two different days for accurate diagnosis. Choice **a**, ceruloplasmin, is incorrect because it is used to diagnose Wilson's disease. Choice **b**, troponin T, is incorrect because it is a cardiac marker used to diagnose myocardial injury. Choice **c**, chest X-ray, is incorrect because it is a non-specific test for lung abnormalities. Choice **d**, electrocardiogram (EKG), is incorrect because it tests cardiac electrical activities.

Task Area: Using Laboratory and Diagnostic Studies
Organ System: Pulmonary

260. d. Choice **d**, Psoas sign, is the correct answer. Choice **a**, Rovsing's sign, is incorrect because this patient does not show RLQ pain with palpation over LLQ. Choice **b**, Collen's sign, is incorrect because the patient does not show periumbilical bluish discoloration from hemoperitoneum. Choice **c**, Obturator sign, is incorrect because the exam does not show RLQ pain with internal rotation of the flexed right thigh. Choice **e**, Grey-Turner's sign, is incorrect because this sign is related to retroperitoneal hemorrhage with discoloration of the flank.

Task Area: History Taking and Performing Physical Examinations
Organ System: Gastrointestinal/Nutritional

261. a. The correct answer is choice **a**. None of the other choices are the correct sequence.

Task Area: Applying Basic Science Concepts
Organ System: Cardiovascular

262. a. The correct answer is choice **a**, joint aspiration showing negatively birefringent, needle-shaped crystals, which is diagnostic of true gout. Choice **e**, none of the above, is therefore incorrect. Choice **b**, joint aspiration showing rhomboidal, positively birefringent crystals, is incorrect because this finding is diagnostic for pseudogout. Choice **c**, joint aspiration positive for *S. aureus*, is incorrect because this finding is consistent with septic joint rather than true gout. Choice **d**, X-ray showing a hairline fracture of the first metatarsal phalangeal joint, is incorrect because it is not consistent with gout.

Task Area: Using Laboratory and Diagnostic Studies
Organ System: Musculoskeletal

263. a. Given the increased FSH and LH, this patient most likely has premature ovarian failure. The correct answer is choice **a**, oral contraceptives, which help to restore estrogen. Choice **b**, oxytocin, is incorrect because it is indicated in treatment of postpartum hemorrhage. Choice **c**, laparoscopic surgery, is incorrect because it is not indicated in this condition. Choices **d**, spironolactone, and **e**, levothyroxine, are incorrect because they are used in treatment of hirsutism and hypothyroidism, respectively.

Task Area: Pharmaceutical Therapeutics
Organ System: Reproductive

264. d. This patient's clinical presentation is typical benign prostatic hyperplasia (BPH) (choice **d**), which is a common condition that affects men over age 50. Choice **a**, urinary tract infection, is incorrect because the urinalysis is within normal limits. Choice **b**, testicular torsion, is incorrect because there is no mention of testicular symptoms. Choice **c**, urinary incontinence, is incorrect because he has increased urgency rather than lack of control. Choice **e**, pyelonephritis, is incorrect because his urinalysis is within normal limits.

Task Area: History Taking and Performing Physical Examinations
Organ System: Genitourinary

265. d. Malignant pleural effusions occur when lung cancer causes abnormal fluid collection to build up between the outside of the lung and the chest cavity. Once the effusions are drained, a procedure called pleurodesis (choice **d**) should be performed. If a malignant pleural effusion is very small, it can sometimes be left alone. Thoracentesis can be performed to drain the fluid, but it frequently returns. To prevent fluid from returning, pleurodesis may be done. In this procedure, a chemical such as talc is inserted between the 2 layers of the pleura so that they stick together, preventing fluid from accumulating. This is successful for 60% to 90% of people. Choice **a**, pericardiocentesis, should not be considered because this procedure is performed to remove excess fluid around the heart. Choice **b**, thoracentesis, is the procedure used to drain pleural effusions; according to the question, this has already been performed, so a pleurodesis procedure should also be performed. Choice **c**, paracentesis, should not be considered as this is the procedure to remove fluid from the abdomen. Choice **e**, amniocentesis, should not be considered as this is used to test for abnormalities during pregnancy.

Task Area: Clinical Intervention
Organ System: Pulmonary

266. d. Ultraviolet light exposure has been linked to increased risk for skin cancer. Patient education is an important part of care for patients with a history of skin cancer. The correct answer is choice **d**, all of the above. Choice **e**, none of the above, is therefore incorrect.

Task Area: Health Maintenance
Organ System: Dermatologic

267. e. The correct answer is choice **e**, increase dietary intake of water, caffeine, and salt. The reason for this is that water, caffeine, and salt will all cause blood pressure to elevate, thus reducing the effects of orthostatic hypotension. Calcium channel blockers (choice **a**), ACE inhibitors (choice **b**), and beta blockers (choice **c**) are effective in treating hypertension; therefore, prescription of these medications can cause already low blood pressure to become dangerously low. Choice **d**, a change in diet to reduce water, caffeine, and salt intake, will cause blood pressure to remain low, and orthostatic hypotension will not be treated.

Task Area: Clinical Intervention
Organ System: Cardiovascular

268. a. The correct answer is choice **a**, lung ventilation and perfusion scan to rule out pulmonary embolism. Pulmonary embolism would be your primary concern in this situation because of the elevated D-dimer, low pulse oximetry reading, and rapid heart rate. Under normal circumstances, choice **b**, CT scan with contrast of the chest to rule out pulmonary embolism, would be the diagnostic study of choice in this situation. However, the elevated BUN and creatinine along with the depressed GFR contraindicates the use of contrast for this patient because it may cause kidney failure. You might think that choice **c**, myocardial perfusion imaging to rule out acute myocardial infarction, would be the most obvious choice. However, the normal troponin level and relatively normal electrocardiogram should rule out a cardiac emergency. Choice **d**, CT scan with contrast of the abdomen to rule out aortic dissection, would also be a valid study to perform. However, the elevated BUN and creatinine along with the depressed GFR should dissuade you from using any contrast material on this patient, as it could cause kidney failure. Choice **e**, cardiac catheterization to assess myocardial ischemia, would not be a viable option because of the relatively normal electrocardiogram and the fact the patient's renal function is suppressed.

Task Area: Using Laboratory and Diagnostic Studies
Organ System: Pulmonary

269. a. Mastoiditis is a condition that is easily treated with a course of intravenous antibiotics (choice **a**) if the infection is recognized in an early stage. Choices **b** and **c**, combined antibiotic therapies with corticosteroids or with anti-inflammatory agents, will generally not assist in the treatment of mastoiditis. (If the condition is not treated with intravenous antibiotics, mastoidectomy would become the only course of treatment.) Choice **d**, biopsy of affected ear, will not add any value to a course of treatment for mastoiditis. Choice **e**, mastoidectomy, is a last recourse for treatment of mastoiditis and should be used only when treatment with intravenous antibiotics has proven ineffective.

Task Area: Clinical Intervention
Organ System: EENT (Eye, Ear, Nose, and Throat)

270. d. Addison's disease (choice **d**) is a disorder characterized by weight loss, muscle weakness, fatigue, and darkening of the skin. It can also cause low blood pressure, and is characterized by abnormal adrenal glands that cannot produce sufficient amounts of cortisol to maintain normal bodily functions such as blood pressure. Choice **a**, pheochromocytoma, is incorrect because it is a rare tumor of the adrenal gland whose characteristics are high blood pressure, heart palpitations, and headache, which the patient does not present. Choice **b**, Wilson's disease, can cause weakness, confusion, and cognitive impairments. In addition, Wilson's disease is characterized by an extremely high level of copper in the blood stream. Choice **c**, Graves' disease, would not be the appropriate diagnosis because the thyroid hormone levels are normal, although this disorder can cause muscle weakness and weight loss. Choice **e**, Huntington's disease, should not be an option at all because this disease classically affects the nervous system.

Task Area: Formulating Most Likely Diagnosis
Organ System: Endocrine

271. e. This patient has a series of contraindications for different antihypertensive drugs. Digoxin toxicity is particularly common in patients with hypokalemia, so thiazides (choice **a**) and loop diuretics (choice **b**) are contraindicated because of their tendency to reduce plasma potassium levels. Beta-blockers (choices **c** and **d**) tend to exacerbate symptoms of COPD. Amiloride (choice **e**) is a more appropriate choice because, unlike thiazides and loop diuretics, it does not cause hypokalemia.

Task Area: Pharmaceutical Therapeutics
Organ System: Cardiovascular

272. a. Stroke therapy with recombinant tissue plasminogen activator is most effective when administered within three hours (choice **a**) after the initial onset of symptoms. Complications associated with this type of medication include an increased risk of bleeding. This type of medication is contraindicated in patients with suspicion of intracranial bleed, recent intracranial surgery, serious head trauma, or previous stroke. With respect to choices **b**, **c**, **d**, and **e**, the longer that has elapsed before stroke treatment with recombinant tissue plasminogen activator, the greater chance there will be for permanent consequences of the stroke.

Task Area: Clinical Intervention
Organ System: Neurologic

273. e. Foods that contain the amino acid tyramine are contraindicated for individuals who are prescribed monoamine oxidase inhibitors (MAOIs) (choice **e**). Treatment with MAOIs adversely affects the body's ability to metabolize the amino acid tyramine. Failure to break down tyramine can lead to a hypertensive crisis and migraine headaches. Serious side effects, such as a hypertensive crisis, may occur if tyramine is ingested while on MAOIs. Some common foods that contain tyramine include wine, beer, nearly all cheeses, aged foods, and smoked meats. Choices **a**, **b**, **c**, and **d** are all incorrect.

Task Area: Pharmaceutical Therapeutics
Organ System: Psychiatry/Behavioral Science

274. b. Rheumatoid arthritis (choice **b**) is an autoimmune condition that causes inflammation in the carpometacarpal joints, the metacarpophalangeal joints, the proximal interphalangeal joints, and occasionally other joints. Stiffness and pain usually increase with lack of movement, including while the patient is sleeping, and consequently improve over the course of the day. This progressive improvement is a classic feature that is highly suggestive of autoimmunity rather than degeneration as the cause of the patient's pain. Osteoarthritis (choice **a**), by contrast, presents with pain in both types of interphalangeal joints along with large weight-bearing joints, and the symptoms tend to *increase* over the course of the day. Carpal tunnel syndrome (choice **c**) is caused by pressure on the median nerve and leads to pain, weakness, and parasthesia in the median nerve distribution (the radial side of the hand). Scleroderma (choice **d**) causes systemic symptoms that include hand pain, but this is a constrictive pain caused by tightening of the surrounding skin. Peripheral neuropathy (choice **e**) would cause pain, weakness, and parasthesia in the distribution of the affected nerve, but it usually presents in the lower limbs before it does in the upper limbs.

Task Area: Formulating Most Likely Diagnosis
Organ System: Musculoskeletal

275. d. A short history of pain, fever, and diarrhea may be caused by several different forms of colitis. The important thing to recognize for this question is the value of the recent antibiotic use; pseudomembranous colitis (choice **d**) is generally caused by overgrowth of *Clostridium difficile* after elimination of other gut bacteria by antibiotic therapy. This is most commonly caused by fluoroquinolones, but other antibiotics can also cause it. Clindamycin, for instance, is noted for causing pseudomembranous colitis with a particularly high frequency (but it is not used often, so fluoroquinolone-induced pseudomembranous colitis is still more common). Because of the possibility of antibiotic cross-reactivity, the patient should also be advised to inform any other clinicians about her history of antibiotic-induced pseudomembranous colitis. Colorectal carcinoma (choice **a**) usually presents with symptoms related to bleeding (anemia or blood in the feces) or obstruction (constipation and incomplete bowel voiding) rather than diarrhea. Colorectal adenoma (choice **b**) is a precursor to colorectal carcinoma and often presents with similar symptoms. Ischemic colitis and ulcerative colitis (choices **c** and **e**) have a clinical appearance similar to pseudomembranous colitis, but the recent history of antibiotic use suggests *C. difficile* overgrowth as a more likely pathophysiological process.

Task Area: Pharmaceutical Therapeutics
Organ System: Gastrointestinal/Nutritional

276. e. While short episodes of dizziness are more commonly caused by orthostatic hypotension and/or presyncope, the feeling of a spinning room with a stationary patient is a classic description of vertigo. The most common cause of vertigo is canalithiasis, a condition in which calcium crystals from the utricle become dislodged and cause a blockage in the semicircular canals. This leads to benign paroxysmal positional vertigo (BPPV); the disturbance in the vestibular system can cause nausea (choice **e**) but not vomiting (choice **b**). Because BPPV episodes are generally associated with changes in position, the presentation may appear to be similar to that of orthostatic hypotension (choice **a**) and presyncope (choice **c**); however, these options are incorrect because they are not associated with vertigo. Vertigo may also be caused by otitis interna, but not by otitis media (choice **d**).

Task Area: History Taking and Performing Physical Examinations
Organ System: EENT (Eye, Ear, Nose, and Throat)

277. a. This patient most likely has androgen insensitivity syndrome (also known as testicular feminization syndrome), a disorder in which a genetically male patient has nonfunctional androgen receptors. The patient still has testes, but they are located within the abdomen; the testes secrete testosterone and mullerian inhibiting factor (MIF), but because the peripheral receptors are insensitive to this testosterone, it is converted to estradiol in peripheral tissues. The presence of estradiol leads to the formation of breasts and a short vagina, but the MIF inhibits the development of ovaries and a uterus. Choice **a** is correct: a hormone test will find that the patient has normal levels of testosterone and dihydrotestosterone (DHT). If both levels are low (choice **b**), the patient may have testicular dysgenesis or Leydig cell aplasia. If DHT is low but testosterone is normal (choice **c**), 5α-reductase deficiency should be suspected; however, this is more likely to present with hirsutism. Choices **d** and **e** are not associated with this sort of clinical picture.

Task Area: Using Laboratory and Diagnostic Studies
Organ System: Reproductive

278. a. This patient's proteinuria, hypoalbuminemia, and hypercholesterolemia are suggestive of a renal insufficiency due to a nephrotic syndrome, the most common of which in children is minimal change disease. While the precise etiology is still not known, it usually involves an immune abnormality that leads to podocyte foot-process effacement, which causes nephrotic syndrome via loss of the charge barrier at the glomerular basement membrane. First-line therapy is usually systemic corticosteroids (choice **a**). Broad-spectrum antibiotics (choice **b**) may be useful in the case of pyelonephritis or other infectious renal disease, but this is more likely to present with fever and dysuria. Plasmapheresis (choice **c**) and hemodialysis (choice **d**) are generally reserved for chronic renal disease that is otherwise irreversible. Some forms of antineoplastic chemotherapy (choice **e**) may be useful for immunosuppression, but this is a very toxic form of therapy that is inadvisable to use when alternatives are available.

Task Area: Clinical Intervention
Organ System: Genitourinary

279. **a.** Cephalexin is a drug that contains a sulfur group, which is a common cause of allergy (choice **a**). Cephalosporins are generally less likely to cause rashes than penicillin-group drugs, but allergic reactions are still fairly common. This allergy generally manifests as an erythematous rash that may present in a variety of different parts of the body. If the symptoms become significant, it is generally advisable to switch the patient to a different antibiotic regimen. Allergies to anesthetic agents (choice **b**) and oxycodone (choice **c**) are possible, but are less likely to result in a rash. Infectious dermatitis (choice **d**) is possible, but does not typically present with such a widespread bilateral rash; furthermore, it is especially unlikely in a patient who is taking prophylactic antibiotics. Autoimmune disorders (choice **e**) such as psoriasis often cause rashes, but are less common than sulfa drug allergies.

Task Area: Pharmaceutical Therapeutics
Organ System: Dermatologic

280. **e.** While most of the spleen's functions can be covered by other organs, it is the main organ responsible for elimination of encapsulated bacteria, which include *Streptococcus pneumoniae, Neisseria meningitidis, Haemophilus influenzae,* and *Salmonella typhi* (choice **e**). A splenectomy is essentially curative for hereditary spherocytosis, but it does cause the side effect of increased susceptibility to these bacteria; 33% of patients will be hospitalized within the next ten years, with the highest risk of hospitalization during the first two years after the procedure. Vaccines are readily available for *S. pneumonia, N. meningitidis,* and *H. influenzae,* but the best way to protect against *S. typhi* is to ensure that all food (especially chicken and pork) is thoroughly cooked. Choices **a**, **b**, **c**, and **d** can also act as food-borne pathogens, but are not likely to occur with increased frequency after a splenectomy.

Task Area: Applying Basic Science Concepts
Organ System: Infectious Diseases

281. **d.** The patient is an intravenous drug user with bacterial endocarditis. She is also in septic shock. The murmur most commonly associated with an intravenous drug user is tricuspid regurgitation (choice **d**). Therefore, aortic regurgitation (choice **a**), aortic stenosis (choice **b**), mitral regurgitation (choice **c**), and pulmonary stenosis (choice **e**) are incorrect.

Task Area: History Taking and Performing Physical Examinations
Organ System: Cardiovascular

282. **a.** The use of cotton swabs (choice **a**) such as Q-tips push the wax farther down the ear canal and prevents its clearance; as does the use of ear buds (choice **e**). Commercial ear drops (choice **d**) can help liquify ear wax. Regular checkups will allow early detection and management. Regular cleaning of the auricle (choice **c**) has no detrimental effect.

Task Area: Health Maintenance

Organ System: EENT (Eye, Ear, Nose, and Throat)

283. **b.** The patient seems to be having an ischemic stroke. A CT brain angiogram (choice **b**) is indicated in hemorrhagic stroke, not in ischemic stroke. All of the other options are appropriate clinical interventions for this patient. Anticoagulation (choice **a**) can be initiated up to four hours after the onset of symptoms. Blood pressure (choice **c**) should be managed both in long-term and short-term settings. Stroke victims are often bedridden for many weeks, and therefore are at risk for developing DVTs (choice **d**). Lipid-lowering agents such as statins have been shown to be effective in preventing strokes (choice **e**).

Task Area: Clinical Intervention

Organ System: Neurologic

284. **e.** Monitoring C-reactive protein (CRP) (choice **e**) would not be useful. All the other options would be, because anemia (checked by full blood count (choice **a**)), nutritional deficencies (check B12/folate (choice **b**)), hypothyroidism (check TSH (choice **c**)), and drugs (checked with blood toxicology screen (choice **d**)) can all cause symptoms of depression.

Task Area: Using Laboratory and Diagnostic Studies

Organ System: Psychiatry/Behavioral Science

285. **c.** Infectious esophagitis (choice **c**) is a rare disorder; however, it is most common in immunosuppressed patients. Patients with infectious esophagitis will complain of difficult and painful swallowing. An endoscopy will reveal lesions in the esophagus that vary according to the causing virus. Infection with the cytomegalovirus will cause large deep ulcers, herpes simplex virus will cause multiple shallow ulcers, and a candidal infection will reveal white plaques. Choice **a**, esophageal varices, is incorrect because of the lack of history of alcoholism and bleeding. Choice **b**, esophageal neoplasm, is incorrect because of the endoscopic evidence of ulcer instead of a tumor; also, the presence of the cytomegalovirus should rule out esophageal varices. Lack of regurgitation, endoscopic evidence of ulcers, and the presence of the cytomegalovirus should rule out choice **d**, esophageal dysmotility, and choice **e**, reflux esophagitis.

Task Area: Formulating Most Likely Diagnosis

Organ System: Gastrointestinal/Nutritional

286. **e.** The patient most likely has iron deficiency anemia as indicated by the low ferritin level. A positive Romberg's sign (choice **e**) is present in B12 deficiency, not in iron deficiency anemia. Anemia in general can cause tachycardia (choice **a**) and dyspnea (choice **b**). Pica (choice **c**), the craving to eat nonorganic materials such as sand or charcoal, can be seen in iron deficiency. Melena (choice **d**) can cause iron deficiency.

Task Area: History Taking and Performing Physical Examinations

Organ System: Hematologic

287. a. Familial hypercholesterolemia is a rare disorder caused by a hereditary deficiency of LDL receptors (choice **a**), which normally mediates the endocytosis of low-density lipoproteins. In the absence of the LDL receptor, a patient's cholesterol levels will continue to increase until coronary atherosclerosis causes significant cardiovascular issues at an early age. Heterozygotes are somewhat common (1 in 500 patients), but the severity of this patient's symptoms suggests that he is a homozygote (1 in 1,000,000 patients). In addition to signs of hypercholesterolemia (such as xanthelasmata), patients often present with angina. Often, there is a family history of unexpected young death. Homozygotes, who generally have a family history on both sides of their family, do not survive past age 40 without intervention; while there is no gold standard for treatment, it is advisable to use drastic measures such as liver transplantation, ileal bypass surgery, or LDL apheresis. Heterozygotes can survive to old age but are at far higher risk of coronary artery disease. Choices **b**, VLDL receptor, and **c**, HDL receptor, are not known receptor deficiencies. Choice **d**, chloride channel, describes the deficiency that is responsible for cystic fibrosis, a hereditary disease that primarily affects the lungs and exocrine glands. Choice **e**, transferrin receptor, suggests hemochromatosis, another hereditary disorder that causes iron overload.

Task Area: Applying Basic Science Concepts
Organ System: Cardiovascular

288. e. This patient may have a Mallory-Weiss tear, a tear of the lower esophagus that is often caused by esophageal acid exposure due to excessive vomiting. A recent history of excessive alcohol consumption (and consequent vomiting) is a major risk factor for a Mallory-Weiss tear. The typical presentation consists of hematemesis, but some patients may also present with melena. Endoscopy (choice **e**) is the only investigation that can be used to confirm the diagnosis. Barium swallow (choice **a**) may demonstrate evidence of an esophageal tear in some cases, but this cannot help establish or exclude a firm diagnosis. A chest X-ray (choice **b**) or CT (choice **c**) may be useful in the case of achalasia, but does not provide a clear diagnosis. A full blood count (choice **d**) will help to grade the level of blood loss, but again does not provide a diagnosis.

Task Area: Using Laboratory and Diagnostic Studies
Organ System: Gastrointestinal/Nutritional

289. **a.** Avascular necrosis is an uncommon cause of hip joint damage, but it is rapidly progressive and can lead to collapse of the femoral head. It is often difficult to distinguish from more common pathological processes based on clinical examination and X-ray findings, but its presenting complaints are somewhat different from those seen in osteoarthritis and osteoporosis. Avascular necrosis generally presents in younger patients (it is most common between the ages of 30 and 50) and is characterized by acute onset of pain (choice **a**). The pain is usually localized to a single joint with no involvement elsewhere in the body. A wide variety of risk factors has been associated with avascular necrosis, but family history (choice **b**) has not been shown to be implicated. Exacerbation with weight bearing (choice **c**) and lessening of symptoms over the course of the day (choice **d**) are features that are common to both avascular necrosis and osteoarthritis, so they are not the most suggestive symptoms for a diagnosis of avascular necrosis. Multiple joint/bone involvement (choice **e**) is unlikely in avascular necrosis, but is common in osteoarthritis and osteoporosis.

Task Area: History Taking and Performing Physical Examinations
Organ System: Musculoskeletal

290. **b.** The correct answer is choice **b**, do not remove object, and arrange for patient to be transported to the nearest emergency room for a consultation with an ophthalmologist. Choice **a** is incorrect because a penetrating trauma to the eye is considered emergent and should be treated immediately in an emergency room by a qualified ophthalmologist. One suggestion for treatment of penetrating trauma is to place an inverted Styrofoam cup over the injured eye, tape it in place, patch the other eye (the patching of the other eye minimizes conjugate movement), then transport to an ophthalmologist stat. Choices **c**, **d**, and **e** are incorrect because you would never want to remove the object yourself, as this has the potential to cause further damage to the eye and increase the risk of vision loss. The object removal should be performed by an ophthalmologist.

Task Area: Clinical Intervention
Organ System: EENT (Eye, Ear, Nose, and Throat)

291. c. Cannabis is one of the most widely used recreational drugs in the United States. In patients with certain genetic risk factors, its regular use has been associated with a significantly increased risk of developing schizophrenia (choice **c**). One large longitudinal study found that patients who have used cannabis on more than 50 occasions are six times more likely to develop schizophrenia than the general population. Some scientists have hypothesized that certain psychological risk factors may independently lead to both schizophrenia and cannabis use. This link has been well established in several studies. Chronic obstructive pulmonary disease (COPD) (choice **a**), asthma (choice **b**), and lung cancer (choice **e**) are possible consequences of regular smoking, but have not been associated with cannabis use; because this patient's smoking history (approximately once per week) is relatively mild in comparison with chronic pack-a-day smokers (who smoke more than 100 cigarettes per week), the risk of respiratory complications is relatively low. Major depressive disorder (choice **d**) may induce a patient to self-medicate with cannabis, but this link is not as well established as the link with schizophrenia.

Task Area: Health Maintenance
Organ System: Psychiatry/Behavioral Science

292. b. A lateral neck radiograph (choice **b**) will differentiate between a diagnosis of croup and epiglottitis. Epiglottitis is characterized radiographically by the "thumb sign," indicating inflammation and enlargement of the epiglottis. Croup will visualize radiographically as subglottic haziness and narrowing as well as distention of the hypopharynx. Choice **a**, posteroanterior X-ray view of the neck, will be of no use for diagnosis of epiglottitis because the cervical spine will obscure the epiglottis. Choice **c**, CT scan of the neck, can indicate airway obstruction; however, it is of little use in differentiating between croup and epiglottitis. Choice **d**, MRI scan of the neck, much like a CT scan, can indicate airway obstruction; however, it is of little use in differentiating between croup and epiglottitis. Choice **e**, ultrasound of the neck, is of no clinical use in differentiating between croup and epiglottitis.

Task Area: Using Laboratory and Diagnostic Studies
Organ System: Pulmonary

293. **d.** Reactive arthritis (choice **d**), formerly known as Reiter's syndrome, presents with urethritis, conjunctivitis, oligoarthritis, and mucosal ulcers. This disorder is often the result of chlamydia infection or gastroenteritis. Patients may present with asymmetric arthritis in the large joints below the waist. Other common presentations are balanitis, stomatitis, urethritis, and conjunctivitis. This disorder affects males more than females. Choice **a**, septic arthritis, is caused by bacterial infections in other parts of the body and spreads to the joints. In addition, septic arthritis is associated with joint redness and low-grade fever, which are not exhibited in this patient. Choice **b**, rheumatoid arthritis, should be excluded because this disorder is primarily symmetric, attacking both sides of the body equally. Choice **c**, psoriatic arthritis, should be excluded because this disorder is associated with psoriasis, or red patches on the skin, which is not presented in this patient. Choice **e**, scleroderma, should be excluded immediately because this condition is characterized by symmetric thickening of the skin.
Task Area: Formulating Most Likely Diagnosis
Organ System: Musculoskeletal

294. **c.** This patient appears to be suffering from dyspareunia, or pain during sexual intercourse. Often, dyspareunia is related to a psychological barrier to sexual contact, and this etiology is particularly likely in a patient who has been abstinent for most of her life, has experienced dyspareunia since her first sexual contact, and has even been reluctant to use tampons. A common cause of dyspareunia is vaginismus, a condition in which the pubococcygeus muscle contracts on vaginal penetration, thereby causing significant pain. Because it is possible for a small amount of penetration to occur in the area distal to the pubococcygeus muscle, patients with very little sexual experience may not be aware that a sexual problem is present; this is a likely explanation for the fact that this patient has presented with concerns about fertility rather than concerns about sexual intercourse. Psychological support (choice **c**) can be initially beneficial, and if the problem persists, it may be treated with progressive vaginal sensitization through the use of progressively larger vaginal dilators. Pain relief (choice **a**) may be somewhat useful for this patient, but it does not provide a long-term solution. Surgical correction (choice **b**) may be necessary if other strategies are unsuccessful and an anatomical abnormality is discovered. Antibiotic therapy (choice **d**) or antifungal therapy (choice **e**) would be beneficial if an infectious etiology could be demonstrated.
Task Area: Clinical Intervention
Organ System: Reproductive

295. c. Minoxidil (choice **c**) is an antihypertensive, vasodilator medication that is known for its ability to slow or stop hair loss and promote regrowth. This medication is the safest, most effective treatment for male pattern baldness. Choice **a**, finasteride, may also be effective to treat male pattern baldness; however, loss of libido and erectile dysfunction may occur with use of finasteride. Choice **b**, vitamin A, can prevent hair loss: however, *overconsumption* of vitamin A can actually *cause* hair loss. Choice **d**, topical steroid creams, may have some hair growth benefits; however, for best results, topical steroid creams should be used in conjunction with minoxidil. Topical antibiotic creams (choice **e**) have not been scientifically proven to promote hair growth.

Task Area: Pharmaceutical Therapeutics
Organ System: Dermatologic

296. b. A time out procedure (choice **b**) is the universal protocol to verify the correct patient, procedure, site, and implants. Choice **a**, HIPAA, is incorrect as this legislation is designed to insure the privacy and security of personal health information. Choice **c**, Safe Medical Devices Act, is incorrect as this legislation requires users of medical devices to report any incidents that could in any way suggest that the device caused death, serious injury, or illness to a patient. Choice **d**, Patient's Bill of Rights, is incorrect as this legislation requires healthcare providers to inform all patients of their rights as patients receiving medical treatment. Choice **e**, EMTALA, is incorrect as this legislation legally obligates healthcare facilities to provide emergent care regardless of citizenship, legal status, or ability to pay.

Task Area: Clinical Intervention
Organ System: Musculoskeletal

297. b. Choice **b**, tubal ligation, is correct because procedure can be reversed; usually there are two remaining fallopian tube segments. Successful fallopian tube repair now occurs in approximately 98 percent of the women who undergo the procedure, although fertility is not guaranteed. Choices **a, c, d**, and **e** are incorrect as all of these procedures are permanent and involve the removal of organs necessary for fertility.

Task Area: History Taking and Performing Physical Examinations
Organ System: Reproductive

298. a. Ice packs and analgesics (choice **a**) are the appropriate treatment measures for orchitis that occurs secondary to the mumps virus. Antibiotics are only indicated if orchitis is caused by a bacterium. Choices **b, c, d**, and **e** are all incorrect as these medications are antibiotics and are only indicated if the orchitis was caused by a bacterial infection.

Task Area: Health Maintenance
Organ System: Genitourinary

299. b. While dryness in the eyes and mouth is a nonspecific set of symptoms, the enlarged parotid glands and elevated levels of rheumatoid factor (an IgM antibody against IgG) suggest a diagnosis of Sjögren's syndrome, an autoimmune deficiency of the exocrine glands. Unless symptoms are severe, Sjögren's syndrome is generally treated with symptomatic management, which involves replacement of the deficient fluids. For this patient, the initial therapy regimen would involve the use of artificial tears and artificial saliva (choice **b**). Fluid replacement (choice **a**) would be beneficial if the patient had dry mucous membranes as a result of hypovolemia. Corticosteroid (choice **c**) or methotrexate (choice **d**) therapy is useful in some autoimmune disorders, but they are not generally recommended as initial therapy in patients with Sjögren's syndrome. Desmopressin (choice **e**) is an antidiuretic hormone (ADH) analog that can be used to treat some forms of hypovolemia.
Task Area: Clinical Intervention
Organ System: Musculoskeletal

300. c. Ceftriaxone (choice **c**) is the treatment of choice for men and women infected with gonorrhea. There is much resistance to other medications such as penicillin, tetracyclines, and fluoroquinolones, so ceftriaxone is the drug of choice. Choices **a**, **d**, and **e** might all be considered for treatment of gonorrhea; however, there are a variety of strains of gonorrhea that are resistant to these medications, so ceftriaxone is the more appropriate choice. Choice **b**, mebendazole, should not be considered as this is an anthelmintic medication.
Task Area: Pharmaceutical Therapeutics
Organ System: Infectious Diseases

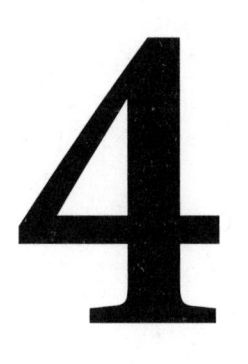 

PRACTICE TEST 2

This is the second of two practice tests included with *PANCE: Power Practice*. Each practice test consists of questions that mirror those you will find on the official PANCE. The 300-question test, separated into 60-question sections, was developed by test experts.

Remember, on test day, you will have 60 minutes to complete each 60-question section. After you finish a section and start the next, you are not allowed to go back to answer questions in a previous section. Try to adhere to test day rules when you take these practice tests so that you have the most authentic practice experience possible.

These tests will show you how much you know and what kinds of problems you still need to study. In the answer explanations that follow the test, you will find which organ system and which task area each question covers. Take note of which question types you tend to get wrong; this will help you focus your study until you take the actual exam.

Mastering these practice tests will allow you to reach your highest potential on the real PANCE. Good luck!

Practice Test 2 Answer Sheet

Section 1

1. ⓐ ⓑ ⓒ ⓓ ⓔ	21. ⓐ ⓑ ⓒ ⓓ ⓔ	41. ⓐ ⓑ ⓒ ⓓ ⓔ
2. ⓐ ⓑ ⓒ ⓓ ⓔ	22. ⓐ ⓑ ⓒ ⓓ ⓔ	42. ⓐ ⓑ ⓒ ⓓ ⓔ
3. ⓐ ⓑ ⓒ ⓓ ⓔ	23. ⓐ ⓑ ⓒ ⓓ ⓔ	43. ⓐ ⓑ ⓒ ⓓ ⓔ
4. ⓐ ⓑ ⓒ ⓓ ⓔ	24. ⓐ ⓑ ⓒ ⓓ ⓔ	44. ⓐ ⓑ ⓒ ⓓ ⓔ
5. ⓐ ⓑ ⓒ ⓓ ⓔ	25. ⓐ ⓑ ⓒ ⓓ ⓔ	45. ⓐ ⓑ ⓒ ⓓ ⓔ
6. ⓐ ⓑ ⓒ ⓓ ⓔ	26. ⓐ ⓑ ⓒ ⓓ ⓔ	46. ⓐ ⓑ ⓒ ⓓ ⓔ
7. ⓐ ⓑ ⓒ ⓓ ⓔ	27. ⓐ ⓑ ⓒ ⓓ ⓔ	47. ⓐ ⓑ ⓒ ⓓ ⓔ
8. ⓐ ⓑ ⓒ ⓓ ⓔ	28. ⓐ ⓑ ⓒ ⓓ ⓔ	48. ⓐ ⓑ ⓒ ⓓ ⓔ
9. ⓐ ⓑ ⓒ ⓓ ⓔ	29. ⓐ ⓑ ⓒ ⓓ ⓔ	49. ⓐ ⓑ ⓒ ⓓ ⓔ
10. ⓐ ⓑ ⓒ ⓓ ⓔ	30. ⓐ ⓑ ⓒ ⓓ ⓔ	50. ⓐ ⓑ ⓒ ⓓ ⓔ
11. ⓐ ⓑ ⓒ ⓓ ⓔ	31. ⓐ ⓑ ⓒ ⓓ ⓔ	51. ⓐ ⓑ ⓒ ⓓ ⓔ
12. ⓐ ⓑ ⓒ ⓓ ⓔ	32. ⓐ ⓑ ⓒ ⓓ ⓔ	52. ⓐ ⓑ ⓒ ⓓ ⓔ
13. ⓐ ⓑ ⓒ ⓓ ⓔ	33. ⓐ ⓑ ⓒ ⓓ ⓔ	53. ⓐ ⓑ ⓒ ⓓ ⓔ
14. ⓐ ⓑ ⓒ ⓓ ⓔ	34. ⓐ ⓑ ⓒ ⓓ ⓔ	54. ⓐ ⓑ ⓒ ⓓ ⓔ
15. ⓐ ⓑ ⓒ ⓓ ⓔ	35. ⓐ ⓑ ⓒ ⓓ ⓔ	55. ⓐ ⓑ ⓒ ⓓ ⓔ
16. ⓐ ⓑ ⓒ ⓓ ⓔ	36. ⓐ ⓑ ⓒ ⓓ ⓔ	56. ⓐ ⓑ ⓒ ⓓ ⓔ
17. ⓐ ⓑ ⓒ ⓓ ⓔ	37. ⓐ ⓑ ⓒ ⓓ ⓔ	57. ⓐ ⓑ ⓒ ⓓ ⓔ
18. ⓐ ⓑ ⓒ ⓓ ⓔ	38. ⓐ ⓑ ⓒ ⓓ ⓔ	58. ⓐ ⓑ ⓒ ⓓ ⓔ
19. ⓐ ⓑ ⓒ ⓓ ⓔ	39. ⓐ ⓑ ⓒ ⓓ ⓔ	59. ⓐ ⓑ ⓒ ⓓ ⓔ
20. ⓐ ⓑ ⓒ ⓓ ⓔ	40. ⓐ ⓑ ⓒ ⓓ ⓔ	60. ⓐ ⓑ ⓒ ⓓ ⓔ

Section 2

61.	ⓐ	ⓑ	ⓒ	ⓓ	ⓔ	**81.**	ⓐ	ⓑ	ⓒ	ⓓ	ⓔ	**101.**	ⓐ	ⓑ	ⓒ	ⓓ	ⓔ
62.	ⓐ	ⓑ	ⓒ	ⓓ	ⓔ	**82.**	ⓐ	ⓑ	ⓒ	ⓓ	ⓔ	**102.**	ⓐ	ⓑ	ⓒ	ⓓ	ⓔ
63.	ⓐ	ⓑ	ⓒ	ⓓ	ⓔ	**83.**	ⓐ	ⓑ	ⓒ	ⓓ	ⓔ	**103.**	ⓐ	ⓑ	ⓒ	ⓓ	ⓔ
64.	ⓐ	ⓑ	ⓒ	ⓓ	ⓔ	**84.**	ⓐ	ⓑ	ⓒ	ⓓ	ⓔ	**104.**	ⓐ	ⓑ	ⓒ	ⓓ	ⓔ
65.	ⓐ	ⓑ	ⓒ	ⓓ	ⓔ	**85.**	ⓐ	ⓑ	ⓒ	ⓓ	ⓔ	**105.**	ⓐ	ⓑ	ⓒ	ⓓ	ⓔ
66.	ⓐ	ⓑ	ⓒ	ⓓ	ⓔ	**86.**	ⓐ	ⓑ	ⓒ	ⓓ	ⓔ	**106.**	ⓐ	ⓑ	ⓒ	ⓓ	ⓔ
67.	ⓐ	ⓑ	ⓒ	ⓓ	ⓔ	**87.**	ⓐ	ⓑ	ⓒ	ⓓ	ⓔ	**107.**	ⓐ	ⓑ	ⓒ	ⓓ	ⓔ
68.	ⓐ	ⓑ	ⓒ	ⓓ	ⓔ	**88.**	ⓐ	ⓑ	ⓒ	ⓓ	ⓔ	**108.**	ⓐ	ⓑ	ⓒ	ⓓ	ⓔ
69.	ⓐ	ⓑ	ⓒ	ⓓ	ⓔ	**89.**	ⓐ	ⓑ	ⓒ	ⓓ	ⓔ	**109.**	ⓐ	ⓑ	ⓒ	ⓓ	ⓔ
70.	ⓐ	ⓑ	ⓒ	ⓓ	ⓔ	**90.**	ⓐ	ⓑ	ⓒ	ⓓ	ⓔ	**110.**	ⓐ	ⓑ	ⓒ	ⓓ	ⓔ
71.	ⓐ	ⓑ	ⓒ	ⓓ	ⓔ	**91.**	ⓐ	ⓑ	ⓒ	ⓓ	ⓔ	**111.**	ⓐ	ⓑ	ⓒ	ⓓ	ⓔ
72.	ⓐ	ⓑ	ⓒ	ⓓ	ⓔ	**92.**	ⓐ	ⓑ	ⓒ	ⓓ	ⓔ	**112.**	ⓐ	ⓑ	ⓒ	ⓓ	ⓔ
73.	ⓐ	ⓑ	ⓒ	ⓓ	ⓔ	**93.**	ⓐ	ⓑ	ⓒ	ⓓ	ⓔ	**113.**	ⓐ	ⓑ	ⓒ	ⓓ	ⓔ
74.	ⓐ	ⓑ	ⓒ	ⓓ	ⓔ	**94.**	ⓐ	ⓑ	ⓒ	ⓓ	ⓔ	**114.**	ⓐ	ⓑ	ⓒ	ⓓ	ⓔ
75.	ⓐ	ⓑ	ⓒ	ⓓ	ⓔ	**95.**	ⓐ	ⓑ	ⓒ	ⓓ	ⓔ	**115.**	ⓐ	ⓑ	ⓒ	ⓓ	ⓔ
76.	ⓐ	ⓑ	ⓒ	ⓓ	ⓔ	**96.**	ⓐ	ⓑ	ⓒ	ⓓ	ⓔ	**116.**	ⓐ	ⓑ	ⓒ	ⓓ	ⓔ
77.	ⓐ	ⓑ	ⓒ	ⓓ	ⓔ	**97.**	ⓐ	ⓑ	ⓒ	ⓓ	ⓔ	**117.**	ⓐ	ⓑ	ⓒ	ⓓ	ⓔ
78.	ⓐ	ⓑ	ⓒ	ⓓ	ⓔ	**98.**	ⓐ	ⓑ	ⓒ	ⓓ	ⓔ	**118.**	ⓐ	ⓑ	ⓒ	ⓓ	ⓔ
79.	ⓐ	ⓑ	ⓒ	ⓓ	ⓔ	**99.**	ⓐ	ⓑ	ⓒ	ⓓ	ⓔ	**119.**	ⓐ	ⓑ	ⓒ	ⓓ	ⓔ
80.	ⓐ	ⓑ	ⓒ	ⓓ	ⓔ	**100.**	ⓐ	ⓑ	ⓒ	ⓓ	ⓔ	**120.**	ⓐ	ⓑ	ⓒ	ⓓ	ⓔ

Section 3

121.	ⓐ	ⓑ	ⓒ	ⓓ	ⓔ	**141.**	ⓐ	ⓑ	ⓒ	ⓓ	ⓔ	**161.**	ⓐ	ⓑ	ⓒ	ⓓ	ⓔ
122.	ⓐ	ⓑ	ⓒ	ⓓ	ⓔ	**142.**	ⓐ	ⓑ	ⓒ	ⓓ	ⓔ	**162.**	ⓐ	ⓑ	ⓒ	ⓓ	ⓔ
123.	ⓐ	ⓑ	ⓒ	ⓓ	ⓔ	**143.**	ⓐ	ⓑ	ⓒ	ⓓ	ⓔ	**163.**	ⓐ	ⓑ	ⓒ	ⓓ	ⓔ
124.	ⓐ	ⓑ	ⓒ	ⓓ	ⓔ	**144.**	ⓐ	ⓑ	ⓒ	ⓓ	ⓔ	**164.**	ⓐ	ⓑ	ⓒ	ⓓ	ⓔ
125.	ⓐ	ⓑ	ⓒ	ⓓ	ⓔ	**145.**	ⓐ	ⓑ	ⓒ	ⓓ	ⓔ	**165.**	ⓐ	ⓑ	ⓒ	ⓓ	ⓔ
126.	ⓐ	ⓑ	ⓒ	ⓓ	ⓔ	**146.**	ⓐ	ⓑ	ⓒ	ⓓ	ⓔ	**166.**	ⓐ	ⓑ	ⓒ	ⓓ	ⓔ
127.	ⓐ	ⓑ	ⓒ	ⓓ	ⓔ	**147.**	ⓐ	ⓑ	ⓒ	ⓓ	ⓔ	**167.**	ⓐ	ⓑ	ⓒ	ⓓ	ⓔ
128.	ⓐ	ⓑ	ⓒ	ⓓ	ⓔ	**148.**	ⓐ	ⓑ	ⓒ	ⓓ	ⓔ	**168.**	ⓐ	ⓑ	ⓒ	ⓓ	ⓔ
129.	ⓐ	ⓑ	ⓒ	ⓓ	ⓔ	**149.**	ⓐ	ⓑ	ⓒ	ⓓ	ⓔ	**169.**	ⓐ	ⓑ	ⓒ	ⓓ	ⓔ
130.	ⓐ	ⓑ	ⓒ	ⓓ	ⓔ	**150.**	ⓐ	ⓑ	ⓒ	ⓓ	ⓔ	**170.**	ⓐ	ⓑ	ⓒ	ⓓ	ⓔ
131.	ⓐ	ⓑ	ⓒ	ⓓ	ⓔ	**151.**	ⓐ	ⓑ	ⓒ	ⓓ	ⓔ	**171.**	ⓐ	ⓑ	ⓒ	ⓓ	ⓔ
132.	ⓐ	ⓑ	ⓒ	ⓓ	ⓔ	**152.**	ⓐ	ⓑ	ⓒ	ⓓ	ⓔ	**172.**	ⓐ	ⓑ	ⓒ	ⓓ	ⓔ
133.	ⓐ	ⓑ	ⓒ	ⓓ	ⓔ	**153.**	ⓐ	ⓑ	ⓒ	ⓓ	ⓔ	**173.**	ⓐ	ⓑ	ⓒ	ⓓ	ⓔ
134.	ⓐ	ⓑ	ⓒ	ⓓ	ⓔ	**154.**	ⓐ	ⓑ	ⓒ	ⓓ	ⓔ	**174.**	ⓐ	ⓑ	ⓒ	ⓓ	ⓔ
135.	ⓐ	ⓑ	ⓒ	ⓓ	ⓔ	**155.**	ⓐ	ⓑ	ⓒ	ⓓ	ⓔ	**175.**	ⓐ	ⓑ	ⓒ	ⓓ	ⓔ
136.	ⓐ	ⓑ	ⓒ	ⓓ	ⓔ	**156.**	ⓐ	ⓑ	ⓒ	ⓓ	ⓔ	**176.**	ⓐ	ⓑ	ⓒ	ⓓ	ⓔ
137.	ⓐ	ⓑ	ⓒ	ⓓ	ⓔ	**157.**	ⓐ	ⓑ	ⓒ	ⓓ	ⓔ	**177.**	ⓐ	ⓑ	ⓒ	ⓓ	ⓔ
138.	ⓐ	ⓑ	ⓒ	ⓓ	ⓔ	**158.**	ⓐ	ⓑ	ⓒ	ⓓ	ⓔ	**178.**	ⓐ	ⓑ	ⓒ	ⓓ	ⓔ
139.	ⓐ	ⓑ	ⓒ	ⓓ	ⓔ	**159.**	ⓐ	ⓑ	ⓒ	ⓓ	ⓔ	**179.**	ⓐ	ⓑ	ⓒ	ⓓ	ⓔ
140.	ⓐ	ⓑ	ⓒ	ⓓ	ⓔ	**160.**	ⓐ	ⓑ	ⓒ	ⓓ	ⓔ	**180.**	ⓐ	ⓑ	ⓒ	ⓓ	ⓔ

Section 4

181.	ⓐ ⓑ ⓒ ⓓ ⓔ		201.	ⓐ ⓑ ⓒ ⓓ ⓔ		221.	ⓐ ⓑ ⓒ ⓓ ⓔ
182.	ⓐ ⓑ ⓒ ⓓ ⓔ		202.	ⓐ ⓑ ⓒ ⓓ ⓔ		222.	ⓐ ⓑ ⓒ ⓓ ⓔ
183.	ⓐ ⓑ ⓒ ⓓ ⓔ		203.	ⓐ ⓑ ⓒ ⓓ ⓔ		223.	ⓐ ⓑ ⓒ ⓓ ⓔ
184.	ⓐ ⓑ ⓒ ⓓ ⓔ		204.	ⓐ ⓑ ⓒ ⓓ ⓔ		224.	ⓐ ⓑ ⓒ ⓓ ⓔ
185.	ⓐ ⓑ ⓒ ⓓ ⓔ		205.	ⓐ ⓑ ⓒ ⓓ ⓔ		225.	ⓐ ⓑ ⓒ ⓓ ⓔ
186.	ⓐ ⓑ ⓒ ⓓ ⓔ		206.	ⓐ ⓑ ⓒ ⓓ ⓔ		226.	ⓐ ⓑ ⓒ ⓓ ⓔ
187.	ⓐ ⓑ ⓒ ⓓ ⓔ		207.	ⓐ ⓑ ⓒ ⓓ ⓔ		227.	ⓐ ⓑ ⓒ ⓓ ⓔ
188.	ⓐ ⓑ ⓒ ⓓ ⓔ		208.	ⓐ ⓑ ⓒ ⓓ ⓔ		228.	ⓐ ⓑ ⓒ ⓓ ⓔ
189.	ⓐ ⓑ ⓒ ⓓ ⓔ		209.	ⓐ ⓑ ⓒ ⓓ ⓔ		229.	ⓐ ⓑ ⓒ ⓓ ⓔ
190.	ⓐ ⓑ ⓒ ⓓ ⓔ		210.	ⓐ ⓑ ⓒ ⓓ ⓔ		230.	ⓐ ⓑ ⓒ ⓓ ⓔ
191.	ⓐ ⓑ ⓒ ⓓ ⓔ		211.	ⓐ ⓑ ⓒ ⓓ ⓔ		231.	ⓐ ⓑ ⓒ ⓓ ⓔ
192.	ⓐ ⓑ ⓒ ⓓ ⓔ		212.	ⓐ ⓑ ⓒ ⓓ ⓔ		232.	ⓐ ⓑ ⓒ ⓓ ⓔ
193.	ⓐ ⓑ ⓒ ⓓ ⓔ		213.	ⓐ ⓑ ⓒ ⓓ ⓔ		233.	ⓐ ⓑ ⓒ ⓓ ⓔ
194.	ⓐ ⓑ ⓒ ⓓ ⓔ		214.	ⓐ ⓑ ⓒ ⓓ ⓔ		234.	ⓐ ⓑ ⓒ ⓓ ⓔ
195.	ⓐ ⓑ ⓒ ⓓ ⓔ		215.	ⓐ ⓑ ⓒ ⓓ ⓔ		235.	ⓐ ⓑ ⓒ ⓓ ⓔ
196.	ⓐ ⓑ ⓒ ⓓ ⓔ		216.	ⓐ ⓑ ⓒ ⓓ ⓔ		236.	ⓐ ⓑ ⓒ ⓓ ⓔ
197.	ⓐ ⓑ ⓒ ⓓ ⓔ		217.	ⓐ ⓑ ⓒ ⓓ ⓔ		237.	ⓐ ⓑ ⓒ ⓓ ⓔ
198.	ⓐ ⓑ ⓒ ⓓ ⓔ		218.	ⓐ ⓑ ⓒ ⓓ ⓔ		238.	ⓐ ⓑ ⓒ ⓓ ⓔ
199.	ⓐ ⓑ ⓒ ⓓ ⓔ		219.	ⓐ ⓑ ⓒ ⓓ ⓔ		239.	ⓐ ⓑ ⓒ ⓓ ⓔ
200.	ⓐ ⓑ ⓒ ⓓ ⓔ		220.	ⓐ ⓑ ⓒ ⓓ ⓔ		240.	ⓐ ⓑ ⓒ ⓓ ⓔ

Section 5

241.	ⓐ	ⓑ	ⓒ	ⓓ	ⓔ	**261.**	ⓐ	ⓑ	ⓒ	ⓓ	ⓔ	**281.**	ⓐ	ⓑ	ⓒ	ⓓ	ⓔ
242.	ⓐ	ⓑ	ⓒ	ⓓ	ⓔ	**262.**	ⓐ	ⓑ	ⓒ	ⓓ	ⓔ	**282.**	ⓐ	ⓑ	ⓒ	ⓓ	ⓔ
243.	ⓐ	ⓑ	ⓒ	ⓓ	ⓔ	**263.**	ⓐ	ⓑ	ⓒ	ⓓ	ⓔ	**283.**	ⓐ	ⓑ	ⓒ	ⓓ	ⓔ
244.	ⓐ	ⓑ	ⓒ	ⓓ	ⓔ	**264.**	ⓐ	ⓑ	ⓒ	ⓓ	ⓔ	**284.**	ⓐ	ⓑ	ⓒ	ⓓ	ⓔ
245.	ⓐ	ⓑ	ⓒ	ⓓ	ⓔ	**265.**	ⓐ	ⓑ	ⓒ	ⓓ	ⓔ	**285.**	ⓐ	ⓑ	ⓒ	ⓓ	ⓔ
246.	ⓐ	ⓑ	ⓒ	ⓓ	ⓔ	**266.**	ⓐ	ⓑ	ⓒ	ⓓ	ⓔ	**286.**	ⓐ	ⓑ	ⓒ	ⓓ	ⓔ
247.	ⓐ	ⓑ	ⓒ	ⓓ	ⓔ	**267.**	ⓐ	ⓑ	ⓒ	ⓓ	ⓔ	**287.**	ⓐ	ⓑ	ⓒ	ⓓ	ⓔ
248.	ⓐ	ⓑ	ⓒ	ⓓ	ⓔ	**268.**	ⓐ	ⓑ	ⓒ	ⓓ	ⓔ	**288.**	ⓐ	ⓑ	ⓒ	ⓓ	ⓔ
249.	ⓐ	ⓑ	ⓒ	ⓓ	ⓔ	**269.**	ⓐ	ⓑ	ⓒ	ⓓ	ⓔ	**289.**	ⓐ	ⓑ	ⓒ	ⓓ	ⓔ
250.	ⓐ	ⓑ	ⓒ	ⓓ	ⓔ	**270.**	ⓐ	ⓑ	ⓒ	ⓓ	ⓔ	**290.**	ⓐ	ⓑ	ⓒ	ⓓ	ⓔ
251.	ⓐ	ⓑ	ⓒ	ⓓ	ⓔ	**271.**	ⓐ	ⓑ	ⓒ	ⓓ	ⓔ	**291.**	ⓐ	ⓑ	ⓒ	ⓓ	ⓔ
252.	ⓐ	ⓑ	ⓒ	ⓓ	ⓔ	**272.**	ⓐ	ⓑ	ⓒ	ⓓ	ⓔ	**292.**	ⓐ	ⓑ	ⓒ	ⓓ	ⓔ
253.	ⓐ	ⓑ	ⓒ	ⓓ	ⓔ	**273.**	ⓐ	ⓑ	ⓒ	ⓓ	ⓔ	**293.**	ⓐ	ⓑ	ⓒ	ⓓ	ⓔ
254.	ⓐ	ⓑ	ⓒ	ⓓ	ⓔ	**274.**	ⓐ	ⓑ	ⓒ	ⓓ	ⓔ	**294.**	ⓐ	ⓑ	ⓒ	ⓓ	ⓔ
255.	ⓐ	ⓑ	ⓒ	ⓓ	ⓔ	**275.**	ⓐ	ⓑ	ⓒ	ⓓ	ⓔ	**295.**	ⓐ	ⓑ	ⓒ	ⓓ	ⓔ
256.	ⓐ	ⓑ	ⓒ	ⓓ	ⓔ	**276.**	ⓐ	ⓑ	ⓒ	ⓓ	ⓔ	**296.**	ⓐ	ⓑ	ⓒ	ⓓ	ⓔ
257.	ⓐ	ⓑ	ⓒ	ⓓ	ⓔ	**277.**	ⓐ	ⓑ	ⓒ	ⓓ	ⓔ	**297.**	ⓐ	ⓑ	ⓒ	ⓓ	ⓔ
258.	ⓐ	ⓑ	ⓒ	ⓓ	ⓔ	**278.**	ⓐ	ⓑ	ⓒ	ⓓ	ⓔ	**298.**	ⓐ	ⓑ	ⓒ	ⓓ	ⓔ
259.	ⓐ	ⓑ	ⓒ	ⓓ	ⓔ	**279.**	ⓐ	ⓑ	ⓒ	ⓓ	ⓔ	**299.**	ⓐ	ⓑ	ⓒ	ⓓ	ⓔ
260.	ⓐ	ⓑ	ⓒ	ⓓ	ⓔ	**280.**	ⓐ	ⓑ	ⓒ	ⓓ	ⓔ	**300.**	ⓐ	ⓑ	ⓒ	ⓓ	ⓔ

Questions

Section 1
Time: 60 minutes

1. A 46-year-old male presents for a yearly examination. Auscultation of the chest reveals a systolic murmur between the second and third left intercostal space radiating to the left shoulder and neck. Auscultation also reveals early pulmonic ejection sound. Based on presentation and physical examination, which of the following is the most likely diagnosis?
   - **a.** pulmonic stenosis
   - **b.** tricuspid regurgitation
   - **c.** mitral stenosis
   - **d.** aortic regurgitation
   - **e.** aortic stenosis

2. A 62-year-old man presents with an acute angle-closure glaucoma. Which of the following is the first-line treatment?
   - **a.** acetazolamide
   - **b.** antibiotic ointment
   - **c.** osmotic diuretics
   - **d.** topical corticosteroids
   - **e.** mast cell stabilizer

3. A 52-year-old man presents to his primary care clinic because of a persistent lump on his left shoulder. He reports that the lump has been present for four months and is not associated with any other symptoms. Physical examination reveals an enlarged and tender left supraclavicular lymph node. Which of the following malignancies is most likely to spread to this lymph node?
   - **a.** right lung squamous cell carcinoma
   - **b.** left forearm melanoma
   - **c.** gastric adenocarcinoma
   - **d.** glioblastoma multiforme
   - **e.** atrial myxoma

4. A 58-year-old woman presents to her primary care clinic with a five-month history of hemoptysis. On further questioning, she reports that she has also experienced chronic fatigue over the same time period. She has been previously healthy and is a nonsmoker. Physical examination and a chest X-ray are unremarkable. A bronchoscopic biopsy reveals a carcinoid tumor with a diameter of 2.5 cm in the right main bronchus. Which of the following interventions is most appropriate?
   - **a.** chemotherapy
   - **b.** radiotherapy
   - **c.** brachytherapy
   - **d.** palliative care
   - **e.** surgical excision

5. Which of the following classes of medication is indicated for maintenance therapy of rheumatoid arthritis?
   - **a.** NSAIDs
   - **b.** SSRIs
   - **c.** MAOIs
   - **d.** DMARDs
   - **e.** antibiotics

6. A 39-year-old female presents with a long history of heartburn, chest pain, and regurgitation. Her symptoms are relieved with the administration of antacids. Electrocardiogram shows normal sinus rhythm with no S-T segment abnormalities. Based on the patient's presentation and physical examination, which of the following is the most likely diagnosis?
   - **a.** reflux esophagitis
   - **b.** gastroesophageal reflux disease
   - **c.** esophageal dysmotility
   - **d.** esophageal neoplasm
   - **e.** gastroparesis

7. A 58-year-old female patient presents to her primary care clinic complaining of a three-day history of significant weakness and fatigue. On further questioning, she reports that she has also experienced palpitations over the same time period. Her past history is significant for hypertension that is currently managed with ramipril, but has been managed with other drugs in the past. She recalls that she recently ran out of ramipril, so she has been taking one of the other drugs that had been used in the past; however, she cannot recall the name of the drug. Physical examination is unremarkable, but an ECG demonstrates a narrow QRS complex and flattened T-waves. Which of the following anti-hypertensive drugs may be causing this presentation?

   a. metoprolol
   b. nifedipine
   c. losartan
   d. spironolactone
   e. furosemide

8. A seven-year-old boy with a history of hay fever is complaining of left ear pain and decreased hearing for the past three days. He denies recent trauma, bleeding, or discharge from his left ear. You examine him with an otoscope, and his left ear canal is patent without exudates. His tympanic membrane appears intact but is bulging and red with some whitish discoloration. Conductive hearing loss is positive in his left ear. Which of the following is the most likely diagnosis?

   a. acute otitis externa
   b. acute otitis media
   c. cerumen impaction
   d. ruptured tympanic membrane
   e. periauricular cellulitis

9. A 66-year-old Asian male presents to your clinic and complains of recent weight loss, fatigue, night sweats, and recurrent cough. You order a chest X-ray and find cavitations in the apex of the right lung. You suspect pulmonary tuberculosis. Which of the following is the most appropriate initial laboratory test to confirm your diagnosis?

   a. repeat chest X-ray
   b. three consecutive morning sputums for culture
   c. lung biopsy
   d. PPD skin test
   e. none of the above

10. A 55-year-old Hispanic woman with a medical history of noninsulin dependent diabetes mellitus and hypertension complains of recurrent chest pain that is relieved by resting. Each episode lasts for less than 30 minutes. She is currently experiencing another episode of chest pain and appears in distress. You suspect that she has angina pectoris. Which of the following is the most likely initial management option?

   a. oxygen
   b. morphine
   c. aspirin
   d. nitroglycerin
   e. all of the above

11. A 33-year-old G1 P1 woman develops postpartum hemorrhage after a successful vaginal delivery. Which of the following is the most appropriate treatment at this time?

   a. clopidogrel
   b. warfarin
   c. vitamin K
   d. oxytocin
   e. surgical intervention

12. A newborn male infant presents with extreme cyanosis, poor feeding, and tachypnea without respiratory distress. Absence of lower extremity pulses is noted on physical examination. Auscultation of the chest reveals a single loud S2 and a systolic murmur. Which of the following is the most likely diagnosis?
   a. hyaline membrane disease
   b. pulmonary atresia
   c. Tetralogy of Fallot
   d. hypoplastic left heart syndrome
   e. transposition of the great vessels

13. A 10-month-old boy is brought to the emergency department by his parents because of inconsolable crying, a rectal temperature of 104°F, and a rapidly growing petechial rash on his feet. On examination, he appears to be irritated by bright lights. He is able to follow a bright object with his eyes, but his head movement is somewhat restricted. A lumbar puncture reveals cerebrospinal fluid (CSF) with low glucose, high protein, and presence of polymorphonuclear cells. Which of the following therapeutic strategies is most likely to be beneficial?
   a. directed antibiotic therapy based on CSF culture results
   b. directed antibiotic therapy based on blood culture results
   c. immediate empirical antibiotic therapy with amoxicillin
   d. immediate empirical antibiotic therapy with ceftriaxone
   e. immediate empirical antibiotic therapy with vancomycin

14. A 20-year-old female presents with a one-week history of fatigue, fevers, night sweats, and poor appetite. She was well prior to this episode. Examination reveals multiple tender lymph nodes in the cervical and axillary areas and splenomegaly palpable 3cm below the costal margin. Which of the following laboratory or diagnostic studies would be most appropriate to investigate her condition?
   a. VDRL test
   b. heterophile serology
   c. C-reactive protein (CRP)
   d. erythrocyte sedimentation rate (ESR)
   e. anti-dsDNA serology

15. A chronically ill, 90-year-old male presents to the emergency room unresponsive and without a pulse. The patient's electrocardiogram is illustrated below. Based on the electrocardiographic findings, which of the following is the most appropriate course of treatment?

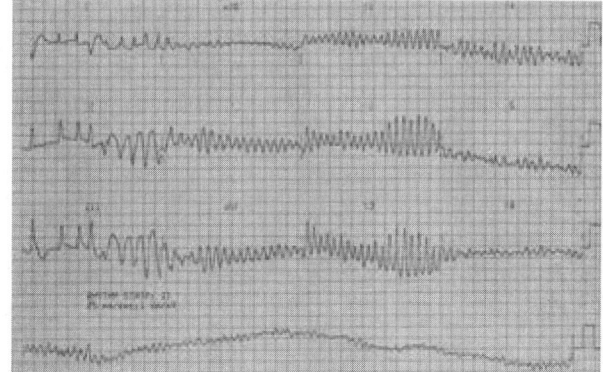

   a. electrical defibrillation
   b. IV lidocaine
   c. IV adenosine
   d. cardiac ablation
   e. cardiac catheterization

16. A 45-year-old male patient presents to his primary care clinic complaining of a four-month history of progressively worsening bilateral flank pain. On further questioning, he recalls that his father died relatively young from kidney problems. Physical examination reveals a blood pressure of 165/105 mmHg. Plasma creatinine and blood urea nitrogen are both mildly elevated. Which of the following is the pattern of inheritance of the most likely diagnosis?

- **a.** autosomal recessive
- **b.** autosomal dominant
- **c.** X-linked recessive
- **d.** X-linked dominant
- **e.** codominant inheritance

17. A 63-year-old man with a history of poorly controlled hypertension, hyperlipidemia, and obesity is brought into the emergency department. He appears lethargic, his speech is slurring, and he has left-sided hemiparesis. His body temperature is 98.0°F; blood pressure is 150/90. Which of the following is the most likely diagnosis?

- **a.** cerebral vascular accident (CVA)
- **b.** Alzheimer's disease
- **c.** Bell's palsy
- **d.** Guillain-Barré syndrome (GBS)
- **e.** meningitis

18. A 22-year-old man presents to the emergency department complaining of extreme pain in his scrotal area for the past two hours. He noticed the pain while he was playing soccer. On exam, he has a left-sided high-riding testis. A color Doppler ultrasound shows undetectable testicular blood flow on the left side. Which of the following is the most appropriate intervention?

- **a.** warm compress and observation
- **b.** manual decompression only
- **c.** surgical exploration
- **d.** acetaminophen
- **e.** oxycodone

19. A 27-year-old woman presents with an itchy rash on her left trunk for a few days. On exam, you find three to four annular lesions of 2 to 3 cm in diameter. Each lesion has a cleared center with a raised, scaly, erythematous border. A KOH preparation shows segmented hyphae. Which of the following is the most appropriate treatment?

- **a.** topical corticosteroid cream
- **b.** topical antibiotic cream
- **c.** topical antifungal cream
- **d.** complete surgical excision
- **e.** none of the above

20. Surgical removal of Morton's neuroma is associated with which of the following permanent side effects?

- **a.** disfigured toes
- **b.** discolored toes
- **c.** pain between the third and fourth toes
- **d.** numbness of the third and fourth toes
- **e.** total foot numbness

21. A 27-year-old man presents with a nodule in his scrotum. On examination the nodule is firm, 1cm in diameter, and attached to the right testicle. An ultrasound of the region suggests that the lesion may be a nonseminomatous germ cell tumor. Which of the following markers is expected to be present?

- **a.** alpha-fetoprotein
- **b.** prostate-specific antigen
- **c.** S-100
- **d.** carcinoembryonic antigen
- **e.** carbohydrate antigen 19-9

22. Which of the following medications is used to decrease the frequency of relapses of moderate or severe attacks stemming from multiple sclerosis?
   a. anti-inflammatory medications
   b. corticosteroids
   c. interferon-β
   d. cyclophosphamide
   e. amantadine

23. A 45-year-old woman presents to the emergency department complaining of a three-hour history of blurred vision, palpitations, and diaphoresis. On further questioning, she mentions that she has also experienced a headache during this time period. She has no significant past medical history. On physical examination, she is found to have a blood pressure of 210/145, a heart rate of 125 bpm, and sweaty and flushed skin. Further investigations reveal normal levels of thyroid hormone and thyroid stimulating hormone along with elevated plasma and urine levels of metanephrine and normetanephrine as well as elevated urine catecholamine levels. Which of the following interventions is most likely to be beneficial?
   a. antithyroid therapy
   b. thyroidectomy
   c. adrenalectomy
   d. parasympathetic stimulation
   e. sympathetic blockade

24. Which of the following conditions is treated with the group of medications called sympathomimetics?
   a. body dysmorphic disorder
   b. bulimia nervosa
   c. anorexia nervosa
   d. binge eating
   a. emaciation

25. A 19-year-old woman is diagnosed with epilepsy. She has a BMI of 30 and smokes 10 cigarettes a day. She has simple partial seizures and is being treated with gabapentin. Which of the following additional lifestyle changes would be most helpful in preventing further seizures?
   a. weight loss
   b. alcohol cessation
   c. smoking cessation
   d. exercise
   e. yoga

26. A 34-year-old woman is diagnosed with eczema and is prescribed a corticosteroid cream. Which of the following is NOT a side effect of long-term use of this medication?
   a. acne
   b. albinism
   c. dry skin
   d. fungal infection
   e. pruritus

27. A 31-year-old woman presents with repeated episodes of bleeding on a background immune thrombocytopenic purpura (ITP). Her ITP has been refractory to medical therapy including steroids, intravenous immunoglobulins, and azathioprine. Which of the following clinical interventions is indicated for this patient?
   a. splenectomy
   b. bone marrow transplant
   c. liver transplant
   d. kidney transplant
   e. ileostomy

28. A 33-year-old obese white female presents with feeling of vaginal fullness, lower abdominal aching, lower back pain, and a sensation of sitting on a ball. Mild dropping of the uterus is appreciated upon physical examination. Which of the following is the most likely diagnosis?
   a. uterine prolapse
   b. leiomyomata
   c. endometriosis
   d. adenomyosis
   e. polycystic ovarian syndrome

29. A 15-month-old infant female presents with a skull deformity and rib-breastbone joint enlargement. The child has developmental issues with delays in sitting, walking, and crawling. Blood work shows decreased calcium and vitamin D. X-rays reveal a flattened skull, bowing of long bones, and dorsal kyphosis. Which of the following is the most likely diagnosis?
   a. osteomalacia
   b. rickets
   c. Paget's disease
   d. osteoporosis
   e. osteomyelitis

30. For which of the following psychological disorders is a CT scan of the brain a useful diagnostic tool?
   a. bipolar disorder
   b. attention deficit disorder
   c. schizophrenia
   d. obsessive-compulsive disorder
   e. anorexia nervosa

31. A 28-year-old pregnant woman at 28 weeks gestation presents to the emergency department with a four-hour history of painful uterine contractions and vaginal bleeding that has required her to use three disposable menstrual pads. On further questioning, she reports that she has noticed a decrease in fetal movement over the same time period. Physical examination reveals uterine tenderness with normal abdominal distention, no cervical dilation, and normal fetal heart sounds. Which of the following is the most likely diagnosis?
   a. premature labor
   b. Braxton-Hicks contractions
   c. vasa previa
   d. placenta previa
   e. abruptio placentae

32. A 31-year-old female presents with persistent mild depression with symptoms including loss of interest, social withdrawal, overeating, oversleeping, and lack of self-esteem for more than two years. The patient states there have not been any psychotic, manic, or hypomanic episodes. Based on the patient's history, which of the following is the most likely diagnosis?
   a. bipolar disorder
   b. dysthymic disorder
   c. cyclothymic disorder
   d. adjustment disorder
   e. narcissistic personality disorder

33. A 75-year-old female with a history of chronic renal disease presents with nausea, vomiting, and difficulty breathing. History obtained from the patient reveals she has been using milk of magnesia for the past few days for an intestinal disorder. Physical exam reveals reduced deep tendon reflexes and low blood pressure. Blood work reveals a plasma magnesium level of 3.1 mEq/L (1.5-2.5 mEq/L), which confirms the diagnosis of hypermagnesemia. Which of the following medications would you administer to this patient to treat her condition?
   a. intravenous sodium chloride
   b. intravenous potassium chloride
   c. intravenous calcium gluconate
   d. intravenous 5% dextrose solution
   e. intravenous heparin

34. Which of the following preventative measures would you advise for an individual concerned with transmission of pediculosis?
   a. wash hair several times per day
   b. shower thoroughly several times per day
   c. stay indoors
   d. avoid sharing contact items
   e. avoid contact with animals

35. A 62-year-old female presents with headache, dizziness, weakness, fatigue, and blurred vision. Systolic hypertension, engorged retinal veins, and splenomegaly are appreciated upon physical examination. Blood work reveals hematocrit of 62%, elevated red cell mass, neutrophilic leukocytosis, increased basophils and eosinophils, and increased numbers of large bizarre platelets. Based on the patient's presentation, physical examination, and lab results, which of the following is the most likely diagnosis?
   a. thrombocytopenia
   b. hemolytic anemia
   c. polycythemia vera
   d. leukemia
   e. hemophilia

36. A 58-year-old woman presents to her primary care clinic complaining of a recent history of polyuria and polydipsia. On further questioning, she reports that she has also been losing some weight recently despite the fact that she feels like she has been eating more than usual. Physical examination is significant for a BMI of 33 kg/m². A random blood sugar test reveals a glucose level of 270 mg/dL (15 mmol/L). Which of the following statements describes this patient's optimal diagnostic strategy?
   a. A diagnosis of diabetes mellitus can be established based on the available information.
   b. A second random blood glucose test is required in order to establish the diagnosis of diabetes mellitus.
   c. A fasting blood glucose test is required in order to establish the diagnosis of diabetes mellitus.
   d. A random HbA1C level is required in order to establish the diagnosis of diabetes mellitus.
   e. A glucose tolerance test is required in order to establish the diagnosis of diabetes mellitus.

37. A cervical cerclage is indicated for which of the following conditions?
   a. cervical dysplasia
   b. cervical insufficiency
   c. induction of labor
   d. cervical neoplasia
   e. none of the above

38. A 62-year-old man complains of worsening ability to keep food or liquid down, with occasional regurgitation of undigested food particles. He denies swallowing any corrosive material. You suspect that this patient may have signs of achalasia. Which of the following imaging studies is the gold standard to confirm achalasia?
   a. chest/abdominal X-ray
   b. upper endoscopy
   c. abdominal ultrasound
   d. esophageal manometry
   e. chest/abdominal CT

39. A 42-year-old woman presents with worsening pain in her right wrist over the past six months. She denies recent injury or any pain above her wrist. The pain is dull, accompanied by occasional paresthesia of her fingers, exacerbated by activity, and relieved by shaking her hand. You suspect that she has carpal tunnel syndrome. If your diagnosis is correct, which of the following is the most likely physical finding on exam?
   a. negative Phalen's test
   b. positive Tinel's sign
   c. positive Heberden's nodes
   d. positive Bouchard's nodes
   e. positive Baker's cyst

40. Which of the following pulmonary conditions requires immediate decompression with a large bore needle?
   a. closed pneumothorax
   b. spontaneous pneumothorax
   c. hemopneumothorax
   d. tension pneumothorax
   e. primary pneumothorax

41. A 38-year-old male presents with swelling in the right eye. The patient states there is no pain or vision loss associated with the swelling. A physical examination of the right eye reveals a yellowish, fleshy conjunctival mass on the sclera. Which of the following is the most likely diagnosis?
   a. blepharitis
   b. viral conjunctivitis
   c. bacterial conjunctivitis
   d. pterygium
   e. pinguecula

42. Individuals in which of the following age groups should receive pyrantel as treatment for hookworms?
   a. 0 to 2 years
   b. 18 months to 3 years
   c. 2 to 4 years
   d. 3 to 5 years
   e. over 5 years

43. A 54-year-old patient with a history of hypercholesterolemia presents to his primary care clinic complaining of a three-month history of occasional crushing chest pain at rest. The pain radiates to his jaw and his left arm, is exacerbated by exertion, and usually continues for a few minutes at a time. Physical examination is unremarkable. Which of the following investigations will help exclude the possibility of coronary artery vasospasm?
   a. electrocardiogram
   b. echocardiogram
   c. exercise stress test
   d. inflammatory markers
   e. coronary angiography

44. A 27-year-old male patient presents to the emergency department with a sudden onset of severe dyspnea after a tackle during a casual football game. Physical examination is significant for reduced breath sounds in the left hemithorax and a tracheal deviation to the right side. Which of the following interventions is most likely to be beneficial?
   a. thrombolytic therapy
   b. inhaled albuterol
   c. inhaled corticosteroids
   d. thoracentesis
   e. blood transfusion

45. A 54-year-old overweight Caucasian woman presents with diffuse abdominal pain that has persisted for approximately three months. On further questioning, she mentions that her appetite has declined over the past month, and she has consequently lost approximately 6 kg (13 lbs), but her bowel habits have not changed, and she has experienced no nausea or vomiting. A fecal occult blood test is positive, and a CBC shows mild microcytic, hypochromic anemia. Which of the following is the most appropriate next step?
   a. sigmoidoscopy
   b. colonoscopy
   c. CT scan
   d. MRI
   e. X-ray

46. A 76-year-old female patient presents to her primary care clinic to request a health assessment for renewal of her driver's license. Her visual acuity is found to be 20/60 in the left eye and 20/40 in the right eye; there is no improvement with the use of a pinhole occluder. She does not use corrective glasses or contact lenses. Slit lamp examination demonstrates a dense clouding in the lens of each eye. Which of the following interventions is most likely to improve this patient's visual acuity?
   a. use of corrective lenses for myopia
   b. medical therapy for glaucoma
   c. cataract surgery
   d. corneal transplant
   e. laser photocoagulation

47. An otherwise healthy 43-year-old man with a 10-pack-year smoking history presents for his regular check-up. He has been anxious since he heard his brother-in-law had a heart attack. He is worried that the same might happen to him. After a careful screen of cardiac risk factors and a physical examination, you conclude that he has no additional risk factors. What should you do next?
   a. offer to examine his brother-in-law
   b. offer him a trial of a nicotine patch
   c. discuss the benefits of varenicline
   d. ask if he has ever tried to stop smoking
   e. try to reduce his anxious state by recommending yoga

48. A 63-year-old man with a history of polymyalgia rheumatica presents to his primary care clinic with a two-day history of pain and stiffness in the shoulder muscles that is most pronounced early in the morning. His condition has been in remission for the past year, and no therapy has been necessary. In addition to pain relief, which of the following drugs is most likely to be beneficial as long-term therapy?
  a. methotrexate
  b. cyclophosphamide
  c. sulfasalazine
  d. infliximab
  e. prednisone

49. A 17-year-old boy with cystic fibrosis wants to know why his mucus is so thick. Which one of the following is the best answer?
  a. defective water channels
  b. defective ion channels
  c. defective sugar metabolism
  d. defective immune system
  e. defective DNA repair mechanism

50. A 25-year-old man is suspected of having Crohn's disease. Which antibody serology would help confirm the diagnosis?
  a. cANCA
  b. pANCA
  c. ASCA
  d. anti-tTG
  e. anti-dsDNA

51. A 15-year-old boy presents with reduced visual acuity and pain in his right eye. The patient claims that he got sand in his eye while playing a baseball game an hour ago. On examination, the patient is determined to have conjunctival infections in both his eyes. Which of the following is the next step in his management?
  a. ciprofloxicin eyedrops
  b. injection of local anesthetic
  c. surgical correction of a lens defect
  d. saline wash of both eyes
  e. removal of the foreign objects using a needle and a slit lamp

52. A 29-year-old female, who is an avid golfer, presents with nagging, chronic pain in her left elbow, with inflammation overlying the olecranon process. Which of the following is the most likely diagnosis?
  a. lateral epicondylitis
  b. medial epicondylitis
  c. olecranon bursitis
  d. avascular necrosis
  e. fibromyalgia

53. Infections of the urinary tract or prostate are appropriately treated by which of the following medications?
  a. fluoroquinolone
  b. ceftriaxone
  c. ACE inhibitors
  d. doxycycline
  e. diuretics

54. A 52-year-old man presents to his primary care clinic complaining of a three-year history of progressive dyspnea and fatigue. On further questioning, he reports that his symptoms are associated with occasional chest discomfort and palpitations. He has a 35-pack-year history of tobacco smoking, a long history of alcohol abuse, and an occasional history of cannabis use. Physical examination reveals a BMI of 28 kg/m², a blood pressure of 135/105 mmHg, and bilateral distention of the jugular veins. A chest X-ray demonstrates cardiomegaly. Which of the following risk factors is likely to be the strongest contributor to this patient's condition?

a. age
b. BMI
c. alcohol abuse
d. tobacco smoking
e. cannabis use

55. A 68-year-old female patient presents to her primary care clinic with a two-year history of progressive dyspnea and dry cough. Her past medical history is significant for a Hodgkin's lymphoma approximately 20 years earlier, which was treated with a standard chemotherapy regimen of doxorubicin, bleomycin, vinblastine, and dacarbazide. She also used hormone replacement therapy for five years after menopause. Physical examination reveals fine crackles at both lung bases along with an FEV$_1$/FVC ratio of 88% on spirometry (normal <80%). A chest CT demonstrates reticular changes with a honeycomb appearance. If her condition is determined to be iatrogenic, which of the following drugs is the most likely cause?

a. doxorubicin
b. bleomycin
c. vinblastine
d. dacarbazide
e. hormone replacement therapy

56. A 23-year-old female patient presents to her primary care clinic with a two-week history of sore throat and fever. She had initially dismissed the symptoms as "just a sore throat," but in the past five days, she has developed a progressively worsening persistent peritonsillar pain as well as vocal distortion. Physical examination is significant for an inability to open the mouth fully, redness and swelling of the left tonsillar area, cervical lymphadenopathy, and difficulty with vocalization. Which of the following is the most likely diagnosis?

a. pharyngitis
b. laryngitis
c. dental abscess
d. peritonsillar abscess
e. mononucleosis

57. A 40-year-old male presents with dizziness and syncopal episodes when transferring from a sitting to a standing position. Blood pressure in the sitting position is 130/80 mmHg. Blood pressure in the standing position is noted to be 80/40 mmHg. It is noticed that his pulse rate in the sitting position is 80 bpm and 105 bpm in the standing position. Based on this information, which of the following is the likely cause of the patient's postural hypotension?

a. medications
b. central nervous system disease
c. depleted blood volume
d. peripheral neuropathy
e. cardiac arrhythmia

58. A 62-year-old male presents with progressive dyspnea. The patient's history reveals that he worked in a coal mine for several years. Physical examination reveals inspiratory crackles. Chest X-ray reveals small opacities in the upper lung fields. Based on the patient's presentation, history, and chest X-ray, which of the following is the most likely diagnosis?
   a. coal worker's pneumoconiosis
   b. cystic fibrosis
   c. sarcoidosis
   d. silicosis
   e. pneumonia

59. Which of the following is a gastrointestinal disorder that is characterized by increased volume and frequency of stool?
   a. malabsorption
   b. diarrhea
   c. volvulus
   d. constipation
   e. obstipation

60. A 66-year-old woman presents with left knee pain after a minor motor vehicle collision. The pain is worse on valgus stress. An X-ray series of the knee reveals minimal displacement of the tibial plateau. Which of the following is the definitive management of this fracture?
   a. full leg cast
   b. arthroscopy
   c. functional cast brace
   d. open reduction
   e. acetaminophen

Section 2
Time: 60 minutes

61. A 27-year-old sexually active woman presents with mucopurulent vaginal discharge with irritation and pain in her vaginal area. Vaginal culture is positive for *Chlamydia trachomatis*. Which of the following is the most appropriate treatment?
   a. abstinence
   b. metronidazole
   c. doxycycline
   d. ciprofloxacin
   e. none of the above

62. Hypertriglyceridemia can be managed effectively with daily consumption of which of the following vitamins?
   a. niacin
   b. vitamin C
   c. vitamin D
   d. riboflavin
   e. thiamine

63. A 31-year-old male presents with anxiety, depression, and irrational fear of contracting a serious illness. He commonly misinterprets normal bodily sensations as manifestations of disease. Which of the following is the most likely diagnosis?
   a. conversion disorder
   b. factitious disorder
   c. hypochondriasis
   d. pain disorder
   e. malingering

64. A 72-year-old male patient with a history of congestive heart failure (managed with digoxin and ramipril) presents to the emergency department with a three-hour history of shortness of breath. On further questioning, he reports that he has experienced mild shortness of breath while lying in bed for the past three nights and has used three pillows in order to ensure adequate ventilation. Which of the following additional physical examination findings would be most suggestive of a pleural effusion?
 a. plural friction rub
 b. decreased breath sounds
 c. crackles at lung bases
 d. hyperresonance to percussion
 e. tachypnea

65. A 19-year-old female presents following a Caribbean vacation, during which she admitted to drinking unbottled water. Since her return, she has had intermittent diarrhea, abdominal cramps, bloating, and flatus. She describes her stool as "very stinky" and greasy. She has lost five pounds and complains of loss of appetite. You diagnose this patient with giardiasis. Based on this patient's presentation, which of the following is the most appropriate medical treatment?
 a. praziquantel
 b. paromomycin
 c. metronidazole
 d. mebendazole
 e. ketoconazole

66. Given the increased cardiovascular and embolic events that are associated with the use of oral contraceptives (OCPs), which of the following is a contraindication for use of OCPs, especially for women ages 35 and older?
 a. lack of physical exercise
 b. cigarette smoking
 c. alcohol use
 d. obesity
 e. stressful lifestyle

67. Gastric ulcers and chronic gastritis are commonly caused by which of the following Gram-negative, spiral-shaped bacillus?
 a. *Lactobacillus rhamnosus*
 b. *Lactobacillus acidophilus*
 c. *Helicobacter pylori*
 d. *Streptococcus agalactiae*
 e. *Legionella pneumophila*

68. A 58-year-old man presents to his primary care clinic for a general checkup. During the consultation, he mentions that he has experienced a mild pulsating pain in his abdomen for the past two months. His past history includes hyperlipidemia (controlled with atorvastatin) and hypertension (controlled with hydrochlorothiazide). Physical examination reveals a stationary pulsating mass near the center of his abdomen. Which of the following is the most likely diagnosis?
 a. umbilical hernia
 b. rhabdomyolysis
 c. gastric carcinoma
 d. ischemic bowel disease
 e. abdominal aortic aneurysm

69. A 60-year-old African-American female presents with pain and swelling in the left eyelid. A physical examination of the left eyelid reveals a palpable, indurate area with a central area of purulence and surrounding redness. Which of the following is the most likely diagnosis?
  a. orbital cellulitis
  b. dacryostenosis
  c. chalazion
  d. hordeolum
  e. blepharitis

70. Pregabalin (Lyrica) is the only FDA-approved medication for the treatment of which of the following conditions?
  a. Huntington's disease
  b. scleroderma
  c. multiple sclerosis
  d. fibromyalgia
  e. systemic lupus erythematosus

71. A 68-year-old female who sustained a myocardial infarction ten days ago presents with fever. An echocardiogram reveals pericarditis. A chest X-ray reveals pleural effusions. Which of the following is the most likely diagnosis?
  a. pulmonary embolism
  b. cardiogenic shock
  c. Dressler's syndrome
  d. cardiac tamponade
  e. congestive heart failure

72. A 23-year-old woman with a body mass index (BMI) of 31 kg/m^2 presents to your clinic for a routine annual physical. Which of the following is the most appropriate health maintenance measure you would discuss with this patient?
  a. maintain a BMI between 25 and 29
  b. maintain a diet with no carbohydrates but high in fat
  c. start regular physical exercise
  d. this patient is still young, so no health maintenance discussions are necessary
  e. none of the above

73. A newborn infant presents with cyanosis, shock, heart failure, and respiratory distress. Auscultation of the chest reveals a single S2 sound. Based on the presentation and physical examination, which of the following is the most likely diagnosis?
  a. pulmonary atresia
  b. Tetralogy of Fallot
  c. hypoplastic left heart syndrome
  d. transposition of the great vessels
  e. patent ductus arteriosus

74. A 46-year-old woman presents for a follow-up after taking two courses of antibiotics for a prophylaxis after a hysterectomy and for an incidental upper respiratory tract infection that occurred subsequently. Recently, she has developed some diarrhea and constipation. Which of the following is the most likely cause of her symptoms?
  a. pseudomembranous colitis
  b. viral gastroenteritis
  c. bacterial gastroenteritis
  d. antibiotic-induced GI upset
  e. irritable bowel syndrome

75. A 62-year-old man presents with worsening toe pain. He rates the pain as 10/10 and states that it woke him up in the middle of the night. Aspiration of the joint fluid reveals rodlike crystals that are blue on parallel light. Which of the following is the most likely diagnosis?
- **a.** gout
- **b.** pseudogout
- **c.** osteoarthritis
- **d.** psoriactic arthritis
- **e.** septic arthritis

76. A 33-year-old physician assistant, who works at a local emergency department and has no significant medical history, presents to your clinic complaining of a fever of 101° to 102°F and chills for the past seven days accompanied by generalized fatigue, muscle aches, and cough with mucopurulent sputum. She recalls multiple sick contacts recently at her job. A chest X-ray confirms your suspicion of left lower lobe pneumonia. Which of the following is the most likely physical finding on exam?
- **a.** decreased breath sound in left lower lobe of lung field
- **b.** pericardial friction rub
- **c.** diastolic decrescendo murmur at left upper sternal border
- **d.** hyperresonance in left lower lung field
- **e.** all of the above

77. A 72-year-old Caucasian man with a history of poorly controlled hypertension is brought to the emergency department complaining of a sudden and severe "ripping" pain in his chest that radiates to his upper back. On exam, he appears in severe distress. Vital signs are: blood pressure of 182/91, heart rate of 66, temperature of 98.9°F, and respiration rate of 24. You also find unequal pulses in his lower extremities. Which of the following is the most likely diagnosis?
- **a.** aortic dissection
- **b.** acute myocardial infarction
- **c.** anxiety attack
- **d.** gastroesophageal reflux disease (GERD)
- **e.** pulmonary embolism

78. A 33-year-old pregnant woman at 37 weeks gestation presents to the emergency department after rupture of membranes. She also reports that she has noticed a decrease in fetal movements over the past few hours. Her cervix is 3cm dilated, and her contractions are still irregular. A cardiotocograph demonstrates fetal tachycardia, and a subsequent fetal scalp sample reveals lactic acidosis. Which of the following management strategies is most appropriate?
- **a.** continued observation
- **b.** emergency caesarean delivery
- **c.** scheduled caesarean delivery in two to three weeks
- **d.** immediate induction of labor
- **e.** administration of epidural analgesia

79. A 57-year-old woman has had recurrent symptoms of dizziness, nausea, and vomiting for the last three years; they have been worse in the morning and seem to be triggered by head movements. She has no symptoms of hearing loss or tinnitus. On examination, the Dix-Hallpike manuever is performed and indicates a horizontal nystagmus beating toward the affected ear. An audiogram detects no hearing loss. Which of the following is the most likely diagnosis?

a. Meniere's disease

b. benign paroxysmal positional vertigo

c. acoustic neuroma

d. schwannoma

e. ear canal foreign body

80. A 25-year-old female patient presents to her primary care clinic for a follow-up after seeing a psychiatrist for the first time. She reports that the psychiatrist has recommended the regular use of haloperidol for the treatment of symptoms that are consistent with schizophrenia. Which of the following abnormalities in this patient is most likely to be corrected by haloperidol?

a. overstimulation of dopamine receptors

b. understimulation of dopamine receptors

c. overstimulation of serotonin receptors

d. understimulation of serotonin receptors

e. overproduction of epinephrine

81. A 12-year-old boy presents with sudden onset of severe right-sided testicular pain after being kicked during a soccer game. Physical exam revealed a swollen scrotum. You suspect testicular torsion. Which of the following is the best diagnostic procedure to confirm this diagnosis?

a. testicular ultrasound

b. nuclear medicine testicular scan

c. CT angiogram of the testicles

d. MRI angiogram of the testicles

e. X-ray of the pelvis

82. A 34-year-old man presents to his primary care clinic complaining of a one-week history of persistent fever and arthralgia. On further questioning, he reports that he recently returned from a hiking trip in the California desert. Physical examination reveals localized areas of red painful rash in his lower limbs as well as dullness to percussion and reduced air entry in the left lung base. Which of the following is the most likely diagnosis?

a. bacterial pneumonia

b. candidiasis

c. histoplasmosis

d. coccidioidomycosis

e. blastomycosis

83. A 43-year-old pregnant woman at 12 weeks gestation presents to her prenatal clinic for a regular review. This is her first pregnancy. Her BMI prior to pregnancy was 31 kg/m², and she has a history of polycystic ovarian syndrome. She has a younger sister with Down syndrome and is concerned about the possibility of similar problems in her child. Which of the following maternal risk factors is most strongly correlated with an increased risk of fetal chromosomal abnormalities?
  a. age over 40
  b. nulliparity
  c. obesity
  d. family history of Down syndrome
  e. history of polycystic ovarian syndrome

84. A 47-year-old male presents with fever, fatigue, weight loss, and bilateral morning stiffness in the neck, shoulders, and pelvis. The patient states that his pain is most severe after rest and in the morning. Which of the following is the most likely diagnosis?
  a. polymyositis
  b. polymyalgia rheumatica
  c. polyarteritis nodosa
  d. systemic sclerosis
  e. fibromyalgia

85. A 17-year-old female presents as being underweight and emaciated. Physical examination reveals orthostatic hypotension, salivary gland hypertrophy, and dental erosion. The patient states she has a normal appetite but doesn't eat much because she is afraid of becoming overweight. Lab work reveals hypokalemia, hypochloremia, and elevated blood urea nitrogen. Based on the patient's history, physical examination, and test results, which of the following is the most likely diagnosis?
  a. binge eating disorder
  b. anorexia nervosa
  c. bulimia nervosa
  d. narcissistic personality disorder
  e. body dysmorphic disorder

86. A 36-year-old male presents with right flank pain and hematuria. You suggest an intravenous pyelogram to rule out kidney stone. During the procedure, the machine malfunctions, thus overexposing the patient to ionizing radiation, which causes skin redness and epilation to the affected area. Which of the following is the federal policy that requires you to report this incident?
  a. HIPAA
  b. MIPPA
  c. EMTALA
  d. Safe Medical Devices Act
  e. Patient's Bill of Rights

87. A 56-year-old female patient presents to her primary care clinic with a small painless round nodule on her right forearm. She first noticed the lesion approximately two years ago, and it appears to have grown over that time period. The nodule now has a diameter of 1.5 cm. Dermatoscopic inspection demonstrates a shiny red appearance with clearly defined margins. Which of the following topical treatments is most likely to be beneficial?

a. prednisone
b. imiquimod
c. erythromycin
d. tetracycline
e. lidocaine

88. A 44-year-old woman inpatient is currently undergoing treatment after an acute event that caused fever, thrombocytopenia, and thrombosis. She was diagnosed with thrombotic thrombocytopenic purpura and treated with plasmapheresis and immunosuppressive therapy. Which of the following molecules is most likely to be abnormal in this patient?

a. tyrosine kinase
b. vitamin K
c. coagulation factor VIII
d. von Willebrand factor
e. tissue factor

89. A 45-year old pregnant female, with six previous childbirths and a 10-pack-year history of cigarette smoking, presents at 32 weeks with painless vaginal bleeding. Ultrasound reveals that the placenta is covering the cervical os. Which of the following is the most likely diagnosis?

a. spontaneous abortion
b. ectopic pregnancy
c. gestational trophoblastic disease
d. abruptio placentae
e. placenta previa

90. A 31-year-old woman with type 2 diabetes is prescribed metformin. Which of the following medical conditions would NOT contraindicate its use?

a. liver failure
b. heart failure
c. alcoholism
d. renal failure
e. osteoporosis

91. An 82-year-old man dies of aspiration pneumonia. He is suspected to have had Alzheimer's disease. Which one of these post-mortem findings would be most consistent with this suspected diagnosis?

a. neurofibrillary tangles
b. Lewis bodies
c. basal ganglion degeneration
d. atherosclerotic change in cerebral arteries
e. hematomas in the subdural space

92. A 12-year-old girl is immunized with the quadrivalent HPV vaccine Gardisil®. Which of the following subtypes of HPV is NOT covered by this vaccine?

a. 6
b. 11
c. 13
d. 16
e. 18

93. A 12-year-old boy is brought in by ambulance with severe third-degree burns on his right arm. He has a pulse of 130/min and a blood pressure of 92/54. His airway has been secured, and fluid resuscitation was started. Which of the following topical treatments would best prevent burn wound infection?

a. topical penicillin
b. topical corticosteroids
c. topical fluconazole
d. topical silver sulfadiazin
e. topical doxycycline

94. A 29-year-old man presents with fever, weight loss, and night sweats. Examination of lymph nodes reveals multiple enlarged, nontender lymph nodes in the neck. A biopsy of a cervical lymph node shows the presence of Reed-Sternberg cells. Which of the following is the most likely diagnosis?
  a. chronic myeloid leukemia
  b. acute myeloid leukemia
  c. chronic lymphocytic leukemia
  d. Hodgkin's lymphoma
  e. non-Hodgkin's lymphoma

95. A 34-year-old female presents to her primary care physician with a six-month history of uncontrollable anxiety. On further questioning, she reports that she has also experienced palpitations, heat intolerance, and 10 kg (22 lbs) of unintentional weight loss. Physical examination shows tachycardia and a mild resting tremor. Thyroid function tests find significantly elevated levels of thyroxine and thyroid stimulating hormone (TSH). Which of the following ophthalmologic symptoms is the most likely consequence of this condition?
  a. homonymous hemianopia
  b. bitemporal hemianopia
  c. binasal hemianopia
  d. exophthalmos
  e. endophtalmos

96. A 58-year-old male patient is brought to the emergency department by his wife after he experiences short-term memory loss and an inability to walk in a straight line. He is unable to give a coherent history, but his wife reports that he has a 24-year history of alcohol abuse. On physical examination, he is found to have nystagmus and gait ataxia. Which of the following initial interventions is most likely to benefit the patient?
  a. IV thiamine infusion
  b. thrombolytic therapy
  c. anticoagulation
  d. craniotomy and drainage
  e. antibiotic therapy

97. A 48-year-old male patient with a history of alcoholic liver disease presents with a five-day history of fever, sore throat, and headache. On examination, he is febrile at 38.5°C (100°F), his cervical lymph nodes are tender, and his tonsils are swollen along with an exudate. During the consultation, he mentions that he had a childhood allergy to penicillin, but he cannot recall the nature of his reaction. Which of the following is the best choice of therapy for this patient?
  a. amoxicillin
  b. ceftriaxone
  c. ceftazidime
  d. erythromycin
  e. azithromycin

98. A 23-year-old woman who is in her third trimester of pregnancy presents with an acute loss of facial muscular tone in her left face since yesterday. She denies history of recent headaches, fever, or change of vision. On exam, she is unable to wrinkle her left forehead or to raise her left eyebrow. When she is asked to smile, the left corner of her mouth remains unmoved. Which of the following is the most likely diagnosis?

a. status epilepticus
b. stroke
c. Guillain-Barré syndrome
d. Bell's palsy
e. migraine headache

99. A 28-year-old male visits his primary care physician complaining of a two-week history of fever, dry cough with very little sputum production, sore throat, and general malaise. Vital signs include a temperature of 39°C (102°F) Physical examination reveals dullness to percussion and reduced air entry in the right lung base in addition to bronchial breathing. A sputum sample is taken for culture, and a course of oral cefixime is prescribed. One week later, the patient returns because his symptoms have not resolved. The sputum culture reports no growth. Which of the following pathogens is the most likely cause of this patient's symptoms?

a. respiratory syncytial virus
b. influenza virus
c. *Candida albicans*
d. *Mycoplasma pneumoniae*
e. *Mycobacterium tuberculosis*

100. A 44-year-old female presents with a seven-month history of lack of energy, difficulty concentrating, and recurrent thoughts of worthlessness. She is diagnosed with major depressive disorder. Which of the following is the most appropriate treatment?

a. lithium
b. sertraline
c. risperidone
d. haloperidol
e. none of the above

101. A 66-year-old Asian woman with a history of type 2 diabetes presents with a rash on her left trunk. The rash is painful and burning. On exam, you find a 2×5 cm, papular, erythematous, pustular lesion along one thoracic dermatome. The patient denies new medication use or other associated symptoms. Which of the following is the most likely diagnosis?

a. tinea corporis
b. psoriasis
c. acanthosis nigricans
d. varicella zoster virus infection
e. rosacea

102. Overdose of which of the following types of medication is effectively treated with calcium gluconate?

a. ACE inhibitors
b. ritodrine
c. magnesium sulfate
d. calcium channel blockers
e. clomiphene citrate

103. Which of the following radiologic modalities is most effective in visualizing white matter lesions in the central nervous system associated with multiple sclerosis?
   a. PET scanning
   b. angiography
   c. CT scanning
   d. nuclear medicine
   e. MRI

104. A 26-year-old man with chronic asthma and tobacco use reports a worsening of symptoms for the past few months. He has been experiencing wheezing attacks at least three times every week but no more than once every day. He also has nighttime symptoms more than twice per month. Which of the following is the most appropriate option regarding health maintenance measures?
   a. none at this time other than using bronchodilators as needed
   b. moderate tobacco use
   c. influenza vaccination during worsening of symptoms
   d. pneumococcal vaccine and annual influenza vaccinations
   e. avoid physical activity

105. A 48-year-old overweight female presents to her primary care clinic with a two-week history of severe abdominal pain. On further questioning, she explains that the pain is sharp and cramping in character, rapidly fluctuates in severity, radiates in the direction of the right scapula, and is most severe after a fatty meal. Physical examination is significant for scleral icterus and significant right upper quadrant tenderness. An abdominal ultrasound demonstrates impaction of the neck of the gallbladder. Which of the following therapeutic interventions is most appropriate at this stage?
   a. endoscopic retrograde cholangiopancreatography (ERCP)
   b. magnetic resonance cholangiopancreatography (MRCP)
   c. cholecystectomy
   d. pancreaticoduodenectomy
   e. antibiotic therapy

106. A 64-year-old female patient presents to her primary care physician for a state-mandated assessment for renewal of her driver's license. Visual field examination demonstrates significant bilateral loss of peripheral vision. Intraocular pressure is measured at 24 mmHg in the right eye and 28 mmHg in the left eye. Ophthalmoscopic examination demonstrates a cup-to-disc ratio of approximately 70%. Three years earlier, an opthalmoscopic examination had found a cup-to-disc ratio of approximately 50%, and no visual field deficit was detected. Which of these features is singlehandedly most suggestive of a diagnosis of glaucoma?
   a. peripheral vision loss
   b. increased intraocular pressure
   c. variation in intraocular pressures between the eyes
   d. increased optic cup size
   e. decreased optic disc size

107. An 89-year-old man with decompensated heart failure is given a drug that will increase the contraction of his heart. Which of the following drugs can perform this function?
a. flecainide
b. verapamil
c. nifedipine
d. dapsone
e. dobutamine

108. An eight-year-old girl is brought in by her parents because she is often short of breath. The child also complains of cough that is brought on by playing in the park. During the physical examination multiple wheezes can be heard on auscultation. She is sent for spirometry. The results can be seen below:

FEV$_1$:2L
FVC:3L

The results become normal after treatment with a beta 2 agonist. Which of the following is the most likely diagnosis?
a. chronic obstructive pulmonary disease (COPD)
b. acute viral bronchitis
c. asthma
d. cystic fibrosis
e. upper respiratory tract infection

109. A 23-year-old athlete presents with an acute left knee pain that occurred during a basketball game about three hours ago. On exam, his left knee is well aligned, and no crepitus is noted with movement. The skin is intact and without edema, ecchymosis, or erythema. Tenderness is elicited on passive flexion and extension. Anterior drawer sign is positive, and posterior drawer sign is negative. There is no focal effusion, and no popliteal lesions are palpable in the knee area. Which of the following is the most likely diagnosis?
a. anterior cruciate ligament (ACL) tear
b. posterior cruciate ligament (PCL) tear
c. Baker's cyst
d. cellulitis
e. genu varum

110. Ventricular tachycardia is most appropriately treated with which of the following medications?
a. lidocaine
b. adenosine
c. diltiazem
d. nitroglycerin
e. furosemide

111. A 7-year-old boy presents to the emergency department with a suspected broken leg. An X-ray is taken and shows a fracture in which one side of the bone is broken while the other side is bent. Which of the following types of fractures is this?
a. transverse fracture
b. greenstick fracture
c. Colles' fracture
d. open fracture
e. comminuted fracture

112. Which of the following eye disorders may be caused by prolonged use of phenothiazine medications such as prochlorperazine maleate?
   a. cataracts
   b. macular degeneration
   c. glaucoma
   d. orbital cellulitis
   e. chalazion

113. A young couple presents to the primary care clinic soon after having a baby boy with cystic fibrosis. During the consultation, they request advice regarding the best way to care for the child. Which of the following is most likely to adversely affect the child's long-term survival?
   a. early pulmonary colonization with *Pseudomonas aeruginosa*
   b. frequent upper respiratory tract infections
   c. continuously clearing the airways of mucus
   d. use of bronchodilator therapy
   e. intussusception

114. A 58-year-old man with a history of hypercholesterolemia presents to his primary care clinic for a routine checkup. Physical examination reveals a blood pressure of 165/95 mmHg; this is the third consecutive time that a high blood pressure has been noted. Which of the following antihypertensive drugs should be avoided in this patient on account of his history of hypercholesterolemia?
   a. hydrochlorothiazide
   b. furosemide
   c. spironolactone
   d. ramipril
   e. metoprolol

115. A 16-year-old boy presents to the primary care clinic complaining of persistent pain from an injury caused by falling onto his outstretched hand while skateboarding. The pain has been present for seven days and appears to limit the movement of his thumb. Which of the following additional physical examination findings would be most suggestive of a scaphoid fracture?
   a. dramatically reduced range of motion at the thumb
   b. dramatically reduced range of motion at the wrist
   c. swelling over the anterior radial aspect of the wrist
   d. swelling over the posterior radial aspect of the wrist
   e. tenderness over the anatomical snuffbox

116. A 72-year-old male presents with lightheadedness when transferring from a sitting position to a standing position. Blood pressure reading in the sitting position is 130/80 mmHg and 90/50 mmHg in the standing position. Based on the patient's presentation and blood pressure readings, which of the following is the most likely diagnosis?
   a. primary hypertension
   b. postural hypotension
   c. malignant hypertension
   d. hypoglycemia
   e. cardiac arrhythmia

117. A 27-year-old, HIV-positive male presents with fever, tachypnea, and nonproductive cough. Chest X-ray reveals perihilar infiltrates but no pleural effusions. Blood work reveals lymphopenia and CD4 count of 144 cells/μL. Based on the patient's presentation and test results, which of the following is the most likely diagnosis?
   a. nosocomial pneumonia
   b. *Pneumocystis* pneumonia
   c. community-acquired pneumonia
   d. tuberculosis
   e. cystic fibrosis

118. A 40-year-old, morbidly obese female presents for consultation for bariatric surgery. She is an acceptable candidate with a history of stable obesity for more than five years, no glandular abnormalities, failure of other weight loss methods, and no dependence on alcohol or drugs. Her surgical options are discussed. Which of the following is a bariatric surgical procedure that involves a circular band implanted around the upper portion of a patient's stomach?
   a. gastric bypass
   b. lap band procedure
   c. liposuction
   d. stomach stapling
   e. partial gastrectomy

119. A 74-year-old woman presents for a hearing test. A Weber test is positive for lateralization to the right ear. A Rinne test reveals AC>BC (sound is heard through air longer than through bone) in the left ear and BC>AC (sound is heard through bone longer than it is through air) in the right ear. Which of the following is the most likely diagnosis?
   a. conductive hearing loss of the right ear
   b. conductive hearing loss of the left ear
   c. sensorineural hearing loss of the right ear
   d. sensorineural hearing loss of the left ear
   e. bilateral sensorineural hearing loss

120. A 21-year-old female presents with headache, sore throat, and postnasal drainage. On physical examination, you find cobblestoning of the posterior oropharynx and pale, "boggy," swollen nasal mucosa. You diagnose allergic rhinitis. Which of the following medications is the appropriate for treatment of this condition?
   a. antibiotics
   b. antihistamines
   c. corticosteroids
   d. NSAIDs
   e. anti-inflammatories

Section 3
Time: 60 minutes

121. A 15-year-old boy is brought to his primary care physician by his mother because she is concerned about a persisting bruise on his left leg that was caused by impact from a baseball during his physical education class three weeks earlier. On further questioning, the boy reveals that he has recently been unusually reticent in athletic situations because of rapid fatigue. Physical examination is significant for general pallor in the face, the mucous membranes, and the palmar creases. He has petechiae and purpura over his arms, legs, and abdomen. In this clinical setting, which of the following tests would be most useful for distinguishing aplastic anemia from acute lymphoblastic leukemia?
   a. white blood cell count
   b. red blood cell count
   c. platelet count
   d. peripheral blood smear
   e. hematocrit

122. A 63-year-old woman presents with worsening joint pain in her hands. She has worked as a seamstress for the last 40 years. A diagnosis of osteoarthritis is considered. Which of the following signs or symptoms would be most consistent with this diagnosis?
   a. joint pain is worse in the morning
   b. joint pain is relieved with movement
   c. ulnar deviation of the fingers
   d. nodules on the DIP and PIP joints
   e. nodules underneath the elbow

123. A fecal fat analysis is performed in order to diagnose the condition of malabsorption. Which of the following is the gold standard method for fecal fat analysis?
   a. D-xylose absorption test
   b. bile acid breath test
   c. microscopic study of stool for increase in fat globules
   d. quantitative measurement of fecal fat
   e. urea breath test

124. A 50-year-old woman presents with progressive shortness of breath. Chest X-ray reveals an area suspicious for tumor in the left lung. PET scan is suspicious for the presence of a malignant single pulmonary lesion. Which of the following types of biopsy would you perform in order to remove this entire lesion?
   a. fine-needle aspiration
   b. incision biopsy
   c. excision biopsy
   d. sentinel node biopsy
   e. endoscopic biopsy

125. A 51-year-old obese female presents in the emergency department with acute myocardial infarction. The patient's initial blood pressure is 130/80 mmHg. Shortly after presentation, the patient's blood pressure drops to 70/30 mmHg, her heart rate is 144 bpm, and she becomes agitated and confused. Based on the presentation and the patient's condition, which of the following is the most likely diagnosis?
   a. congestive heart failure
   b. orthostatic hypotension
   c. cardiogenic shock
   d. cardiac arrest
   e. septic shock

126. Which of the following medications is indicated for maintenance therapy of Crohn's disease?
  a. antacids
  b. mesalamine
  c. aminosalicylates
  d. immunodilators
  e. prednisone

127. A 36-year-old woman presents to her primary care clinic with a four-month history of polyarthritis in various joints including the wrists, metacarpophalangeal joints, and knees. She has also experienced a fluctuating fever over the same time period. Physical examination reveals tenderness and swelling in the affected joints as well as an erythematous rash over the nose and cheeks. Which of the following positive laboratory tests would be most suggestive of a diagnosis of systemic lupus erythematosus (SLE)?
  a. antineutrophil cytoplasmic antibody
  b. antinuclear antibody
  c. anti-dsDNA antibody
  d. rheumatoid factor
  e. C-reactive protein

128. A 75-year-old woman presents to the emergency department with sudden onset of severe abdominal pain. Which of the following physical examination findings would be most suggestive of a gastrointestinal perforation?
  a. diffuse abdominal tenderness
  b. hypotension
  c. guarding
  d. boardlike rigidity
  e. high-pitched bowel sounds

129. A 28-year-old female presents with difficulty focusing, hearing loss in the right ear, dizziness, and vertigo. Inflammation of the inner ear and involuntary eye movements are appreciated upon physical examination. Which of the following is the most likely diagnosis?
  a. central vertigo
  b. labyrinthitis
  c. barotrauma
  d. tympanic membrane rupture
  e. otitis media

130. A 26-year-old man with chronic asthma reports a worsening of symptoms for the past few months. He is not taking any medication at this time. He has been experiencing wheezing attacks at least three times every week but no more than once every day. He also has nighttime symptoms more than twice per month. Which of the following is the most appropriate treatment regimen for him at this time?
  a. a short-acting bronchodilator as needed
  b. a daily short-acting bronchodilator
  c. daily anti-inflammatory agent (either inhaled corticosteroid or cromolyn)
  d. daily anti-inflammatory agent (either inhaled corticosteroid or cromolyn) plus a daily short-acting bronchodilator
  e. none of the above

131. A 32-year-old woman complains of worsening chest pain for the past week that is relieved by sitting. She reports shortness of breath and pain upon deep inspiration. Her vital signs are normal except for a temperature of 100°F. Your physical exam reveals pericardial friction rub. An electrocardiogram (EKG) shows diffuse ST elevation. Which of the following is the most likely diagnosis?
a. gastroesophageal reflux disease (GERD)
b. mitral valve stenosis
c. acute myocardial infarction
d. pericarditis
e. anxiety attack

132. Which of the following is the most accurate description of the underlying disease process in osteoporosis?
a. autoimmune disorder
b. infectious process
c. inflammatory process
d. metabolic disorder
e. genetic disorder

133. A 55-year-old male presents to the emergency room with disorientation and convulsions. A physical exam reveals tachycardia, hypotension, fever, and dry mucous membranes. Lab work reveals a plasma sodium level of 218 mEq/L. The patient's renal panel revealed a BUN of 38mg/dL, creatinine of 2.2mg/dL, and GFR of 27ml/min. With a plasma sodium elevation of this nature, what course of treatment would you prescribe to regulate this condition?
a. drink plenty of water
b. intravenous 5% dextrose solution
c. intravenous saline solution
d. dialysis
e. intravenous potassium

134. A 48-year-old obese male patient presents to his primary care clinic along with his wife, who complains that he has appeared increasingly sleepy and lethargic in recent months. He still sleeps eight hours every night, but he often falls asleep during meetings at work. On further questioning, his wife reports that his snoring appears to have been progressively worsening. Which of the following is the most likely diagnosis?
a. narcolepsy
b. idiopathic hypersomnolence
c. chronic insufficient sleep
d. central sleep apnea
e. obstructive sleep apnea

135. A 35-year-old woman presents to her primary care clinic complaining of abdominal pain and constipation. She has presented with similar complaints several times in the past, although the character and the location of the pain are often variable. Which of the following additional findings is most suggestive of a diagnosis of somatization disorder rather than irritable bowel syndrome?
a. normal laboratory findings
b. no physical examination abnormalities
c. recent diagnosis of colorectal cancer in patient's mother
d. exacerbation of symptoms with stress
e. past history of major depressive disorder

136. A four-year-old male presents with fever, headache, lethargy, and bone pain in the sternum, tibia, and femur. Blood work reveals pancytopenia with circulating blasts and terminal deoxynucleotidyl transferase. Which of the following is the most likely diagnosis?
a. cystic fibrosis
b. polycythemia vera
c. thrombocytopenia
d. acute lymphocytic leukemia
e. acute myelogenous leukemia

137. A classic "crescent sign" on a hip X-ray is an indication for which of the following conditions?
   a. avascular necrosis
   b. septic arthritis
   c. Osgood-Schlatter disease
   d. slipped capital femoral epiphysis
   e. acute hip fracture

138. Prior to a surgical procedure of a radial nephrectomy, the performing physician has a conversation with the patient that encompasses the procedure being performed, the reason the procedure is being performed, the benefits of the procedure being performed, and the risks of the procedure being performed. Which of the following is the medical term for this conversation?
   a. HIPAA
   b. time out
   c. Safe Medical Devices Act
   d. Patient's Bill of Rights
   e. informed consent

139. A G2 P1001 woman in her second trimester presents with an acute right upper quadrant (RUQ) pain that radiates to her right shoulder area. She reports intolerance to fatty foods. She appears jaundiced. Her lab test shows increased liver enzymes and bilirubin. Which of the following is the most likely diagnosis?
   a. gastroesophageal reflux disease (GERD)
   b. appendicitis
   c. cholecystitis
   d. acute gastroenteritis
   e. gastric ulcer disease

140. A 43-year-old man with a history of type 2 diabetes presents with a rash on his left trunk. The rash is very itchy. Over-the-counter hydrocortisone creams have worsened the symptom. On exam, you find three to four annular lesions of 2 to 3 cm in diameter. Each lesion has a cleared center with a raised, scaly, erythematous border. A potassium hydroxide (KOH) preparation shows segmented hyphae. Which of the following is the most likely diagnosis?
   a. folliculitis
   b. psoriasis
   c. actinic keratosis
   d. varicella-zoster
   e. tinea corporis

141. A 58-year-old female presents with exertional dyspnea, nonproductive cough, and fatigue. Auscultation of the chest reveals basilar rales and cardiac gallops. Chest X-ray reveals cardiomegaly, bilateral pleural effusions, and perivascular edema. Based on the patient's presentation, physical exam, and test results, which of the following is the most likely diagnosis?
   a. primary pneumothorax
   b. tension pneumothorax
   c. cystic fibrosis
   d. congestive heart failure
   e. pulmonary embolism

142. A 19-year-old female presents with fever, headache, and a stiff neck. A petechial rash is noticed upon physical examination. You suspect meningitis. Which of the following clinical interventions must be performed to confirm the diagnosis?

   a. insert pledgets in the nose to evaluate cerebrospinal fluid (CSF)
   b. lumbar puncture to evaluate cerebrospinal fluid (CSF)
   c. MRI with gadolinium to confirm meningeal inflammation
   d. angiogram to confirm meningeal inflammation
   e. CT scan with contrast to confirm meningeal inflammation

143. Through which of the following mechanisms do calcium channel blockers treat pre-term uterine contractions?

   a. decrease estrogen levels
   b. inhibit myometrial contractility mediated by calcium
   c. stimulate β-receptors to relax smooth muscle
   d. increase intracellular magnesium ions
   e. decreases the influx of intracelluar calcium ions

144. A 39-year-old man with a history of chronic sinusitis presents with hematuria. A differential of Wegener's granulomatosis is considered. Which of the following serology results would be most consistent with this diagnosis?

   a. ANCA positive
   b. ANCA negative
   c. anti-dsDNA positive
   d. anti-dsDNA negative
   e. anti-BM positive

145. A 65-year-old female presents with body aches, nausea, loss of appetite, and increased thirst. Blood work reveals an elevated blood calcium level. Which of the following is the most likely diagnosis?

   a. hypothyroidism
   b. hyperthyroidism
   c. hyperparathyroidism
   d. hypoparathyroidism
   e. diabetes mellitus

146. Which of the following muscles is affected with tennis elbow?

   a. extensor carpi radialis brevis
   b. extensor carpi radialis longus
   c. pronator teres
   d. flexor digitorum
   e. palmaris longus

147. Which of the following antiseizure medications is used primarily when patients are unresponsive to other antiseizure medications?

   a. carbamazepine
   b. valproic acid
   c. phenytoin
   d. felbamate
   e. gabapentin

148. A 36-year-old female presents with nonproductive cough, shortness of breath, fever, sore throat, headache, and body aches. Auscultation of the chest reveals expiratory rhonchi and wheezes. A chest X-ray is negative. Which of the following is the most likely diagnosis?

   a. chronic obstructive pulmonary disease (COPD)
   b. acute bronchitis
   c. acute epiglottitis
   d. tuberculosis
   e. pneumonia

149. A 30-year-old primigravid woman presents for a regular prenatal checkup. She states she has a pet cat. You advise her to avoid contact with the litter. What infection is the patient at risk of contracting if she does not follow this advice?

a. toxoplasmosis
b. herpes
c. influenza
d. sarcoidosis
e. syphilis

150. A 17-year-old boy presents with galactorrhea and decreased libido. He has only recently noticed the galactorrhea but has had a continuous decline in his libido over the last three months. He also complains of headaches and denies any trauma to the head. He is otherwise well. On examination he is of normal stature and pubescent. He is noted to have bitemporal hemianopia. Based on these findings, which of the following is the most likely diagnosis?

a. McCune-Albright syndrome
b. macroscopic adenoma
c. microscopic adenoma
d. craniopharyngioma
e. berry aneurysm

151. A potassium hydroxide preparation is commonly used to rule out which of the following skin conditions?

a. contact dermatitis
b. seborrheic dermatitis
c. lichen simplex chronicus
d. pityriasis rosea
e. psoriasis

152. A 75-year-old woman presents with new onset confusion. She has recently been started on a new set of medications. Which of the following medications is most likely to be responsible for her delirium?

a. acetaminophen
b. atorvastatin
c. oxybutynin
d. ramipril
e. metformin

153. A 71-year-old man presents for his annual checkup. Although he is able to maintain attention, he is noted to have some decreased cognitive function. He is not currently on any anticholinergic medication. He has not suffered from any head trauma and has no other neurological symptoms. Which of the following would be recommended for this patient?

a. increased social interaction
b. antioxident supplements
c. physical exercise
d. memory training
e. all of the above

154. A 63-year-old man presents with symptoms of gradually increasing urinary frequency, urgency, hesitancy, and a feeling of incomplete voiding. The patient also comments on decreased stream flow and dribbling. The patient denies type 2 diabetes or any previous history of renal stones. He is otherwise well. A digital rectal exam reveals prostate width of three finger breadths. Urinalysis reveals no abnormality. There is no major elevation of prostate-specific antigen (PSA). No malignant changes are seen on the biopsy of his prostate tissue. Which of the following is the most likely diagnosis?

   a. urinary tract infection

   b. nephrolithiasis

   c. acute prostatitis

   d. prostate cancer

   e. benign prostatic hyperplasia

155. Which antiarrhythmic drug binds to open sodium channels, prevents sodium influx, and treats supraventricular tachycardia?

   a. lidocaine

   b. quinidine

   c. mexiletine

   d. verapamil

   e. adenosine

156. An HIV-positive 53-year-old man is diagnosed with AIDS. He develops a tumor after being infected with HHV-8. Which of the following signs or symptoms is most consistent with this lesion?

   a. diarrhea

   b. leukoplakia

   c. scleral icterus

   d. jaundice

   e. macular lesions

157. A 44-year-old man complains of recurrent epigastric area pain that is worst on an empty stomach and is relieved by food. He is subsequently diagnosed with duodenal ulceration on an upper endoscopy. Which of the following medications is the most appropriate for this patient?

   a. aspirin

   b. clopidogrel

   c. ciprofloxacin

   d. acetaminophen

   e. omeprazole

158. A 37-year-old woman with a history of rheumatic heart disease presents with exertional dyspnea. Her dyspnea is associated with chest pain. She complains of swelling in her legs. On physical examination, she is noted to have a raised jugular venous pressure, bibasal crackles in her lungs, a displaced apex beat, and a systolic murmur radiating to her axilla. She is thought to have heart failure associated with left ventricular dilatation. Which investigation will best confirm and quantify the anatomical changes in her heart?

   a. electrocardiogram

   b. chest X-ray

   c. CT angiogram

   d. echocardiogram

   e. MRI

159. A 41-year-old female presents to her primary care clinic complaining of erratic menstrual periods and vaginal irritation. She expresses concerns that she is relatively young for the onset of menopause and mentions that she has heard that early menopause is a sign of shorter life expectancy. After she is reassured about her potential to live a long and healthy life, she requests information regarding the implications of early menopause. Which of the following diseases is she at increased risk of developing in the future?
a. osteoarthritis
b. osteoporosis
c. osteomalacia
d. breast cancer
e. ovarian cancer

160. A 58-year-old man presents to his primary care clinic with a five-month history of progressive anterior neck enlargement. He has also noticed a feeling of tightness in his throat. He has noticed no concurrent cardiovascular or neurological symptoms. Physical examination of the anterior neck reveals a solitary nodule with hard consistency and ill-defined borders over the cricothyroid cartilage. The nodule is on the right side of the anterior neck, and it elevates when the patient swallows. The examination is otherwise normal. Laboratory investigations show normal levels of thyroid hormone and thyroid stimulating hormone along with elevated levels of carcinoembryonic antigen. A Tc-99m scan demonstrates increased uptake in the thyroid. Which of the following interventions is most likely to be beneficial?
a. surgical excision
b. antithyroid therapy
c. thyroid hormone supplementation
d. radioiodine therapy
e. observation

161. A 22-year-old man presents with a painless, rubbery, firm nodule on his upper eyelid. The lesion is nonexudative, and there is no significant discoloration or ulceration. He denies vision changes. You suspect the lesion to be chalazion. Which of the following is the most likely underlying cause of this condition?
a. bacterial infection of the meibomian gland
b. obstruction of the meibomian gland
c. basal cell carcinoma of the eyelid
d. increased intraocular pressure
e. vascular occlusion

162. Which of the following diagnostic imaging modalities can be useful in the diagnosis of schizophrenia?
a. electroencephalogram (EEG)
b. MRI of the brain
c. CT scan of brain
d. SPECT scan of the brain
e. cerebral angiogram

163. Intravenous amphotericin B combined with oral flucytosin has been proven to be an effective treatment for which of the following infectious diseases?
a. malaria
b. cryptococcosis
c. shigellosis
d. salmonellosis
e. botulism

164. A 31-year-old pregnant woman at 29 weeks gestation presents to her primary care clinic with a five-hour history of vaginal bleeding. This is her first pregnancy, and it has been uncomplicated thus far. Which of the following additional findings would be most consistent with a provisional diagnosis of placenta previa?

a. painful uterine contractions
b. generalized abdominal pain
c. generalized pelvic pain
d. no pain
e. blood found on digital examination

165. A 59-year-old woman is recently diagnosed with type 2 diabetes mellitus. Which of the following treatment options may cause lactic acidosis?

a. glipizide (sulfonylurea)
b. metformin (biguanide)
c. acarbose (alpha-glucosidease inhibitor)
d. insulin
e. all of the above

166. A 35-year-old male presents with sudden onset of shortness of breath and dizziness. An electrocardiogram reveals the following rhythm:

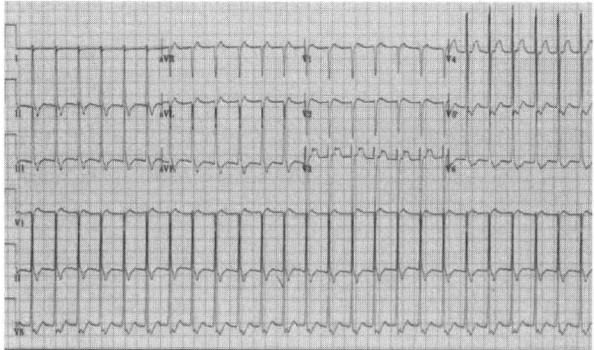

Which of the following describes this cardiac arrhythmia?

a. atrial flutter
b. supraventricular tachycardia
c. ventricular tachycardia
d. atrial fibrillation
e. sinus tachycardia

167. Which of the following conditions is most effectively treated with meclizine?

a. barotrauma
b. acute vertigo
c. motion sickness
d. labyrinthitis
e. presbycusis

168. A 32-year-old man visits his primary care clinic for a routine physical examination. His past medical history is unremarkable, but he reports a few recent paroxysmal episodes that include dyspnea and palpitations. On further questioning, he reports that he also feels dizzy during the episodes; he is unable to identify any triggers. A physical examination is normal, but the EKG reveals a normal sinus rhythm at 72 bpm despite a shortened PR interval, a lengthened QRS complex, and a slurring in the upstroke of the QRS complex. Which of the following is most likely to benefit this patient?

a. daily therapy with amiodarone
b. daily therapy with adenosine
c. daily therapy with metoprolol
d. cardioversion
e. catheter ablation

169. A 56-year-old woman with a 40-pack-year cigarette smoking history presents for a regular checkup. She mentions that she has a mild chronic productive cough and occasional exertional dyspnea, but she is not currently in respiratory distress. On spirometry, her FEV_1/FVC ratio is found to be 65% (normal range 70% to 80%). Which of the following actions is most likely to independently improve her long-term prognosis with regard to respiratory function?

a. smoking cessation
b. aerobic exercise program
c. bronchodilator therapy
d. inhaled corticosteroid therapy
e. chemotherapy

170. A 58-year-old woman presents to her primary care clinic with a three-year history of gnawing stomach pain. This has been associated with unexplained fatigue, unintentional weight loss, and unusually early satiety. Despite two years of therapy with proton pump inhibitors and antibiotics for peptic ulcer disease, the pain and weight loss have continued. Recently, she has also experienced pain on defecation and during sexual intercourse. Which of the following is the most likely diagnosis?

a. gastric adenocarcinoma
b. chronic gastritis
c. resistant *Helicobacter pylori*
d. pelvic inflammatory disease
e. cervical squamous cell carcinoma

171. A 67-year-old man presents to the emergency department with a one-hour history of a tearing chest pain. The pain appeared suddenly and feels very sharp and severe. He has a history of hypertension that is managed with furosemide, but he admits that he only usually takes the drug when he feels sick. Physical examination reveals a diminished pulse in the right arm and a blood pressure of 175/110 mmHg in the left arm. A chest X-ray demonstrates mediastinal widening and tracheal deviation to the right. Which of the following interventions is most likely to be beneficial?

a. thrombolytic therapy
b. immediate surgical intervention
c. angiogram and stenting
d. thoracentesis
e. pain relief

172. A 27-year-old man who is an IV drug user is brought in by ambulance after being found unconscious by his friends. Respiratory depression secondary to opioid overdose is suspected. Which diagnostic test best determines whether hypoxia is present in this patient?

   a. venous blood gas
   b. arterial blood gas
   c. full blood count
   d. spirometry
   e. pulse oximetry

173. A 45-year-old woman presents with muscle fatigue that worsens throughout the day. After a careful work-up, she is diagnosed with myasthenia gravis. Which of the following best represents the pathophysiology of her disease?

   a. IgG against acetylcholine receptors
   b. IgG against calcium channels
   c. demyelination of Schwan cells
   d. demyelination of astrocytes
   e. T-cell inflammation of myocytes

174. Which of the following types of medication is the most effective treatment for congestive heart failure?

   a. ACE inhibitors
   b. diuretics
   c. β-adrenergic antagonists
   d. calcium channel blockers
   e. corticosteroids

175. A 45-year-old African-American male presents with sudden onset of crushing substernal chest pain and shortness of breath. An electrocardiogram reveals normal sinus rhythm at 78 bpm with no ST segment abnormality. Pulse oximetry reveals a level of 86% on room air. Troponin level is >0.1. D-dimer level is 0.92. BUN is 44. Creatinine is 2.2. GFR is 28. A lung V/Q scan is obtained and shows unmatched perfusion defects in the apicoposterior segment of the left upper lobe and the anteriomedial basilar segment of the left lower lobe. Based on the patient's presentation and the test results, which of the following is the most likely diagnosis?

   a. lung cancer with metastases
   b. pneumonia
   c. pulmonary embolism
   d. bilateral pleural effusions
   e. congestive heart failure

176. A 62-year-old man presents to his primary care clinic because of a three-day history of persistent weakness in his left foot. He reports that the symptoms started after he experienced a one-hour episode of severe pain. His past medical history is significant for a myocardial infarction five years earlier. Physical examination reveals absent pulses below the left femoral artery. Additionally, his left lower leg is considerably colder and paler than his right lower leg. Which of the following definitive interventions is most likely to be beneficial?

   a. femoral embolectomy
   b. thrombolytic therapy
   c. anticoagulant therapy
   d. pain relief
   e. amputation

177. A 48-year-old woman presents to the emergency department with a 24-hour history of severe abdominal pain. On further questioning, she reports that she has also experienced two instances of passing dark-colored urine over the same time period. Physical examination reveals a temperature of 101°F and marked tenderness in the right upper quadrant. Abdominal ultrasound demonstrates dilation of the common bile duct. Which of the following is the most likely diagnosis?
   a. cholecystitis
   b. cholelithiasis
   c. cholangitis
   d. cholangiocarcinoma
   e. appendicitis

178. A 22-year-old woman presents with a two-month history of amenorrhea. Her BMI is 14. She reports intense anxiety about gaining too much weight. She prefers low-calorie foods and exercises after each meal. She frequently becomes frustrated with herself for overeating. Which of the following is the most appropriate treatment for this patient?
   a. diet counseling
   b. psychotherapy
   c. anxiolytic medications
   d. rehabilitation facilities
   e. all of the above

179. A three-year-old girl is brought to the emergency department with stridor, dysphagia, and drooling since this morning. On exam, the girl is in moderate distress. Oral exam is grossly benign. An X-ray of the neck is positive for the "thumb sign." Which of the following is the most likely diagnosis?
   a. tonsillitis
   b. foreign body obstruction of the oral pharynx
   c. scarlet fever
   d. epiglottitis
   e. none of the above

180. Which of the following treatment options would you suggest for a patient who has been diagnosed with pulmonary embolism?
   a. surgical clot removal
   b. vena cava interruption
   c. anticoagulation
   d. hyperbaric treatment
   e. lithotripsy

Section 4
Time: 60 minutes

181. A 65-year-old man with a history of chronic hepatitis B is found to have the following signs on exam: palmar erythema, spider nevi, mild abdominal distention, and caput medusae (distended and engorged periumbilical veins). Which of the following is the most likely diagnosis?
   a. common bile duct stone obstruction
   b. acute hepatitis flare
   c. inflammatory bowel disease
   d. toxic megacolon
   e. liver cirrhosis

182. A 14-year-old male patient is brought to the primary care clinic by his mother for a regular review of his asthma management. During the consultation, he inquires about the meaning of the elevated white blood cell count in a recent test. Which of the following types of white blood cells is most likely to be present in larger quantities during an asthma exacerbation?
   a. neutrophil
   b. basophil
   c. B-lymphocyte
   d. giant cell
   e. mast cell

183. Which of the following medications that are used for cardioversion is contraindicated in a patient with atrial fibrillation and associated heart failure?
   a. amiodarone
   b. dofetilide
   c. digoxin
   d. propafenone
   e. adenosine

184. Which of the following lifestyle habits is most critical to prevent progression of retinopathy?
   a. low-fat diet
   b. controlled blood glucose
   c. stop tobacco use
   d. decrease stress
   e. avoid sunlight

185. A 24-year-old female presents with abdominal pain, heartburn, bloating, and nausea. Blood work reveals a fasting gastrin level of 286 pg/mL which is indicative of hypergastrinemia. Endoscopy reveals a gastrinoma in the duodenum. Based on the patient's presentation and test results, which of the following is the most likely diagnosis?
   a. Zollinger-Ellison syndrome
   b. gastric adenocarcinoma
   c. carcinoid stomach tumor
   d. gastric lymphoma
   e. gastroparesis

186. Which of the following medications is effective in lowering serum glucose, serum triglycerides, and promoting weight loss without risk of hypoglycemia?
   a. glimepiride
   b. glyburide
   c. metformin
   d. exenatide
   e. glipizide

187. An 18-month-old infant presents with runny nose, sneezing, wheezing, and low-grade fever. Physical examination reveals nasal flaring, tachypnea, and retractions indicating respiratory distress. CBC and chest X-ray are normal. Nasal washing is positive for respiratory syncytial virus. You diagnose this child with bronchiolitis. Which of the following medications would you prescribe to treat this condition?
a. sulfamethoxazole/trimethoprim
b. erythromycin
c. ribavirin
d. cyclosporine
e. ciprofloxacin

188. A 62-year-old woman presents with osteoarthritis. She has worsening knee pain. She has a BMI of 29. She asks about lifestyle changes that may improve her condition. Which of the following is NOT a valid recommendation?
a. weight loss
b. physical therapy
c. occupational therapy
d. weight-bearing exercise
e. heat pads

189. A 32-year-old man with a family history of hypertension presents to have his blood pressure measured. His blood pressure is taken and gives a reading of 150/80. He is given an experimental antihypertensive that acts solely by vasodilating major arteries. What would be expected to happen to his pulse over time?
a. increase
b. decrease
c. remain the same
d. increase and then decrease
e. decrease and then increase

190. For which of the following conditions are pregabalin, milnacipran, and duloxetine hydrochloride the only FDA-approved medications?
a. multiple sclerosis
b. scleroderma
c. fibromyalgia
d. systemic lupus erythematosus (SLE)
e. multiple myeloma

191. An 85-year-old diabetic woman is transferred to the emergency department from a nursing home because of a recurrent fever of 101°F to 102°F for the past three days, accompanied by complaints of malaise, muscle aches, and cough with mucopurulent sputum. A chest X-ray confirms left lower lobe pneumonia. Which of the following is the most appropriate treatment?
a. broad-spectrum fluoroquinolones
b. acetaminophen
c. isonizide
d. metronidazole
e. none of the above

192. A 65-year-old Asian man with a history of hyperlipidemia and diabetes mellitus presents to the emergency department complaining of acute chest pain that started during his Sunday brunch four hours ago. He appears in severe distress and is diaphoretic. You order a 12-lead electrocardiogram (EKG), which shows sinus tachycardia at 105 bpm, ST segment elevation in V1, and reciprocal ST segment depression in V5 and V6. Which of the following is the most likely diagnosis?
a. acute anteroseptal infarct
b. acute lateral wall infarct
c. acute inferior myocardial infarction
d. pericarditis
e. none of the above

193. A 44-year-old man presents to his primary care clinic with a two-week history of lower back pain that seems to have started the day after he engaged in a great deal of heavy lifting while moving to a new house. On further questioning, he reports that the pain often shoots into the back of his right leg and is generally worst after a full day of activity. Which of the following additional physical examination findings would be most consistent with a diagnosis of S1 nerve sciatica?
   a. exaggerated ankle jerk reflex
   b. diminished ankle jerk reflex
   c. exaggerated knee jerk reflex
   d. diminished knee jerk reflex
   e. uniformly exaggerated lower limb reflexes

194. Peripheral vasodilatation is best achieved by administration of which of the following classes of antihypertensive medications? These medications are also most effective among the African-American and elderly populations.
   a. diuretics
   b. β-adrenergic antagonists
   c. calcium channel blockers
   d. ACE inhibitors
   e. corticosteroids

195. A 29-year-old male presents with painful, burning urination associated with a profuse, creamy, bloody, yellow urethral discharge. Which of the following is the most likely diagnosis?
   a. epididymitis
   b. gonorrhea
   c. syphilis
   d. chlamydia
   e. HIV

196. A 26-year-old female patient presents to her primary care clinic complaining of a six-month history of pain in her fingers and toes. The pain has progressively increased in severity and is most pronounced when she wakes up in the morning. Physical examination is significant for tenderness in the metacarpophalangeal joints and the proximal interphalangeal joints as well as for rashes on her elbows. Which of the following features of the rash would suggest a diagnosis of psoriatic arthritis?
   a. asymmetry
   b. redness
   c. tenderness
   d. silvery scale
   e. raised areas

197. A 53-year-old man presents with dull chest pain that radiates to his left arm and jaw. His pain started an hour ago and is associated with shortness of breath and diaphoresis. He states that he has never had this pain before. On examination, he is tachycardic and hypertensive. He has a history of hypertension, hypercholesterolemia, and a 34-pack-year smoking history. He is otherwise well. An electrocardiogram shows ST elevations in leads V1 and V2 with reciprocal changes in 2, 3, and aVF. Which one of the following is NOT indicated for immediate management of his ST elevation myocardial infarction (STEMI)?
   a. morphine
   b. oxygen
   c. metoprolol
   d. aspirin
   e. warfarin

198. A 12-year-old boy is brought to the primary care clinic by his parents for investigation of a truncal rash. On further questioning, his parents report that two other children in his class had recently suffered from a similar illness. Physical examination reveals a temperature of 98.5°F in addition to a maculopapular rash with multiple burrows and pustules. Which of the following is the most likely diagnosis?
  a. dermatitis
  b. atopic eczema
  c. scabies
  d. chickenpox
  e. measles

199. A 34-year-old G4 P3003 pregnant woman presents for her first trimester checkup. Her laboratory result shows hemoglobin (g/dl): 9 (10–13), hematocrit (%): 29 (30–39), normal red blood cell count, MCV (mean corpuscular volume, f/L): 93 (70–90), reticulocyte count (%): 1.5 (1–2), serum iron (ug/dl): 55 (30–100), serum folate (ng/ml): 3 (4–10), and serum vitamin B12 (ng/ml): 80 (70–500). Which of the following is the most likely diagnosis?
  a. folate deficiency anemia
  b. thalassemia trait
  c. iron deficiency anemia
  d. hemachromatosis
  e. mixed anemia

200. A 24-year-old man with a history of what his family describes as "troubled childhood" presents for an evaluation. His record shows multiple arrests for petty theft, physical fights, and destruction of public properties. He has been fired from numerous jobs in the past. However, he does have stable friends. Which of the following is the most likely diagnosis?
  a. delusional disorder
  b. antisocial personality disorder
  c. borderline personality disorder
  d. narcissistic personality disorder
  e. schizoid personality disorder

201. A 43-year-old male patient presents to his primary care clinic for a routine physical examination as required by his insurance company. The only noted abnormality is a heart rate of 54 bpm. Which of the following pulse findings would be most suggestive of second-degree atrioventricular block?
  a. increased pulse pressure
  b. decreased pulse pressure
  c. regularly regular rate
  d. irregularly irregular rate
  e. regularly irregular rate

202. A 26-year-old female, who was a victim of a motor vehicle accident, presents with bright red blood coming from both nostrils. Bright red blood is also seen in the posterior pharynx. Which of the following is the most likely diagnosis?
  a. fractured sinus
  b. epistaxis from the Kiesselbach's plexus
  c. epistaxis from the Woodruff's plexus
  d. epiglottitis
  e. sinusitis

203. A 44-year-old woman presents with increased fatigability, constipation, and dry skin. Her lab result shows normal plasma TSH and low plasma free T4. Which of the following is the most likely diagnosis?
a. primary hypothyroidism
b. secondary hypothyroidism
c. euthyroid goiter
d. primary hyperthyroidism
e. secondary hyperthyroidism

204. A 55-year-old HIV-negative woman with a history of poorly controlled type 2 diabetes presents with a rash on her left trunk for the past few days. The rash is painful and "burning." On exam, you find a 2×5 cm, papular, erythematous, pustular lesion along one thoracic dermatome. The patient denies new medication use or other associated symptoms. Which of the following is the most appropriate treatment?
a. topical antibiotic cream
b. topical antifungal cream
c. surgical excision
d. fluconazole
e. famciclovir

205. A 13-year-old boy is diagnosed with asthma. Which of the following signs or symptoms is NOT consistent with this diagnosis?
a. shortness of breath
b. nasal polyps
c. atopy
d. wheeze
e. cough

206. A 19-year-old female patient presents to her primary care clinic complaining of an oral cold sore on the posterior aspect of her lower lip. She was recently told by a friend that this implies herpes infection, and she is concerned about the implications of such an infection. Which of the following is the most likely pathogen causing the sore?
a. herpes simplex virus, type 1
b. herpes simplex virus, type 2
c. Epstein-Barr virus
d. rhinovirus
e. *Streptococcus pneumoniae*

207. A 49-year-old female presents with memory loss, social withdrawal, and poor personal hygiene. A physical exam reveals muscle rigidity and diminished coordination. An MRI reveals atrophy in the anterior temporal lobe. Which of the following in the most likely diagnosis?
a. pseudodementia
b. frontotemporal dementia
c. vascular dementia
d. Alzheimer's disease
e. Huntington's disease

208. Which of the following medications, used to slow or stop pre-term labor, is no longer available for use in the United States?
a. nifedipine
b. ritodrine
c. magnesium sulfate
d. indocin
e. ketorolac

209. A 24-year-old man presents to the emergency department with a two-day history of nausea, loss of appetite, and lower abdominal pain. His pain started in the periumbilical area and traveled to the right lower quadrant (RLQ). He denies other associated symptoms. An abdominal CAT scan confirms appendicitis. Which of the following is the most appropriate clinical intervention?
a. give antibiotic treatment and observe
b. appendectomy
c. give acetaminophen for pain
d. observe and repeat abdominal CAT scan in one week to confirm
e. perform a colonoscopy

210. If cerebrospinal fluid obtained from a lumbar puncture is *negative* for subarachnoid hemorrhage, what color is the cerebrospinal fluid?
a. clear
b. yellowish
c. cloudy
d. milky
e. bloody

211. A 21-year-old woman presents with primary amenorrhea. On examination she is observed to have a webbed neck and short stature. Her karyotype is 45XO. Which of the following is the most likely diagnosis?
a. Down syndrome
b. Klinefelter syndrome
c. Turner syndrome
d. Noonan syndrome
e. Marfan syndrome

212. An 18-year-old Caucasian male presents for a routine physical exam. His blood pressure has been routinely elevated with little or no reduction in response to diet adjustments, weight loss, or diuretic therapy. Which of the following is the class of medications you would prescribe for this patient to control his blood pressure?
a. higher dose of diuretics
b. β-andrenergic antagonists
c. ACE inhibitors
d. calcium channel blockers
e. nitrates

213. A 30-year-old man presents with complaints of increasing shoe size. The patient also complains about an enlarging fleshy nose when compared to old photographs. A diagnosis of acromegaly is considered. Which of the following hormones would most likely be elevated in this condition?
a. somatostatin
b. erythropoetin
c. dopamine
d. growth hormone
e. thyroxine

214. A 56-year-old man with a history of hypertension presents with pain in his left toe for the past two days. On exam, you find a tender, red, warm lesion on the first metatarsal phalangeal joint of his left foot. Joint aspiration confirms acute gouty attack. Which of the following is the most appropriate treatment at this time?
a. allopurinol
b. colchicine
c. acetaminophen
d. oxycodone
e. omeprazole (proton pump inhibitor)

215. A 43-year-old male patient with alcoholic liver disease asks about preventing further deterioration of his liver. In addition to total cessation of alcohol, which of the following interventions would be best for this patient?

   a. increase salt intake

   b. hepatitis B vaccination

   c. hepatitis C vaccination

   d. increase protein intake

   e. decrease protein intake

216. A 41-year-old woman presents with visual field disturbances. She reports difficulty driving as she cannot see the whole road at once. She also reports an episode of temporary leg paralysis that occurred two months ago. A diagnosis of relapsing-remitting multiple sclerosis is considered. Which of the following diagnostic tests would be most consistent with this diagnosis?

   a. spinal cord lesion detected by CT

   b. spinal cord lesion detected by MRI

   c. multiple central nervous system (CNS) lesions detected by CT

   d. multiple CNS lesions detected by MRI

   e. monoclonal serum IgM

217. A 55-year-old man presents to his primary care clinic with a three-day history of a drooping left eyelid. His past history is significant for a 40-pack-year history of cigarette smoking. Physical examination reveals anhidrosis on the left forehead and miosis in the left eye. Which of the following additional findings would be most suggestive of a lung tumor?

   a. left shoulder pain

   b. left chest pain

   c. right shoulder pain

   d. right chest pain

   e. central back and chest pain

218. A 37-year-old married woman is brought in by ambulance after being awake for five days. During that time she had intercourse with three different partners, bought two cars, and started work on three different screenplays. She also reported an episode of depression that happened two weeks ago. Prior to these events her condition was well controlled with medication. She reportedly stopped taking her drugs about a month ago because she noticed she was urinating more often and had increased thirst. She has no history of diabetes, and her serum and urine glucose levels are normal. Which medication was she most likely taking?

   a. haloperidol

   b. valproate

   c. carbamazepine

   d. clozapine

   e. lithium

219. A 51-year-old man with type 2 diabetes presents for a regular checkup. A urinalysis indicates +++ protein. A diagnosis of diabetic nephropathy is considered. Which of the following signs or symptoms is most consistent with this diagnosis?

   a. Kausmaul breathing

   b. hematuria

   c. dysuria

   d. edema

   e. melena

220. A genetic study on a 43-year-old African-American woman indicates that she has a single copy of the sickle cell trait. She has been asymptomatic her whole life. Which of the following conditions is she most likely to develop as a result of this condition?
  a. sickle cell anemia
  b. bone marrow expansion
  c. peripheral neuropathy
  d. hematuria
  e. obesity

221. A hysterosalpingography is a useful exam for the evaluating which of the following?
  a. ovulation
  b. sperm survival
  c. sperm penetration
  d. tubal patency
  e. sperm count

222. A 24-year-old competitive swimmer presents with his third episode of otitis externa for this year. Which of the following is the most appropriate patient education to prevent repeat infections?
  a. keep the ear canal dry
  b. shake off excess water from ears after swimming
  c. wear protective ear gear
  d. do not clean earwax yourself
  e. all of the above

223. A 28-year-old male, with a respiratory tract infection, presents with a herald patch on the abdomen with an associated rash. Which of the following is the most likely diagnosis?
  a. seborrheic keratosis
  b. dermatophytosis
  c. pityriasis rosea
  d. scabies
  e. vitiligo

224. Which of the following endocrine disorders is classically diagnosed by the presence of hypercalcemia?
  a. hypoparathyroidism
  b. hyperparathyroidism
  c. hypothyroidism
  d. hyperthyroidism
  e. euthyroidism

225. A 21-year-old female patient presents to her primary care clinic after an episode of fainting. This is the third such episode in the past two weeks. Witnesses have told her that she appeared to experience a complete loss of consciousness with rapid onset and rapid recovery, while she seems to feel a general weakness and faintness immediately beforehand. The first episode occurred as she was walking into her college calculus class on the day of an exam that had caused her a great deal of stress; since then, two similar episodes have occurred in the same room, although she was able to complete the exam successfully after arranging to take it in a different room. On further questioning, she reports that she has also experienced a great deal of financial stress related to the possibility of losing her scholarship. Physical examination is unremarkable. Which of the following is the most likely diagnosis?
  a. somatization disorder
  b. malingering
  c. vasovagal response
  d. epilepsy
  e. normal response to stress

226. A 34-year-old man presents to his primary care clinic with a six-month history of progressive scrotal enlargement with no pain and no history of notable trauma. His past medical history is significant for cryptorchidism at birth, which resolved spontaneously. Physical examination reveals a firm scrotal mass with no transillumination. Which of the following further investigations is most appropriate at this stage?
a. ultrasound
b. X-ray
c. MRI
d. fine-needle aspiration biopsy
e. inguinal orchiectomy and biopsy

227. The type of shock that is the result of hemorrhage, loss of plasma, or loss of fluid and electrolytes is accurately defined by which of the following?
a. cardiogenic shock
b. hypovolemic shock
c. obstructive shock
d. septic shock
e. neurogenic shock

228. A 38-year-old pregnant female, who was diagnosed with severe preeclampsia, has blood work that reveals hemolysis, elevated liver enzymes, and low platelet count. Based on the patient's history and lab results, which of the following is the most likely diagnosis?
a. chronic hypertension
b. eclampsia
c. HELLP syndrome
d. pre-term labor
e. leiomyomata

229. A 16-year-old female presents as being underweight and emaciatied. Physical examination reveals dental erosion, esophagitis, calluses on her knuckles, and atrophy of her salivary glands. Blood work reveals hypochloremic hypokalemic alkalosis and hypomagnesemia. Based on the patient's history, physical examination, and test results, which of the following is the most likely diagnosis?
a. binge eating disorder
b. anorexia nervosa
c. bulimia nervosa
d. narcissistic personality disorder
e. body dysmorphic disorder

230. A 60-year-old male presents with dull, aching discomfort in the right hemiscrotum. Physical exam reveals a markedly swollen, very tender scrotal mass. Ultrasound exam confirms a diagnosis of epididymitis. Which of the following medications would you prescribe to treat this condition?
a. ACE inhibitors
b. ceftriaxone
c. tolterodine
d. ciproflaxin
e. warfarin

231. A healthy 27-year-old female presents for her annual physical. The patient does not complain of any symptoms. Her electrocardiogram is normal. Blood pressure is normal. Auscultation of the heart reveals a "swishing" sound. Which of the following diagnostic procedures would you order to evaluate the "swishing" sound?

  a. echocardiogram to assess valvular function
  b. cardiac catheterization to assess for ischemia
  c. 24-hour Holter monitor to rule out cardiac arrhythmia
  d. cardiac stress test to assess for ischemia
  e. cardiac PET scan to evaluate myocardial viability

232. A 22-year-old, slightly built male presents with acute chest pain, shortness of breath, and one-sided chest expansion. Auscultation of the chest reveals diminished breath sounds on the right side. A chest X-ray reveals a visceral pleural line. Which of the following is the most likely diagnosis?

  a. bronchiectasis
  b. pulmonary embolism
  c. pleural effusion
  d. pulmonary hypertension
  e. pneumothorax

233. Which of the following conditions is often treated with scopolamine?

  a. barotrauma
  b. acute vertigo
  c. motion sickness
  d. labyrinthitis
  e. presbycusis

234. A 67-year-old woman presents with several recent episodes of blurred vision in her left eye. On further questioning, she mentions that she has also experienced occasional jaw claudication and some tenderness in her left temporal region. Which of the following conditions is she at greatest risk of developing in the future?

  a. polymyalgia rheumatica
  b. rheumatoid arthritis
  c. Wegener's granulomatosis
  d. sarcoidosis
  e. systemic lupus erythematosus

235. A 58-year-old female comes to the emergency department with acute onset of severe abdominal pain accompanied by urgent bowel movements and bloody diarrhea. She reports no past history of gastrointestinal disease or abdominal trauma, but she is currently taking atorvastatin for management of hypercholesterolemia. She has a 40-pack-year smoking history and no significant history of excessive alcohol consumption. Physical examination reveals mild epigastric tenderness with no change in vital signs and no abnormalities on pelvic examination. If there is no further modification of her lifestyle or her drug regimen, which of the following conditions is she most likely to develop in the future?

  a. chronic pancreatitis
  b. pancreatic carcinoma
  c. colorectal carcinoma
  d. ruptured abdominal aortic aneurysm
  e. ischemic heart disease

236. A 55-year-old female presents to her primary care physician because of a 12-month history of progressively increasing diffuse pain in her fingers. She describes the pain as a general tightness and stiffness that is more prominent in more peripheral areas. On further questioning, she reports that she has recently started to wear thicker gloves because she finds her hands to be more sensitive to cold temperatures. On physical examination, she appears to have tightened and thickened skin over her hands and her face. Additionally, she has reduced movement in her fingers. Which of the following antibodies is most likely to be found on a blood test?
   a. anti-Scl-70
   b. anti-dsDNA
   c. antihistone
   d. antineutrophil
   e. anti-IgG

237. Which of the following medications would be prescribed in order to reduce systemic arterial pressure for patients who have been diagnosed with pulmonary hypertension?
   a. beta blockers
   b. bronchodilators
   c. calcium channel blockers
   d. corticosteroids
   e. diuretics

238. A 33-year-old patient presents with abdominal pain, distention, fever, and tachycardia. Abdominal tympany is appreciated upon physical examination. Abdominal X-ray reveals colonic distention confirming the diagnosis of volvulus. Which of the following clinical procedures would you use to treat this disorder?
   a. surgical correction
   b. endoscopic decompression
   c. colon cleansing
   d. abdominal angiogram
   e. partial colectomy

239. A 23-year-old male presents with pain and tenderness in the fourth and fifth metacarpals of the right hand following a boxing match. Physical examination reveals loss of prominence to the affected knuckles and puncture wounds in the affected knuckles. An X-ray reveals boxer's fractures to the fourth and fifth metacarpal necks. Because of the puncture wounds, which of the following additional treatments is necessary other than splinting the affected fingers?
   a. anti-inflammatories
   b. corticosteroids
   c. antibiotics
   d. opiate pain medication
   e. sutures

240. A ten-year-old uncircumcised boy presents with a retracted foreskin behind the glans penis that cannot be returned to normal position. Physical exam is otherwise unremarkable. He is complaining of pain for the past two days. He denies injury, insect bite, or swelling in other areas of the body. Which of the following is the correct diagnosis?
   a. phimosis
   b. testicular torsion
   c. cryptorchidism
   d. paraphimosis
   e. varicocele

Section 5
Time: 60 minutes

241. A 55-year-old male presents with progressive hearing loss, tinnitus, and dizziness for the past several weeks. Patient also complains of nausea and vomiting associated with the hearing loss. You diagnose this patient with Meniere's disease. Which of the following treatment options would you prescribe for treatment of this disorder?
   a. diuretics and salt restriction
   b. oral antibiotics
   c. over-the-counter antibacterial drops
   d. intravenous antibiotics
   e. oral corticosteroids

242. A 74-year-old woman is currently undergoing inpatient treatment for an infective exacerbation of her chronic obstructive pulmonary disease (COPD). After three days of antibiotic therapy, she still requires delivery of oxygen via nasal prongs. Before admission, she was able to function comfortably on room air. Which of the following measurements is likely to provide the best assessment of her current respiratory status?
   a. current oxygen requirement (FiO_2)
   b. arterial blood gas levels on room air
   c. pulse oximetry on room air
   d. arterial blood gas levels with nasal prongs
   e. pulse oximetry with nasal prongs

243. A 44-year-old male presents with shortness of breath on exertion, fatigue, and sudden nocturnal dyspnea. Auscultation of the chest reveals a mid-diastolic murmur at the apex with little radiation. Auscultation also reveals S1 accentuated opening snap following S2. Based on the presentation and physical examination, which of the following is the most likely diagnosis?
   a. aortic stenosis
   b. aortic regurgitation
   c. mitral stenosis
   d. pulmonic stenosis
   e. tricuspid regurgitation

244. The most common injury of the wrist is a fracture that results from a fall onto a dorsiflexed hand. The X-ray of this fracture is characterized by a silver fork deformity, as seen in the illustration below. Which of the following types of fracture is illustrated in this X-ray?

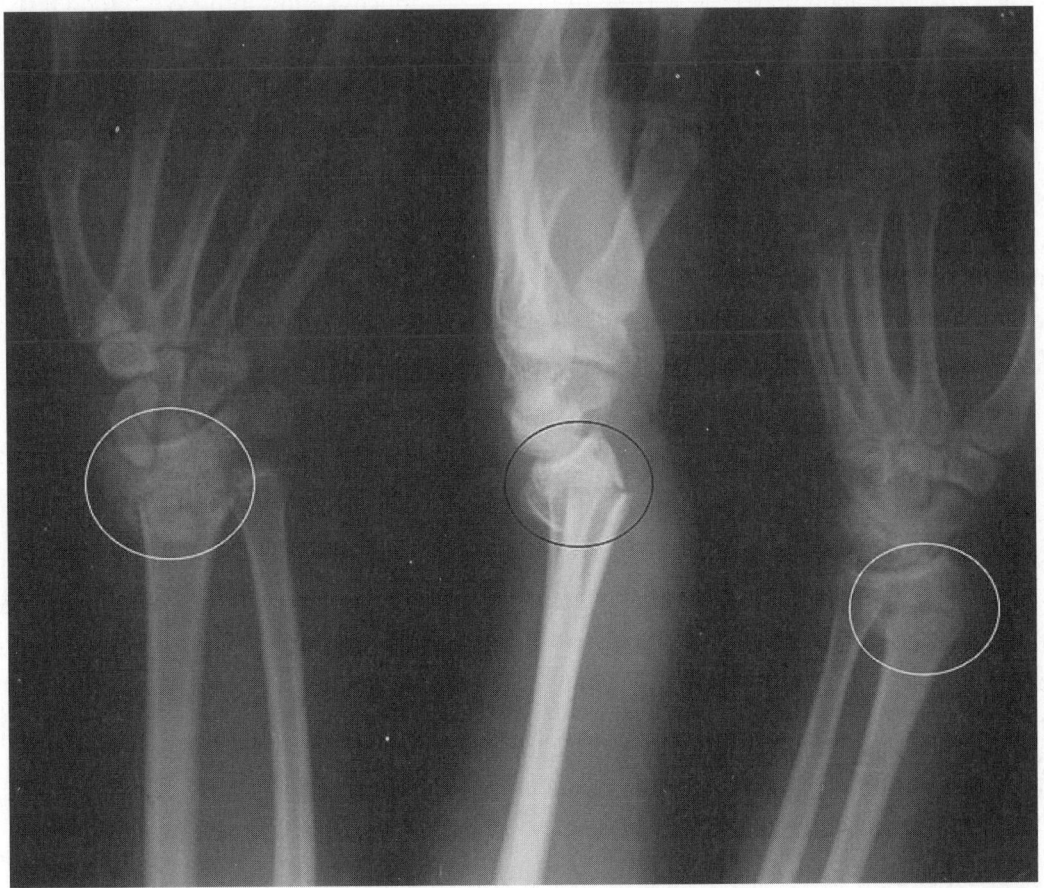

a. buckle (torus) fracture
b. greenstick fracture
c. Colles' fracture
d. open fracture
e. compound fracture

245. A 26-year-old female presents with diarrhea, weight loss, weakness, and abdominal distention. The patient's history and physical exam is very common for celiac disease. Which of the following clinical procedures would you perform to confirm the diagnosis?
a. CT scan of the abdomen
b. barium enema
c. small bowel biopsy
d. gastrointestinal bleeding study
e. endoscopy

246. Maintenance therapy of chronic obstructive pulmonary disease (COPD) is commonly achieved by administration of which of the following medications?
a. antibiotics
b. anticholinergics
c. inhaled corticosteroids
d. β-adrenergic agonists
e. diuretics

247. The clinical condition of severe cardiovascular failure caused by poor blood flow, inadequate distribution of blood flow, and inadequate oxygen delivery to the tissues is accurately defined by which of the following?
a. cardiac arrest
b. hypovolemia
c. shock
d. congestive heart failure
e. myocardial infarction

248. Chronic thrombocytopenia secondary to systemic lupus erythematosus (SLE) is most effectively treated by which of the following?
a. erythropoietin
b. prednisone
c. folic acid
d. vitamin B12
e. vitamin K

249. A 22-year-old woman presents with anal bleeding, left-sided abdominal pain, and tenesmus. A colonoscopy reveals a continuous lesion spanning from the distal colon to the rectum. Biopsies of the lesion reveal nongranulomatous inflammation limited to the mucosa and submucosa. Blood tests reveal an elevated CRP and erythrocyte sedimentation rate, and the presence of pANCA. Which of the following is the most likely diagnosis?
a. bowel cancer
b. irritable bowel syndrome (IBS)
c. Crohn's disease
d. ulcerative colitis
e. celiac disease

250. A 72-year-old female presents with progressive shortness of breath, excessive cough, and sputum production. Decreased breath sounds and early inspiratory crackles are noticed on physical examination. Percussion yields increased resonance. Chest X-ray reveals hyperinflation of the lungs and a flat diaphragm. Which of the following is the most likely diagnosis?
a. alveolitis
b. bronchiectasis
c. pulmonary hypertension
d. pulmonary embolism
e. chronic obstructive pulmonary disease (COPD)

251. A 52-year-old male presents with chronic peritonsillar cellulitis. His symptoms include severe sore throat pain and an airway obstruction that has progressed to the point where he now suffers from sleep apnea. A physical examination of the throat reveals persistent, marked asymmetry of the tonsils. Which of the following would be the most appropriate course of treatment for this patient?
   a. treat medically with oral penicillin or erythromycin
   b. hospital admission in order to treat with intravenous antibiotics
   c. aspiration of the tonsils followed by antibiotics
   d. surgical incision and drainage of the tonsils followed by a course of antibiotics
   e. tonsillectomy

252. A 13-year-old overweight teenage boy presents with a limping gait. He complains of intermittent, dull pain in his left hip without radiation for the past week. He denies previous trauma. All other work-ups are normal, including vitals and blood work. X-rays of his hips and knees show a positive posterior displacement of the left femoral epiphysis with an appearance of "ice cream slipping off a cone." A follow-up MRI shows a widening of the physis with surrounding edema of the left femoral head without bone density changes. Which of the following is the most likely diagnosis?
   a. septic hip
   b. avascular necrosis of the left hip
   c. malignant tumor of the femur
   d. slipped capital femoral epiphysis (SCFE)
   e. none of the above

253. A 66-year-old Asian man with a history of alcoholic liver cirrhosis, splenomegaly, and mild abdominal ascites presents complaining of one episode of hemoptysis two days ago. He denies recent injury, chest pain, nausea, or vomiting, He has clear lung sounds bilaterally. A chest X-ray is negative for focal lesions. Which of the following is the most likely diagnosis?
   a. Mallory-Weiss tear
   b. esophageal varices
   c. lung cancer
   d. hemothorax
   e. tuberculosis

254. A 63-year-old HIV-negative woman with a history of chronic obstructive pulmonary disease (COPD) and poorly controlled type 2 diabetes mellitus presents with a complaint of odynophagia for the past few weeks. Oral exam shows white plaques on her buccal mucosa, palate, and oropharynx, which are consistent with thrush. Which of the following is the most appropriate treatment?
   a. amoxicillin/clavulanate
   b. ciprofloxacin
   c. penicillin VK
   d. esomeprazole
   e. fluconazole

255. A 62-year-old Asian female presents to your clinic and complains of recent weight loss, fatigue, night sweats, and recurrent cough. You order a chest X-ray and find cavitations in the apex of the right lung. An acid-fast bacilli on smear of sputum is positive. Which of the following is the most likely diagnosis?
   a. acute asthma exacerbation
   b. pneumonia
   c. pulmonary tuberculosis
   d. cystic fibrosis
   e. chronic obstructive pulmonary disease (COPD)

256. A 29-year-old Hispanic female with a history of childhood rheumatic fever is found to have abnormal heart sounds on a routine physical exam. She is otherwise healthy. You order an echocardiography, which confirms your suspicion of tricuspid stenosis. Which of the following is the most typical physical finding?

   a. prominent S1 heart sound with an opening snap

   b. S3 heart sound and pansystolic murmur at the apex that radiates into the axilla

   c. soft, absent S2 heart sound

   d. systolic murmur along the left sternal border

   e. diastolic rumble along the lower left sternal border

257. A 63-year-old man presents with a narrow band of lesions on his right chest along the T5 dermatome. The lesions, which are described as "painful" and "burning," are observed to be in different stages of development. The patient cannot remember whether he has had chickenpox. Scrapings from the lesions reveal multinucleated giant cells. Which of the following best describes the infectious agent?

   a. a misfolded protein inducing conformational change in its neighbours

   b. an ATP-dependent intracellular bacterium

   c. a dormant virus in the dorsal root ganglion

   d. an RNA virus containing a reverse transcriptase

   e. a DNA virus containing a reverse transcriptase

258. A 37-year-old woman presents to the primary care clinic because of a long history of periodic severe headaches. The headaches appear suddenly with no warning signs, peak after about 10 to 15 minutes, and gradually decrease in severity over the next half hour. She typically experiences daily episodes for one- to two-month periods, followed by complete remission for several months to years. During the episodes, she feels a characteristic boring pain in one eye along with ipsilateral lacrimation. Which of the following is the most likely diagnosis?

   a. intracerebral aneurysm

   b. migraine

   c. temporal arteritis

   d. cluster headache

   e. chronic sinusitis

259. A 42-year-old man with rheumatoid arthritis is treated with infliximab. Which of the following is a contraindication for its use?

   a. renal failure

   b. positive interferon-γ release assay

   c. regular aspirin use

   d. opioid use

   e. BCG vaccination

260. A 34-year-old woman presents complaining of vaginal itching and increased vaginal discharge for the past one week. You confirm a diagnosis of *Candida* vaginitis. Which of the following is most consistent with this condition?

   a. vaginal pH > 4.5 (normal: 3.8–4.2)

   b. green-yellow frothy discharge

   c. fishy odor on KOH whiff test

   d. positive bacterial culture

   e. none of the above

261. A 45-year-old woman without significant past medical history complains of increasing fatigue for the past few months. She denies change in her normal routine or new medication use. She reports feeling cold easily, being frequently constipated, and having dry skin. Her lab work is significant for elevated TSH level. Which of the following is the most likely diagnosis?
  a. premenopausal syndrome
  b. fibromyalgia
  c. hyperthyroidism
  d. hypothyroidism
  e. depression

262. A 26-year-old woman presents with an acute loss of facial muscular tone in her left face since yesterday. On exam, she is unable to wrinkle her left forehead or raise her left eyebrow. She is able to close her eyelids fully. When asked to smile, the left corner of her mouth remains unmoved. Which of the following nerve groups is involved?
  a. central sensory system
  b. central motor system
  c. peripheral sensory system
  d. peripheral motor system
  e. none of the above

263. A 55-year-old woman has her lab results as follows: arterial pH: 7.30 (7.36 to 7.44); HCO_3 concentration: 25 meq/L (21 to 27); arterial PCO_2: 66 mmHg (36 to 44). Which of the following is the most likely diagnosis based on the findings?
  a. metabolic acidosis
  b. metabolic alkalosis
  c. respiratory acidosis
  d. respiratory alkalosis
  e. mixed alkalosis

264. An 18-year-old female presents with episodes of unexplained muscle weakness and muscle fatigue that varies throughout the day. The patient states her symptoms are alleviated with rest. She also complains of double vision and difficulty chewing. Lab work reveals elevated levels of circulating acetylcholine receptor antibodies. A physical examination reveals bilateral ptosis, normal sensation in the limbs, and no reflex changes. Which of the following is the most likely diagnosis?
  a. Guillain-Barré syndrome
  b. myasthenia gravis
  c. Bell's palsy
  d. diabetic peripheral neuropathy
  e. multiple sclerosis

265. A 35-year-old woman who recently immigrated to the United States from Tibet presents for advice about pregnancy. She has already had a child that was developmentally delayed, and on inspection she has a visible goiter. Supplementation with which of the following nutrients would most likely prevent her next child from also being developmentally delayed?
  a. ascorbic acid
  b. thiamine
  c. folate
  d. iodine
  e. iron

266. Which of the following is the most appropriate treatment for keratoderma?
  a. topical corticosteroids
  b. permethrin
  c. lindane
  d. fluconazole
  e. liquid nitrogen

267. A 68-year-old male with a history of portal hypertension from chronic viral hepatitis presents with hematemesis. Endoscopy reveals dilation of the veins of the esophagus. Based on the patient's presentation and test results, which of the following is the most likely diagnosis?
a. Mallory-Weiss tear
b. esophageal varices
c. Budd-Chiari syndrome
d. esophageal neoplasm
e. reflux esophagitis

268. A 44-year-old female patient with a history of injecting drug use presents to the emergency department with a six-hour history of diffuse chest pain and shortness of breath. She has also experienced a four-day history of low-grade fever, malaise, and myalgia. Physical examination is significant for a temperature of 39°C (103°F). Two separate blood cultures are taken at 12-hour intervals; Gram stains of both cultures reveal Gram-positive cocci in clusters. Which of the following additional investigations is most appropriate if a diagnosis of infective endocarditis is suspected?
a. electrocardiogram
b. echocardiogram
c. angiogram
d. chest CT
e. mitral valve biopsy

269. A 23-year-old woman with a previous history of pelvic inflammatory disease presents with severe abdominal pain and vaginal bleeding. She is not taking any contraceptive pills and has been amenorrheic for the last two months. On examination, she is hypotensive and tachycardic. Her urine is positive for β-hCG. An ultrasound of her abdomen suggests a mass present in her left fallopian tube. The patient is given appropriate fluid resuscitation. Which of the following is the definitive management for this patient?
a. methotrexate
b. patient-controlled analgesia
c. immediate surgical resection of the lesion
d. CT-guided biopsy of the tumor
e. clomiphene

270. A 50-year-old female presents with dull pain, swelling, redness, and tenderness of the left leg. A venous Doppler exam of the lower extremities is positive for deep venous thrombosis. Which of the following is the proper treatment for maintenance therapy of deep venous thrombosis?
a. anti-inflammatories
b. corticosteroids
c. antibiotics
d. warm compresses
e. anticoagulant therapy

271. A 19-year-old man is involved in a motor vehicle accident and is brought in by ambulance to the emergency room. During the secondary survey he has paralysis in one of his legs, associated with ipsilateral dysesthesia. Babinski's reflex is present on the right and absent on the left. The rest of his neurological exam is unremarkable. Which of the following is the most likely site of the lesion?

   a. right side of C1
   b. left side of C1
   c. right side of L1
   d. left side of L1
   e. right side of parietal lobe

272. A 45-year-old Indian female presents to your clinic for a complete physical. She has a family history of congestive heart diseases. She has a BMI of 35. Her blood pressure today is 139/89. Which of the following lifestyle modifications would you recommend at this time?

   a. weight reduction
   b. diet low in fat and sodium but rich in fruits and vegetables
   c. physical activity
   d. moderation of alcohol consumption
   e. all of the above

273. A 23-year-old man is brought in by ambulance after attempted suicide. He is stabilized but is considered to be in imminent risk of self-harm. The patient refuses to stay in the hospital and wants to go home so he can "finish the job." Which of the following is the most appropriate next step?

   a. let him leave as he is a competent adult
   b. let him leave but refer him for psychological consult
   c. begin electroconvulsive therapy immediately
   d. detain him, by force if nessecary
   e. commence a course of outpatient cognitive behavioral therapy

274. Miglitol is a member of the class of medications called α-glucosidase inhibitors. This class of medications lowers blood glucose by which of the following mechanisms?

   a. decreases production of hepatic glucose
   b. stimulates insulin secretion
   c. delays absorption of carbohydrates from the intestine
   d. decreases gastric emptying
   e. increases gastric emptying

275. A 34-year-old Caucasian male patient presents to his primary care clinic with a two-year history of progressive exertional dyspnea in addition to a chronic cough associated with considerable amounts of sputum production. His past medical history is unremarkable, but he has a 15-pack-year smoking history. His FEV_1/FVC ratio is 65% (normal >70%) with no bronchodilator reversibility, while a chest X-ray demonstrates hyperinflation of the lungs. Which of the following additional pathological processes is most likely to be present in this patient?

   a. bronchitis
   b. bronchiectasis
   c. bronchiolitis
   d. asthma
   e. pneumothorax

276. A 64-year-old Caucasian with a history of multiple squamous cell carcinomas (SCCs) asks about steps he can take to prevent further skin cancers. He uses a tanning bed once a month and is a smoker. Which of the following suggestions would be LEAST useful?

   a. regular checkups
   b. use of sunscreen
   c. decreased use of tanning beds
   d. smoking cessation
   e. sunbathing on cloudy days

277. A 27-year-old woman is diagnosed with CML. Fluorescence in situ hybridization (FISH) analysis reveals a 9/22 recombination. She is prescribed imatinib mesylate. What is the mechanism of action of this drug?
a. DNase inhibitor
b. TNF blocker
c. tyrosine kinase inhibitor
d. Cox-4 inhibitor
e. phospholipase A2 inhibitor

278. A 58-year-old male, with a history of diabetes and hypertension, presents with progressive loss of vision. Venous dilatation and retinal edema is noticed upon physical examination. Which of the following is the most likely diagnosis?
a. glaucoma
b. retinopathy
c. orbital cellulitis
d. dacryostenosis
e. viral conjunctivitis

279. A woman who has been treated for breast cancer is at increased risk of developing which of the following forms of cancer?
a. endometrial cancer
b. uterine cancer
c. cervical cancer
d. ovarian cancer
e. bladder cancer

280. Which of the following spinal disorders is most frequently treated with lumbar epidural injections?
a. spinal bony metastases
b. scoliosis
c. kyphosis
d. spinal stenosis
e. ankylosing spondylitis

281. A 27-year-old female presents with weight loss, insomnia, exophthalmos, and a visible goiter. Her chest X-ray is normal. CT scan and ultrasound exams of the abdomen both reveal abnormalities of the adrenal glands. Which of the following is the most likely diagnosis?
a. Addison's disease
b. Graves' disease
c. Wilson's disease
d. pheochromocytoma
e. Wilms' tumor

282. A 48-year-old man with a history of schizophrenia and alcoholism presents to his primary care clinic with a five-day history of a noticeable resting tremor. His wife has also told him that he appears to be moving more slowly than usual. He has been taking haloperidol for the past three months for successful management of his schizophrenia. Physical examination reveals muscle rigidity and resting tremor. Which of the following is the most likely cause of his symptoms?
a. Parkinson's disease
b. complication of schizophrenia
c. hyperthyroidism
d. alcohol withdrawal
e. adverse effects of haloperidol

283. A 32-year-old female patient presents to the emergency department with a nine-hour history of high fever and right flank pain. On further questioning, she reports that she has also experienced dysuria for the past three days. Physical examination reveals a temperature of 40°C (104°F) and tenderness over the right flank; pelvic examination and β-hCG levels are normal. Which of the following is the most likely cause of her acute presentation?
   a. cystitis
   b. lower urinary tract infection
   c. nephrolithiasis
   d. urolithiasis
   e. pyelonephritis

284. A 40-year-old female, experiencing her first pregnancy, presents in week 25 of gestation with swelling of the face and hands, sudden weight gain, headache, visual disturbances, nausea, and decreased urine output. Physical examination reveals high blood pressure, proteinuria, and hyperreflexia. Based on the patient's presentation and physical examination, which of the following is the most likely diagnosis?
   a. eclampsia
   b. preeclampsia
   c. chronic hypertension
   d. premature labor
   e. leiomyomata

285. Which of the following personality disorders is characterized by procrastination, stubbornness, and negative attitudes? Patients with this disorder may also be sullen, argumentative, and resentful of those more fortunate.
   a. passive-aggressive disorder
   b. depressive disorder
   c. sadomasochistic disorder
   d. sadistic disorder
   e. narcissistic personality disorder

286. An 18-year-old athletic male presents with dull, aching discomfort in the left hemiscrotum. Physical exam reveals a markedly swollen, very tender scrotal mass. The patient was recently diagnosed with gonorrhea. Ultrasound exam confirms a diagnosis of epididymitis. Which of the following medications would you prescribe to treat this condition?
   a. ACE inhibitors
   b. ceftriaxone
   c. tolterodine
   d. ciproflaxin
   e. warfarin

287. A 48-year-old woman presents with recent-onset alcohol-induced dilated cardiomyopathy. She is currently well managed symptomatically. Which lifestyle modification would give her the best long-term chance of survival?
   a. training for a marathon
   b. meditation
   c. ceasing all alcohol consumption
   d. cessation of smoking
   e. positive thinking

288. Which of the following is the clinical term for a deep-seated infection of a single hair follicle, commonly known as a boil?
   a. pimple
   b. furuncle
   c. carbuncle
   d. abscess
   e. eczema

289. A 26-year-old man complains of right lower quadrant (RLQ) pain, chronic loose stool with occasional mucus in stool, and significant weight loss during the past year. His stool culture tests negative for infectious organisms. Given his chronic symptoms, he is referred to a gastrointestinal specialist and subsequently undergoes a colonoscopy. The colonoscopy shows aphthoid ulcers of terminal ileum with active cryptitis on biopsy. Which of the following is the most likely diagnosis?
a. Crohn's disease
b. colon carcinoma
c. ulcerative colitis
d. diverticulitis
e. *C. difficile* colitis

290. An overweight 63-year-old man with a 45-pack-year smoking history and a 15-year history of hypertension presents with acute-onset chest pain. An EKG shows ST elevation. Which of the following signs, if present, is most suggestive of a diagnosis of pericarditis?
a. dyspnea
b. systolic murmur
c. diastolic murmur
d. pain relieved by leaning forward
e. pain exacerbated by activity

291. A 28-year-old female presents to her primary care clinic complaining of a three-month history of lethargy, dry hacking cough, and dyspnea. Physical examination is normal. Which of the following chest X-ray findings would be most suggestive of a diagnosis of sarcoidosis?
a. calcification in the lung fields
b. cardiomegaly
c. increased vascular markings
d. bilateral hilar lymphadenopathy
e. basal consolidation

292. An 18-month-old boy is brought to the emergency department by his mother after she noticed a significant amount of bright red blood in his stools. On further questioning, she reports that he has been unusually irritable over the past four days, but often feels better after vomiting or passing small amounts of stool. Vital signs are normal, but abdominal examination is significant for a sausagelike mass in the right lower quadrant. A radionuclide scan demonstrates the presence of gastric tissue in the distal ileum. Which of the following is most likely responsible for his symptoms?
a. diverticulitis
b. appendicitis
c. intussusception
d. upper GI hemorrhage
e. colitis

293. A 62-year-old male presents to his primary care clinic for a regular checkup. During the consultation, he mentions that he has experienced increasing nasal congestion and believes that his sense of smell may be affected. Intranasal examination reveals translucent masses obstructing both sides of the nasal cavity. If the masses are removed surgically, which of the following is the most likely to be found on follow-up?
a. recurrence
b. infection
c. local malignancy
d. excessive bleeding
e. metastasis

294. A 65-year-old man presents with chest pain three days after his first myocardial infarction. On examination he is hypertensive (140/100) and tachycardic (109/min). He has an elevated jugular venous pressure, and on auscultation, a pericardial friction rub is heard. An electrocardiogram shows scooping ST segment elevations on all leads. His physician does not consider this to be life threatening, and he is treated with analgesia. Which of the following descriptions of his chest pain would best fit the clinical scenario?

   a. dull central pain radiating to the arm and jaw

   b. persistent tearing pain radiating to the back

   c. pleuritic pain relieved by leaning forward

   d. chest pain associated with dyspnea

   e. pain that spans across a specific dermatome

295. A 73-year-old man with a history of osteoporosis presents to his primary care clinic with a six-month history of progressive back pain. He recently heard about the option of vertebroplasty, a procedure in which a synthetic cement is injected into a fractured vertebra. Which of the following potential benefits is most likely associated with this procedure?

   a. pain relief

   b. compression fracture repair

   c. prevention of further compression fractures

   d. improved joint mobility

   e. reduction in referred pain to lower limbs

296. After a one-week history of sepsis that is mostly resolved with a course of intravenous antibiotics, a 48-year-old male patient develops left eye pain and blurry vision. Ophthalmic examination reveals diffuse redness in the left eye along with the presence of a small purulent collection in the anterior chamber. His visual acuity is normal in the right eye, but is limited to hand movements in the left eye. Which of the following additional investigations would help to confirm a diagnosis of endophthalmitis?

   a. retinal photography

   b. vitreous humor biopsy

   c. aqueous humor biopsy

   d. intraocular pressure measurement

   e. ophthalmoscopic examination

297. Which of the following class of medications is the gold standard for the medicinal treatment of sarcoidosis?

   a. diuretics

   b. antibiotics

   c. corticosteroids

   d. anti-inflammatories

   e. bronchodilators

298. A 62-year-old male presents with morning joint stiffness and swelling in the hands, wrists, and ankles for approximately three months. Blood work reveals elevated levels of erythrocyte sedimentation rate and C-reactive protein. Blood work is also positive for anticyclic citrullinated peptide antibodies. Which of the following is the most likely diagnosis?

   a. septic arthritis

   b. rheumatoid arthritis

   c. psoriatic arthritis

   d. reactive arthritis

   e. scleroderma

299. Epididymitis that occurs as a result of a sexually transmitted disease such as gonorrhea or chlamydia is effectively treated by the combination of doxycycline and which of the following medications?
a. ceftriaxone
b. ACE inhibitors
c. tolterodine
d. ciprofloxacin
e. diuretics

300. A 46-year-old male presents with a persistent nonspecific headache. Physical examination reveals his blood pressure to be 240/126 mmHg. His mental status and neurolgical exams are unremarkable. Which of the following refers to the disorder that is characterized by blood pressure readings of this range?
a. primary hypertension
b. malignant hypertension
c. hypertensive urgency
d. hypertensive emergency
e. pheochromocytoma

Answers and Explanations

Section 1

1. a. Pulmonic stenosis (choice **a**) is a congenital anomaly that usually presents during infancy or childhood. Adults will present with stenosis resulting from rheumatic scarring or connective tissue disease. Adults with pulmonic stenosis will complain of exercise intolerance. Auscultation will reveal a systolic murmur between the second and third left intercostal space radiating to the left shoulder and neck. Auscultation also reveals early pulmonic ejection sound. Choice **b**, tricuspid regurgitation, is incorrect as this condition is associated with soft holosystolic murmur that increases in intensity with inspiration or pressure on the liver. Choice **c**, mitral stenosis, is incorrect as this condition is associated with a mid-diastolic murmur at the apex with little radiation. Auscultation also reveals S1 accentuated opening snap following S2. Choice **d**, aortic regurgitation, is incorrect as this condition is associated with a soft systolic and diastolic decrescendo from the second to the fourth left intercostal space radiating to the apex and right sternal border. Choice **e**, aortic stenosis, is incorrect as this condition is associated with a mid-systolic murmur at the second right intercostal space radiating to the neck and the left sternal border.
Task Area: Formulating Most Likely Diagnosis
Organ System: Cardiovascular

2. a. This question tests your knowledge of acute angle-closure glaucoma treatment. The primary goal is to control intraocular pressure. The correct answer is choice **a**, acetazolamide, which is usually given via IV followed by oral dosing. Choice **b**, antibiotic ointment; choice **d**, topical corticosteroids; and choice **e**, mast cell stabilizer, are incorrect because they are not indicated in this case. Choice **c**, osmotic diuretics, is incorrect because it is not the first-line treatment.

Task Area: Pharmaceutical Therapeutics
Organ System: EENT (Eye, Ear, Nose, and Throat)

3. c. Virchow's node, one of the left supraclavicular lymph nodes, is unique in the fact that it drains several of the abdominal organs rather than the organs that are physically closer to the node. Enlargement of the node may indicate the presence of a gastrointestinal malignancy such as a gastric adenocarcinoma (choice **c**). While there is also a wide range of other differential diagnoses, it is important to consider the possibility of an abdominal cancer in a patient with supraclavicular lymphadenopathy. A right lung cancer (choice **a**) may drain to one of the right supraclavicular nodes, but it is more likely to drain to the hilar lymph nodes. A left forearm melanoma (choice **b**) is unlikely because the forearm mostly drains into one of the many lymph nodes of the arm. Glioblastoma multiforme (choice **d**) is unlikely to metastasize, and in the rare event that it does, it is more likely to drain into one of the lymph nodes of the head and neck. Heart tumors (choice **e**) usually drain to the mediastinal or hilar lymph nodes.

Task Area: Applying Basic Science Concepts
Organ System: Gastrointestinal/Nutritional

4. e. Carcinoid tumor is a neuroendocrine lesion that is often not associated with a history of smoking. It is most commonly found in the gastrointestinal tract, but also often appears in the respiratory tract. Most carcinoid tumors are asymptomatic, but respiratory tumors may present with hemoptysis and anemia. Surgical excision (choice **e**) is the only curative treatment option if the disease has not metastasized. Chemotherapy (choice **a**) is useful if the tumor is metastatic, but surgery is still the first-line option. Radiotherapy (choice **b**) may be used as an adjuvant to surgery. Brachytherapy (choice **c**) is not usually a part of the treatment regimen. Palliative care (choice **d**) may be used in an older patient with widely metastatic disease, but when only a single lesion is present, surgical excision can be curative.

Task Area: Clinical Intervention
Organ System: Pulmonary

5. d. DMARDs (choice **d**), or disease-modifying antirheumatic drugs, are indicated immediately following the diagnosis of rheumatoid arthritis. These medications will slow down the progression of rheumatoid arthritis. Methotrexate, cyclosporin, rituximab, and sulfasalazine are all examples of disease-modifying antirheumatic drugs. Choice **a**, NSAIDs, is incorrect as these are effective in treating the inflammation associated with rheumatoid arthritis but not the underlying disease. Choices **b**, SSRIs, and **c**, MAOIs, are incorrect as they are commonly prescribed as antidepressants. Choice **e**, antibiotics, is incorrect as they are commonly prescribed to treat infections; however, studies have shown that they may have a use for the treatment of rheumatoid arthritis if the disease is triggered by infection.

Task Area: Health Maintenance
Organ System: Musculoskeletal

6. b. The correct answer is choice **b**, gastroesophageal reflux disease. Otherwise referred to as GERD, this disease is characterized by heartburn, regurgitation, and dysphagia. Other symptoms could include hoarseness, halitosis, cough, hiccups, and chest pain. Classic diagnosis of GERD is made if symptoms are relieved with antacids. If patient presents with chest pain, an electrocardiogram is warranted to rule out any potential cardiac abnormality. Choice **a**, reflux esophagitis, is incorrect as this condition is characterized by painful swallowing, excessive belching, hoarseness, and chest pain that is worse when lying flat. Choice **c**, esophageal dysmotility, is incorrect as this condition is characterized by painful swallowing and a constant feeling of a lump in the throat. Choice **d**, esophageal neoplasm, is incorrect as this condition is associated with difficulty swallowing, weight loss, and excessive choking. Choice **e**, gastroparesis, is incorrect as this condition is associated with nausea, vomiting, and feeling full after eating just a few bites.

Task Area: History Taking and Performing
 Physical Examinations
Organ System: Gastrointestinal/Nutritional

7. e. This patient's presentation is typical of hypokalemia, which may present with weakness, fatigue, and palpitations. The typical EKG finding associated with hypokalemia is a flattened T-wave and, in some cases, a narrow QRS complex. Hypokalemia is often caused by thiazide diuretics and loop diuretics such as furosemide (choice **e**). Consequently, regular electrolyte monitoring is important for patients taking a thiazide diuretic or a loop diuretic. Beta blockers such as metoprolol (choice **a**) may cause heart block, but this produces a very different EKG picture. Calcium channel blockers such as nifedipine (choice **b**) are known for drug interactions, tachycardia, and a variety of other cardiovascular effects. Losartan (choice **c**) is an angiotensin receptor blocker that is fairly similar to ramipril in its effect profile. Spironolactone (choice **d**) is a potassium-sparing diuretic; although it may cause hyperkalemia, it does not cause hypokalemia.

Task Area: Pharmaceutical Therapeutics
Organ System: Cardiovascular

8. b. This patient has hay fever, which is a common cause of acute otitis media (AOM) (choice **b**). He appears to have infectious AOM given his physical findings. Choice **a**, acute otitis externa, is incorrect because the external ear canal is without exudates. Choices **c**, cerumen impaction; **d**, ruptured tympanic membrane; and **e**, periauricular cellulitis, are incorrect because they are all inconsistent with the physical findings.

Task Area: History Taking and Performing Physical Examinations
Organ System: EENT (Eye, Ear, Nose, and Throat)

9. b. The correct answer is choice **b**, three consecutive morning sputums for culture. This is the definitive test for presence of *M. tuberculosis*. Therefore, choice **e**, none of the above, is incorrect. Choice **a**, repeat chest X-ray, is incorrect because it is nonspecific, although strongly suggestive. Choice **c**, lung biopsy, is an invasive procedure not indicated for initial diagnosis. Choice **d**, PPD skin test, is incorrect because it only indicates history of exposure to the organism, but does not confirm active disease.

Task Area: Using Laboratory and Diagnostic Studies
Organ System: Pulmonary

10. e. The correct answer is choice **e**, all of the above. Choices **a**, oxygen; **b**, morphine; **c**, aspirin; and **d**, nitroglycerin, are all correct answers and are part of the initial intervention used for patients with chest pain whose origin is likely cardiac.

Task Area: Clinical Intervention
Organ System: Cardiovascular

11. d. This correct answer is choice **d**, oxytocin, which promotes contraction of the uterus and decreases uterine atony. Choices **a**, clopidogrel; **b**, warfarin; and **c**, vitamin K, are incorrect because they are not indicated in this condition. Choice **e**, surgical intervention, is incorrect because the immediate treatment is oxytocin, and surgical intervention, although it may become necessary, is not necessary at this time.

Task Area: Clinical Intervention
Organ System: Reproductive

12. e. The correct answer is choice **e**, transposition of the great vessels, a congenital abnormality in which the aorta and the pulmonary artery are transposed, or switched. Patients with this condition present with blue skin, clubbing of fingers and toes, poor feeding, and shortness of breath. Auscultation of the chest will reveal a single loud S2 and a systolic murmur. Choice **a**, hyaline membrane disease, is associated with rapid, labored grunting respirations, retractions above and below the breastbone, and flaring of the nostrils occurring shortly after delivery. Choice **b**, pulmonary atresia, a form of congenital heart disease in which the pulmonary valve does not form properly, might be a viable option; however, auscultation of the chest should reveal a hyperdyanamic apical impulse and a single S1 and S2 sound. Choice **c**, Tetralogy of Fallot, is often associated with shortness of breath, agitation, dizziness, and fainting. Choice **d**, hypoplastic left heart syndrome, is associated with lethargy, poor pulse, liver enlargement, and tachycardia.

Task Area: History Taking and Performing Physical Examinations

Organ System: Cardiovascular

13. d. This patient has a classic presentation of meningitis, an infection of the cerebrospinal fluid (CSF) that is known to cause fever, headache, and neck stiffness. In infants, neck stiffness often manifests as reduced head movements when visually following a bright object, while headache presents as general irritability. The petechial rash is typical of meningococcal infection, suggesting that the offending pathogen is *Neisseria meningitidis*. In order to reduce the chances of complications, empirical therapy must be started immediately; third-generation cephalosporins (choice **d**) are generally used because of their broad spectrum and their known activity against *Neisseria*. A CSF culture (choice **a**) should be used to help direct antibiotic therapy when it becomes available, but in the meantime, empirical therapy must be used. Blood culture (choice **b**) may be useful in the case of systemic disease, but it is less sensitive than CSF culture. Amoxicillin (choice **c**) is a good option for empirical therapy but is more likely to encounter bacterial resistance. Vancomycin (choice **e**) is particularly effective against Gram-positive bacteria but is not as useful for *Neisseria*.

Task Area: Clinical Intervention

Organ System: Neurologic

14. b. This patient most likely has glandular fever caused by Epstein-Barr virus (EBV). This causes heterophile antibody seroconversion, which is tested for using heterophile serology (choice **b**). The VDRL test (choice **a**) is a test for early stage syphilis. Anti-dsDNA antibodies (choice **e**) are found in lupus. C-reactive protein (choice **c**) and erythrocyte sedimentation rate (choice **d**) are nonspecific inflammatory markers.

Task Area: Using Laboratory and Diagnostic Studies

Organ System: Infectious Diseases

15. a. The correct answer is choice **a**, electrical defibrillation. The rhythm shown on this patient's electrocardiogram is ventricular fibrillation. Ventricular fibrillation is an extreme medical emergency, and electrical defibrillation must be attempted as soon as the defibrillator is available. Choice **b**, IV lidocaine, is routinely used to treat ventricular tachycardia and would not be effective for this ventricular arrhythmia. Choice **c**, IV adenosine, is incorrect as this medication is used to treat supraventricular tachycardia. Choice **d**, cardiac ablation, would not be appropriate as this particular arrhythmia is an extremely emergent condition, and electrical defibrillation is the only appropriate treatment. Choice **e**, cardiac catheterization, is not appropriate as this treatment option is used to assess blockage of coronary arteries and would be ineffective for treatment of ventricular tachycardia.

Task Area: Clinical Intervention
Organ System: Cardiovascular

16. b. The most common inherited cause of chronic renal failure is polycystic kidney disease, which often carries an initial presentation including hypertension, flank pain, and elevated urea and creatinine levels. The diagnosis can usually be confirmed with a renal ultrasound, which will demonstrate a kidney that is littered with cysts of various sizes. Most patients will experience renal failure and require dialysis. Inheritance is autosomal dominant (choice **b**), so it is important to counsel this patient that any of his children will have a 50% chance of developing the disease. Choices **a**, autosomal recessive; **c**, X-linked recessive; **d**, X-linked dominant; and **e**, codonomant inheritance, are not the patterns of inheritance for polycystic kidney disease, but they may describe a variety of other genetic disorders.

Task Area: Applying Basic Science Concepts
Organ System: Genitourinary

17. a. The correct answer is choice **a**, cerebral vascular accident (CVA). This patient's medical history puts him at high risk for CVA. Choice **b**, Alzheimer's disease, is incorrect because there should not be focal neurological deficits as seen in this patient. Choice **c**, Bell's palsy, is incorrect because it is a palsy of facial nerves, and there should not be any central neurological deficits or speech impairment. Choice **d**, Guillain-Barré syndrome (GBS), is incorrect because it usually presents with symmetrical weakness of distal extremities. Choice **e**, meningitis, is incorrect because this patient is afebrile and has focal neurological deficits.

Task Area: Formulating Most Likely Diagnosis
Organ System: Neurologic

18. c. This patient has a classic presentation of testicular torsion, which is an emergent case requiring surgical intervention because of the risk of tissue ischemia. The correct answer is choice **c**, surgical exploration, which should occur within six hours of onset of symptoms to preclude tissue ischemia. Choice **a**, warm compression and observation, is incorrect because this is a surgical emergency. Choice **b**, manual decompression only, is incorrect. Although this may alleviate the pain temporarily, surgery is still indicated to prevent recurrence. Choices **d**, acetaminophen, and **e**, oxycodone, are incorrect because pain medications are not the standard of treatment for this condition.

Task Area: Clinical Intervention
Organ System: Genitourinary

19. c. The KOH preparation showing hyphae is diagnostic for tinea corporis, a fungal skin condition. The correct answer is choice **c**, topical antifungal cream. Choice **e**, none of the above, is therefore incorrect. Choice **a**, topical corticosteroid cream, is incorrect because this will make the lesion worse by facilitating fungal growth. Choice **b**, topical antibiotic cream, is incorrect because tinea corporis is fungal in nature. Choice **d**, complete excision, is incorrect because tinea corporis is nonmalignant and can be treated with topical antifungal medication.

Task Area: Pharmaceutical Therapeutics
Organ System: Dermatologic

20. d. The correct answer is choice **d**, numbness of the third and fourth toes. Morton's neuroma is an abnormal thickening of the nerve tissue that commonly occurs between the third and fourth toes. The pain associated with this disorder can commonly be treated with soft metatarsal pads in the shoes or steroid injections in the affected area. If conservative treatment fails, surgical removal of the neuroma is warranted; however, this may cause permanent numbness of the third and fourth toes. Choices **a**, disfigured toes; **b**, discolored toes; **c**, pain between the third and fourth toes; and **e**, total foot numbness, are all incorrect as these are not permanent side effects of surgical removal of Morton's neuroma.

Task Area: Clinical Intervention
Organ System: Musculoskeletal

21. a. Alpha-fetoprotein (choice **a**) is usually elevated in nonseminomas. Prostate-specific antigen (choice **b**) is elevated in BPH and prostate cancer. S-100 (choice **c**) is elevated in tumors of the neural crest. Carcinoembryonic antigen (choice **d**) is a tumor marker for many cancers, including colorectal and medullary thyroid cancer. Carbohydrate antigen 19-9 (choice **e**) is a marker for colon and pancreatic cancer.

Task Area: Using Laboratory and Diagnostic Studies
Organ System: Reproductive

22. c. The correct answer is choice **c**, Interferon-β, which is the medication primarily used to prevent relapses of moderate or severe attacks stemming from multiple sclerosis. Choice **a**, anti-inflammatory medications, can be used to relieve pain associated with spasticity that can lead to muscle cramping or tight, aching joints associated with multiple sclerosis, but they are generally ineffective in preventing an attack from the disease. Choice **b**, corticosteroids, are used periodically to treat symptoms associated with multiple sclerosis, but they do not prevent relapses of attacks. Choice **d**, cyclophosphamide, is a chemotherapeutic drug used to treat several types of cancers and is believed to have positive effects for multiple sclerosis patients, but proper clinical evidence is not available to warrant the use of this medication for multiple sclerosis patients. Choice **e**, amantadine, is used to relieve fatigue associated with multiple sclerosis but is ineffective in preventing an attack from the disease.

Task Area: Pharmaceutical Therapeutics
Organ System: Neurologic

23. c. This patient's symptoms would normally be suggestive of hyperthyroidism; however, due to normal levels of thyroid hormone and TSH, excessive sympathetic stimulation appears to be more likely. Because of the excess levels of catecholamines and epinephrine derivatives, it is reasonable to believe that the patient has a pheochromocytoma, an epinephrine-secreting tumor of the adrenal glands. Pheochromocytoma is very difficult to treat with medical therapy, and the treatment of choice is surgical removal of the adrenal gland (choice **c**). Antithyroid therapy (choice **a**) and thyroidectomy (choice **b**) may be options if the patient's symptoms were caused by hyperthyroidism, but this is unlikely due to the normal thyroid hormone levels. Parasympathetic stimulation (choice **d**) and sympathetic blockade (choice **e**) may help to improve her symptoms, but neither will provide a long-term solution.

Task Area: Clinical Intervention
Organ System: Endocrine

24. d. The correct answer is choice **d**, binge eating. Sympathomimetic drugs have an anorexic effect in humans, which makes them a preferred treatment for binge eating. Medications included in this class of drugs are amphetamine, detxroamphetamine, phentermine, phendimetrazine, and bezphetamine. Sympathomimetic drugs are substances that mimic the effects of the sympathetic nervous system. As such, they are also commonly used to treat cardiac arrest and low blood pressure and to delay preterm labor. Choice **a**, body dysmorphic disorder, is a form of obsessive-compulsive disorder that is commonly treated with cognitive behavioral therapy. Choice **b**, bulimia nervosa, is commonly treated with drugs such as Prozac, Topamax, and Effexor. Choice **c**, anorexia nervosa, is commonly treated with buproprion because sympathomimetics may exacerbate the anorexic condition and lower the seizure threshold for patients with anorexia. Choice **e**, emaciation, is incorrect because sympathomimetic drugs have an appetite suppression quality, which would worsen emaciation instead of treating this disorder.
Task Area: Pharmaceutical Therapeutics
Organ System: Psychiatry/Behavioral Science

25. b. Alcohol can excerbate and trigger seizures, so alcohol cessation (choice **b**) would be most helpful for this patient's condition. There is no evidence supporting weight loss (choice **a**), smoking cessation (choice **c**), exercise (choice **d**), or yoga (choice **e**) as treatments for epilepsy.
Task Area: Health Maintenance
Organ System: Neurologic

26. b. Long-term topical corticosteroid use has many local side effects resulting from protein breakdown and immune suppression. These include acne (choice **a**), dry skin (choice **c**), fungal infection (choice **d**), and pruritus (choice **e**), but not albinism (choice **b**).
Task Area: Pharmaceutical Therapeutics
Organ System: Dermatologic

27. a. Immune thrombocytopenic purpura (ITP) causes an immune-mediated sequestration and subsequent destruction of circulating platelets within the spleen. This condition is usually treated with immunosuppressive medications. If medical therapy fails, splenectomy (choice **a**) is indicated. Bone marrow transplant (choice **b**) can cause graft-versus-host disease and worsen ITP. Liver transplant (choice **c**), kidney transplant (choice **d**), and ileostomy (choice **e**) have no effect on ITP.
Task Area: Clinical Intervention
Organ System: Hematologic

28. a. Uterine prolapse (choice **a**) is more common among Caucasian women than among those of African-American or Asian descent. Conditions that increase intra-abdominal pressure, such as obesity and chronic cough, may facilitate prolapse. Symptoms associated with prolapse are vaginal fullness, lower abdominal aching, low back pain, and the sensation of sitting on a ball. Choice **b**, leiomyomata (benign fibroids in the uterine wall), may be associated with painful, abnormal heavy bleeding between menstrual periods. Choice **c**, endometriosis, might be considered; however, the finding of a dropped uterus should rule this out. Choice **d**, adenomyosis, should be excluded because this disorder is associated with painful sexual intercourse, painful periods, and prolonged menstrual bleeding. Choice **e**, polycystic ovarian syndrome, should be excluded based on symptoms, as this disorder is associated with hirsutism, infertility, truncal obesity, irregular menstruation, and skin discoloration.
Task Area: Formulating Most Likely Diagnosis
Organ System: Reproductive

29. b. Rickets (choice **b**) is a disease of defective bone mineralization that occurs in children. Children can present with skull deformity and rib-breastbone joint enlargement, and can have developmental issues such as delays in sitting, walking, and crawling. Blood work will reveal decreased calcium and vitamin D. X-rays can reveal flattened skull, bowing of long bones, and dorsal kyphosis. Choice **a**, osteomalacia, should be considered because the presentation is identical to rickets; however, this condition primarily affects the adult population. Choice **c**, Paget's disease, should not be a consideration because the X-rays would show bone enlargements. Paget's disease is also associated with an elevated alkaline phosphatase blood level. Choice **d**, osteoporosis, should be ruled out simply based on the age of the patient. Choice **e**, osteomyelitis, should be ruled out because this disease is associated with fever and redness and swelling over the painful bony area.
Task Area: History Taking and Performing Physical Examinations
Organ System: Endocrine

30. c. Individuals who suffer from schizophrenia (choice **c**) may show enlarged ventricles and cortical atrophy on a CT scan that may be indicative of chronic schizophrenic disease. Choice **a**, bipolar disorder, is incorrect as CT scanning has no value in the diagnosis of this condition. Bipolar disorder is diagnosed by physical examination and by medical and psychiatric history. Choice **b**, attention deficit disorder (ADD), is incorrect as CT scanning will have no diagnostic value in the diagnosis of this disorder. ADD is diagnosed by physical exam, history, and symptoms. Choices **d**, obsessive-compulsive disorder, and **e**, anorexia nervosa, are incorrect as CT scanning will have no diagnostic value for this disorder. Diagnosis of these conditions is based on medical history, symptoms, and the patient's behavior.

Task Area: Using Laboratory and Diagnostic Studies

Organ System: Psychiatry/Behavioral Science

31. e. Abruptio placentae (choice **e**), or placental abruption, is a condition in which the placenta prematurely separates from the uterus. It occurs in approximately 1% of pregnancies and leads to painful uterine contractions along with bleeding. In some cases, the fetus is already dead upon presentation; however, the presence of a normal fetal heartbeat suggests that this fetus is viable. In most cases, the patient should be managed with an emergency cesarean delivery and hemorrhage control. Premature labor (choice **a**) is unlikely to cause vaginal bleeding and will usually lead to cervical dilation. Braxton-Hicks contractions (choice **b**), or "false labor," are also unlikely to cause bleeding or changes in fetal movement. Placenta previa (choice **d**), a condition in which the placenta obstructs the path between the fetus and the cervix, usually causes painless vaginal bleeding. Vasa previa (choice **c**) is a similar condition in which the obstruction is caused by the fetal vessels, leading to a presentation that is similar to that of placenta previa.

Task Area: Formulating Most Likely Diagnosis

Organ System: Reproductive

32. b. Dysthymic disorder (choice **b**) is characterized by a patient being in a depressed mood for most of the day, more days than not, for a period exceeding over two years. Symptoms may include poor concentration, indecisiveness, hopelessness, poor appetite, overeating, insomnia, hypersomnia, low energy, fatigue, and lack of self-esteem. Choice **a**, bipolar disorder, is incorrect as this condition is characterized by mood swings from excessively high periods or mania to excessively low periods or depression. Choice **c**, cyclothymic disorder, is incorrect as this condition is a milder form of bipolar disorder, with the symptoms being less dramatic than those of bipolar disorder. Choice **d**, adjustment disorder, is incorrect as this condition is characterized by agitation and depression that occurs within three months of a stressor such as divorce or the death of a loved one. Choice **e**, narcissistic personality disorder, is incorrect as this condition is characterized by increased self-importance, need for admiration, and self-absorption.

Task Area: History Taking and Performing Physical Examinations

Organ System: Psychiatry/Behavioral Science

33. c. The correct answer is choice **c**, intravenous calcium gluconate. Intravenous administration of 10–20 mL of 10% calcium gluconate over ten minutes should remedy this situation. Calcium directly antagonizes the neuromuscular and cardiovascular effects of magnesium. Use for patients with symptomatic hypermagnesemia that is causing cardiac effects or respiratory distress. Choices **a**, intravenous sodium chloride; **b**, intravenous potassium chloride; **d**, intravenous 5% dextrose solution; and **e**, intravenous heparin, are all incorrect as these will have no therapeutic effects on hypermagnesemia.

Task Area: Pharmaceutical Therapeutics

Organ System: Genitourinary

34. d. The correct answer is choice **d**, avoid sharing contact items. To avoid transmission of pediculosis (or lice infestation), one must avoid sharing contact items such as hats, hairbrushes, and combs. If transmission is suspected, all shared items should be examined for infestation. Choices **a**, **b**, **c**, and **e** are all incorrect as the majority of cases of pediculosis are transmitted through the sharing of contact items such as hats, combs, and hairbrushes. None of the other answer options would eliminate the transmission of pediculosis.

Task Area: Health Maintenance

Organ System: Dermatologic

35. c. Polycythemia vera (choice **c**) is classically associated with splenomegaly, normal arterial oxygen saturation, and elevated red cell mass. Patients with this disorder may present with headache, dizziness, weakness, fatigue, tinnitus, and blurred vision. Physical examination will reveal flushing, systolic hypertension, engorged retinal veins, and splenomegaly. Choice **a**, thrombocytopenia, is incorrect as this condition is characterized by a low platelet level, and patients experience excessive bleeding and bruising. Choice **b**, hemolytic anemia, is incorrect as this condition is characterized by abnormal paleness of the skin, jaundice of the skin, eyes, and mouth, and a brownish color to the urine, all due to the breakdown of RBCs. Choice **d**, leukemia, is incorrect as individuals with this condition experience not only fatigue, but also susceptibility to infection, fever, chills, and unexplained weight loss. Choice **e**, hemophilia, is incorrect as this condition is characterized by excessive bleeding, excessive deep bruising, and joint pain.

Task Area: History Taking and Performing Physical Examinations

Organ System: Hematologic

36. a. Diabetes mellitus is a strikingly common disease that is often diagnosed and managed in the primary care setting. For this reason, the American Diabetes Association has established a clear set of diagnostic criteria. In a patient with the classic diabetic triad of polyuria, polydipsia, and weight loss (and, in some cases, polyphagia), the diagnosis can be established with a single random blood glucose level over 200 mg/dL (11 mmol/L) (choice **a**), a single fasting plasma glucose level of over 125 mg/dL (7 mmol/L), or a glucose tolerance test result of over 200 mg/dL (11 mmol/L). Choices **b**, **c**, **d**, and **e** are incorrect because no additional information is necessary in order for this patient's diagnosis to be confirmed.

Task Area: Using Laboratory and Diagnostic Studies

Organ System: Endocrine

37. b. This question tests your knowledge of indication for a cervical cerclage. The correct answer is choice **b**, cervical insufficiency. Cerclage, also known as a cervical stitch, is a surgical procedure used to reinforce the cervix to prevent the risk of miscarriage. All the other options are incorrect because cervical cerclage is only indicated in cervical insufficiency.

Task Area: Clinical Intervention

Organ System: Reproductive

38. d. The correct answer is choice **d**, esophageal manometry. Achalasia is a motility disorder of the esophagus. Typical findings of achalasia include complete absence of peristalsis; swallowing results in simultaneous waves of low amplitude and incomplete lower esophageal sphincteric relaxation with swallowing. Choice **a**, chest/abdominal X-ray, is incorrect because it can be inconclusive, although it may show air-fluid level. Choice **b**, upper endoscopy, is incorrect because it is not the best option to access motility disorders. Choices **c**, abdominal ultrasound, and **e**, chest/abdominal CT, are incorrect because they are also not optimal to access motility disorders.

Task Area: Using Laboratory and Diagnostic Studies

Organ System: Gastrointestinal/Nutritional

39. b. This question tests your knowledge of physical exam findings in carpal tunnel syndrome (CTS). CTS is a condition caused by compression of the median nerve as it travels through the carpal tunnel. The correct answer is choice **b**, positive Tinel's sign. A physical exam is usually positive for Phalen's test and Tinel's sign. Choice **a**, negative Phalen's test, is incorrect because the most likely finding is a positive Tinel's sign and a positive Phalen's test. Choice **c**, positive Heberden's nodes, and choice **d**, positive Bouchard's nodes, are incorrect because they are found in arthritis. Choice **e**, positive Baker's cyst, is incorrect because it pertains to the popliteal area of the knee.

Task Area: History Taking and Performing Physical Examinations

Organ System: Musculoskeletal

40. d. The correct answer is choice **d**, tension pneumothorax. A tension pneumothorax is a medical emergency. If a tension pneumothorax is suspected, immediate decompression with a large bore needle is required to allow air to move out of the chest so the lung can re-expand. Once the tension pneumothorax has been decompressed, a chest tube should be inserted to insure proper inflation of the lung. Choice **a**, closed pneumothorax, may simply be treated with oxygen breathing in an attempt to reinflate the lung; if this fails, chest tube insertion may be required. Choice **b**, spontaneous pneumothorax, is treated with chest tube insertion to reinflate the lung. Choice **c**, hemopneumothorax, is treated with a chest tube in order to drain the blood from the cavity and to reinflate the lung. Choice **e**, primary pneumothorax, is classically treated with chest tube insertion.

Task Area: Clinical Intervention

Organ System: Pulmonary

41. e. The correct answer is choice **e**, pinguecula. This disorder is characterized by a yellowish, fleshy mass on the conjunctiva adjacent to the cornea. In addition, pinguecula can lead to painless inflammation. Choice **a**, blepharitis, is incorrect because this disorder is characterized by redness around the rims of the eyelid and possible scaly, dandruff-like deposits. Choice **b**, viral conjunctivitis, can be ruled out because this disorder is characterized by redness of the conjunctiva and watery discharge in the affected eye. Choice **c**, bacterial conjunctivitis, can be ruled out because this disorder is characterized by a purulent discharge in one or both eyes. Choice **d**, pterygium, might be a possibility. However, this is a vascular, triangular-shaped mass that can interfere with vision if it crosses the corneal limbus.

Task Area: History Taking and Performing Physical Examinations

Organ System: EENT (Eye, Ear, Nose, and Throat)

42. e. The correct answer is choice **e**, over 5 years. For individuals who have been diagnosed with hookworms, pyrantel is an effective medication for any patient over 5 years of age. Pyrantel should not be administered to individuals under the age of 5. Individuals under the age of 5 who contract hookworms should be treated with mebendazole or albendazole. Choices **a**, **b**, **c**, and **d** are all incorrect.

Task Area: Pharmaceutical Therapeutics

Organ System: Infectious Diseases

43. e. This patient's pain appears to be ischemic in nature. Because the pain seems to appear at rest, the most likely diagnosis is unstable angina. However, it is important to exclude the possibility of coronary artery vasospasm (also known as Prinzmetal's angina), which requires a different treatment regimen. It is very difficult to make this distinction clinically, but the presence of significant atherosclerotic plaques on coronary angiography (choice **e**) is strongly suggestive of unstable angina rather than coronary vasospasm. Electrocardiogram (choice **a**) may demonstrate ischemic changes in either condition, but it cannot be used to distinguish unstable angina from coronary artery vasospasm. Echocardiogram (choice **b**) is used to study the heart's flow dynamics and is not useful to test for coronary artery disease. An exercise stress test (choice **c**) is somewhat more specific for unstable angina, but may still be abnormal in cases of Prinzmetal's angina. Inflammatory markers (choice **d**) may be elevated if a vasculitis is implicated in this patient's condition, but they are not specific for either condition.

Task Area: Using Laboratory and Diagnostic Studies
Organ System: Cardiovascular

44. d. In a young patient with sudden onset of dyspnea following blunt trauma, it is important to consider the possibility of tension pneumothorax due to a rib fracture. Furthermore, the presence of reduced air entry and contralateral tracheal deviation are fairly specific signs of tension pneumothorax. Thoracentesis (choice **d**) is usually an effective intervention to provide a route for excess air to escape the pleural cavity. Thrombolytic therapy (choice **a**) would be useful for a pulmonary embolism, which is unlikely in this case based on the physical examination findings. Inhaled albuterol (choice **b**) or corticosteroids (choice **c**) are useful options for an asthma attack, which is likely to present with a bilateral wheeze and no tracheal deviation. A blood transfusion (choice **e**) may be an option if the patient's dyspnea is related to anemia, possibly due to blood loss, but this is unlikely to appear so rapidly.

Task Area: Clinical Intervention
Organ System: Pulmonary

45. b. The correct answer is choice **b**, colonoscopy. The key differential diagnosis in this case is colorectal cancer, the third most common cancer and the second most common cause of cancer deaths in the United States. It is particularly common in patients over 50 years of age and often presents with generalized abdominal pain. A positive FOBT (fecal occult blood test) alone is often an adequate indication for a colonoscopy; the patient's symptoms make the presence of a cancer fairly likely. Cancer in the right (proximal) colon generally causes weight loss and blood loss anemia, while cancer in the left (distal) colon or the rectum is more likely to cause symptoms associated with bowel obstruction. Because this patient's symptoms are mostly related to bleeding, the obstruction is most likely to be in the proximal colon; consequently, a sigmoidoscopy (choice **a**) is unlikely to detect the pathological process. Imaging (choices **c**, **d**, and **e**) is fairly insensitive and nonspecific.

Task Area: Using Laboratory and Diagnostic Studies
Organ System: Gastrointestinal/Nutritional

46. c. A cataract is a dense clouding in the lens that generally causes a reduction in visual acuity that cannot be improved with corrective lenses. This is a fairly common condition that can only be treated with surgical replacement of the old lens with an artificial implant, a procedure that is commonly known as cataract surgery (choice **c**). If left untreated, the cataract progressively increases in density and continues to reduce the patient's visual acuity. Myopia (choice **a**) is another very common cause of reduced visual acuity that is usually corrected with glasses or contact lenses, but symptoms of myopia are usually improved with the use of a pinhole occluder. Glaucoma (choice **b**) is an optic neuropathy caused by increased intraocular pressure, but this affects visual fields rather than visual acuity. Corneal transplant (choice **d**) does not provide any benefit for a patient with cataracts. Laser photocoagulation (choice **e**) is usually used for diabetic eye disease and other retinal conditions.

Task Area: Clinical Intervention
Organ System: EENT (Eye, Ear, Nose, and Throat)

47. d. You should first gauge the patient's willingness to stop smoking (choice **d**) before you offer potential strategies (choices **b** and **c**). His anxiety is most likely affected by the fear of a myocardial infarction, which can be alleviated simply with reassurance. Yoga (choice **e**) is not necessary. The health of your patient should be your main concern, not his brother-in-law (choice **a**).

Task Area: Health Maintenance
Organ System: Cardiovascular

48. e. Polymyalgia rheumatica is a self-limiting condition that usually resolves after a few years, but 25% of patients eventually experience a resurgence of symptoms. Most patients will benefit from non-steroidal anti-inflammatory drugs (NSAIDs) for pain relief, but corticosteroids such as prednisone (choice **e**) are also known to be useful for long-term therapy. Because long-term systemic corticosteroid therapy has been associated with a wide range of adverse effects, it is important to reduce the dosage or slowly taper then stop the treatment after the patient's condition eventually improves. Unlike other autoimmune conditions, polymyalgia rheumatica does not usually respond well to therapy with other immunosuppressive drugs such as methotrexate (choice **a**) and cyclophosphamide (choice **b**). Sulfasalazine (choice **c**) is generally only used for ankylosing spondylitis and inflammatory bowel disease. Infliximab (choice **d**) is a monoclonal antibody that is an excellent (but expensive) therapeutic option for other rheumatoid conditions because of its small side effect profile, but it is not useful for polymyalgia rheumatica.
Task Area: Pharmaceutical Therapeutics
Organ System: Musculoskeletal

49. b. Cystic fibrosis is caused by a mutation in the CFTR gene, which codes for chlorine ion channels (choice **b**). Defective water channels (choice **a**) are seen in some congenital cardiomyopathies. Defective sugar metabolism (choice **c**) can describe diabetes. Many diseases can have defective immune systems (choice **d**) and defective DNA repair mechanisms (choice **e**), but neither is characteristic of cystic fibrosis.
Task Area: Applying Basic Science Concepts
Organ System: Pulmonary

50. c. ASCA (choice **c**) is more commonly found in Crohn's disease than in any other condition. cANCA (choice **a**) is not associated with a gastrointestinal disease. pANCA (choice **b**) is found in ulcerative colitis. Anti-tTG (choice **d**) is found in celiac disease. Anti-dsDNA (choice **e**) is found in systemic lupus erythematosus (SLE).
Task Area: Using Laboratory and Diagnostic Studies
Organ System: Gastrointestinal/Nutritional

51. d. The first step in the management of any foreign body in the eye is a saline washout (choice **d**). Use of a slit lamp to detect and remove remaining foreign objects (choice **e**) should be done after the washout and requires both antibiotics (choice **a**) and local anesthesia (choice **b**). Surgical correction of a lens defect (choice **c**) should only be performed if there is evidence of a lens defect.
Task Area: Clinical Intervention
Organ System: EENT (Eye, Ear, Nose, and Throat)

52. c. Olecranon bursitis (choice **c**) is caused by an acute injury or repetitive trauma to the olecranon bursa. The most common finding is inflammation overlying the olecranon bursa. There may or may not be pain associated with this condition. Choices **a**, lateral epicondylitis, and **b**, medial epicondylitis, might also be a considered; however, in either case the swelling would be appreciated in the epicondyle area instead of the olecranon area. Choice **d**, avascular necrosis, is normally associated with severe disease, injury, or trauma to the area that has affected the blood supply to the area. Choice **e**, fibromyalgia, should be excluded because in order to be diagnosed with this disorder, the patient must have pain in at least 11 of 18 areas including buttocks, chests, thighs, and ribcage for a duration of at least three months.

Task Area: Formulating Most Likely Diagnosis
Organ System: Musculoskeletal

53. a. Fluoroquinolone medications (choice **a**) such as norfloxacin are antibiotic medications that are used commonly for first-line defense against infections of the urinary tract and prostate. Choice **b**, ceftriaxone, is incorrect as these antibiotics are most used to prevent infections during surgical procedures, as well as for treating conditions such as osteomyelitis and otitis media. Choice **c**, ACE inhibitors, is incorrect as these medications are taken to establish protection of the heart muscle, particularly in patients with congestive heart failure. Choice **d**, doxycycline, is incorrect as these antibiotics are used to treat disorders such as acne, malaria, and anthrax. Choice **e**, diuretics, is incorrect as these medications are used to rid the body of excess fluids and have no antibiotic effect.

Task Area: Pharmaceutical Therapeutics
Organ System: Genitourinary

54. c. This patient's presentation is typical of dilated cardiomyopathy, a common nonischemic cardiomyopathy that involves stretching of the myocardium as it fails to accommodate the demands of the systemic circulation. In particular, the low pulse pressure (small difference between systolic and diastolic blood pressures), the jugular venous distention, and the demonstrated cardiomegaly are highly suggestive of dilated cardiomyopathy. Although this condition is often idiopathic, one of the most common causes is a long history of excessive alcohol consumption (choice **c**). Age (choice **a**) is not a critical risk factor for dilated cardiomyopathy; it presents in patients of a wide variety of ages. BMI (choice **b**) may be a contributing risk factor, but is less likely to contribute to nonischemic heart disease. Tobacco smoking (choice **d**) promotes coronary atherosclerosis, but again, it is less likely to cause nonischemic disease. Occasional cannabis use (choice **e**) is not clearly associated with any significant cardiovascular risk.

Task Area: History Taking and Performing Physical Examinations
Organ System: Cardiovascular

55. b. This patient's presentation is typical of pulmonary fibrosis, a group of restrictive lung diseases caused by alveolar deposition of foreign substances that cannot be effectively removed by the immune system. Pulmonary fibrosis usually presents with a chronic cough associated with dyspnea, bibasal crackles, and a honeycomb appearance on a chest CT. Restrictive lung diseases also feature an increased FEV_1/FVC ratio. While the disease is usually idiopathic, there are a few known iatrogenic causes; the most significant of these are bleomycin (choice **b**) and amiodarone. Patients who have been on regular therapy with either of these drugs are at a very high risk of developing pulmonary fibrosis later in life. Choices **a**, **c**, and **d** are incorrect because these drugs are not associated with an increased incidence of pulmonary fibrosis. Hormone replacement therapy (choice **e**) is believed to lead to a slight increase in the risk of breast and ovarian cancer, which may present with lung metastases, but this is uncommon and is not consistent with this patient's presentation.
Task Area: Pharmaceutical Therapeutics
Organ System: Pulmonary

56. d. In the presence of a sore throat and a fever, tonsillar inflammation is generally suggestive of a diagnosis of tonsillitis. However, because of the exacerbation of this patient's symptoms after a week of apparent tonsillitis, it is reasonable to believe that the infection has spread. The inability to open the mouth fully, also known as trismus, is fairly specific for a peritonsillar abscess (choice **d**), a purulent abscess that often forms in the space posterior to the tonsil. Vocal distortion is also a common feature of a peritonsillar abscess. Pharyngitis (choice **a**) is likely to present with difficulty swallowing, along with fever and lymphadenopathy as initial signs and symptoms. Laryngitis (choice **b**) generally presents with vocal changes early on and may develop into tonsillitis later. A dental abscess (choice **c**) is likely to be localized to the teeth and gingiva. Mononucleosis (choice **e**) is a systemic infection that includes lymph node swelling, but it is unlikely to feature the other symptoms mentioned.
Task Area: Formulating Most Likely Diagnosis
Organ System: EENT (Eye, Ear, Nose, and Throat)

57. c. The correct answer is choice **c**, depleted blood volume, in this case (with no evidence of blood loss) possibly due to dehydration or to the vasodilative effect of medications, such as ACEIs or CCBs, which can cause a relative hypovolemia. Relative hypovolemia, also known as distributive shock, is hypotension caused by excessive blood vessel dilation, which results in tissue hypoxia. If a patient who is diagnosed with postural hypotension experiences a pulse rate increase of more than 15 bpm moving from a sitting to a standing position, depleted blood volume is the cause of postural hypotension. If the patient experiences no change in pulse rate, the cause of postural hypotension may include medications, central nervous system disease, or peripheral neuropathy. Choices **a**, **b**, and **d** are incorrect because postural hypotension caused by these conditions is not associated with increase in pulse rate. Choice **e**, cardiac arrhythmia, may be a consideration; however, dizziness caused by cardiac arrhythmia is generally not associated with transition from sitting to standing position.
Task Area: Applying Basic Science Concepts
Organ System: Cardiovascular

58. a. The correct answer is choice **a**, coal worker's pneumoconiosis. Pneumoconiosis is an occupational, restrictive lung disease caused by the inhalation of dust, which is very common among coal miners. This disorder is characterized by progressive shortness of breath with inspiratory crackles. A chest X-ray will reveal small opacities in the upper lung fields. Choice **b**, cystic fibrosis, is incorrect because of the age of the patient; cystic fibrosis patients typically have a life expectancy of much less than 60 years, so it would be extremely unlikely that a 62-year-old patient would have cystic fibrosis. The lack of symptoms such as distended abdomen and persistent cough also rule this out. Choice **c**, sarcoidosis, is incorrect because of the lack of symptoms such as fatigue, weight loss, fever, and skin lesions. Choice **d**, silicosis, might be a consideration; however, this condition is often associated with cough, fever, cyanosis, and pulmonary edema. Choice **e**, pneumonia, should be excluded due to lack of symptoms such as productive cough, fever, and chest pain.
Task Area: Formulating Most Likely Diagnosis
Organ System: Pulmonary

59. b. Diarrhea (choice **b**) is the gastrointestinal disorder that is characterized by increased volume and frequency of stool. Diarrhea may be caused by infectious, toxic, or dietary agents. Typically, diarrhea is diagnosed after a period of two to three days of three or more liquid or semisolid stools per day. Choice **a**, malabsorption, is incorrect as this condition is characterized by the body's inability to absorb nutrients from food. Choice **c**, volvulus, is incorrect as this condition is characterized by a bowel obstruction caused by a twist in the intestine. Choice **d**, constipation, is incorrect as this condition is characterized by infrequent and difficult bowel movements. Choice **e**, obstipation, is incorrect as this condition is characterized by severe constipation or intestinal blockage.

Task Area: Applying Basic Science Concepts
Organ System: Gastrointestinal/Nutritional

60. c. A minimally displaced tibial fracture can be treated conservatively with a functional cast brace (choice **c**). A full leg cast (choice **a**) is considered to be less beneficial since it causes muscle weakness and increases the risk of a pulmonary embolism. Acetaminophen (choice **e**) may help with the pain caused by the fracture, but it is not the definitive managment. Arthroscopy (choice **b**) and open reduction (choice **d**) are interventions reserved for severely displaced fractures of the tibial plateau.

Task Area: Clinical Intervention
Organ System: Musculoskeletal

Section 2

61. c. This question tests your knowledge of the treatment of pelvic inflammatory disease (PID). The appropriate treatment for PID is an antibiotic, so the correct answer is choice **c**, doxycycline. Therefore, choice **e**, none of the above, is incorrect. Choice **a**, abstinence, is incorrect because abstaining from sex will not treat PID. Choices **b**, metronidazole, and **d**, ciprofloxacin, are incorrect because they are ineffective in treating *Chlamydia trachomatis*.

Task Area: Pharmaceutical Therapeutics
Organ System: Reproductive

62. a. The correct answer is choice **a**, niacin. The B-complex vitamin niacin has been proven clinically effective for treatment of hypertriglyceridemia. Administration of at least 1.5 grams/day can reduce triglyceride levels by up to 50%. Note, however, that niacin is contraindicated in patients with active peptic ulcer disease. Choices **b**, **c**, **d**, and **e** are all incorrect, as consumption of any of these vitamins will have little to no benefit for treatment of hypertriglyceridemia.

Task Area: Health Maintenance
Organ System: Endocrine

63. c. Hypochondriasis (choice **c**) is a disorder in which a patient has an irrational fear of contracting a serious illness. This disorder is commonly associated with anxiety and depression. The patient continues to have fear of disease even though a physical examination reveals no cause. Choice **a**, conversion disorder, should be ruled out because this disorder is characterized by an unexplained condition of the nervous system such as blindness, numbness, or paralysis. Choice **b**, factitious disorder, should not be considered because this disorder is characterized by an individual falsely claiming to suffer from various medical conditions in order to gain hospital admission and medical treatment. Choice **d**, pain disorder, should be ruled out because this disease is characterized by an individual experiencing chronic pain without explanation. Choice **e**, malingering, should be ruled out because this disorder is characterized by an individual exaggerating or fabricating pain or illness for secondary purposes such as avoiding school, avoiding work, obtaining drugs, or obtaining a lighter criminal sentence.

Task Area: Formulating Most Likely Diagnosis
Organ System: Psychiatry/Behavioral Science

64. a. A pleural effusion occurs when excess fluid accumulates in the pleural cavity. Based on this patient's history of congestive heart failure, this is likely due to pressure buildup in the pulmonary vasculature. While the pleural fluid usually provides a smooth lubrication for movement of the parietal pleura and the visceral pleura, disruption of the normal composition of pleural fluid leads to disruption of its lubricating effect. The consequence is a breath sound known as a pleural friction rub (choice **a**), which is generated by the force of friction between the two layers of pleura. Decreased breath sounds (choice **b**) can also be found in a pleural effusion, but this is a very nonspecific sign that can suggest almost any pulmonary diagnosis. Basal crackles (choice **c**) are another nonspecific sign that may signify pulmonary edema, pneumonia, pulmonary fibrosis, or a range of other possibilities. Hyperresonance to percussion (choice **d**) is unlikely to be found in a pleural effusion; percussion is more likely to reveal dullness because of fluid buildup. Tachypnea (choice **e**) is likely to be present in any patient with shortness of breath, so this sign would not provide a great deal of additional information.

Task Area: History Taking and Performing Physical Examinations
Organ System: Pulmonary

65. c. Metronidazole (choice **c**) is a medication with antibiotic, antiprotozoal, and amebicide properties, which makes it the most appropriate medical treatment for giardiasis. Choice **a**, praziquantel, is incorrect as this medication is the most appropriate treatment for schistosomiasis, which is a parasitic infection characterized by fever, chills, and enlargement of the liver, spleen, and lymph nodes. This condition is uncommon in the United States. Choice **b**, paromomycin, is incorrect as this medication is used to treat amoebiasis, which is associated with bloody and mucus-filled diarrhea. Choice **d**, mebendazole, is incorrect as this medication is used for treatment of roundworm, hookworm, and pinworm. Choice **e**, ketoconazole, is incorrect as this medication is most commonly used to treat yeast infections of the skin, mouth, blood, and urinary tract.

Task Area: Pharmaceutical Therapeutics
Organ System: Gastrointestinal/Nutritional

66. b. This question tests your knowledge of side effects of OCPs. The correct answer is choice **b**, cigarette smoking, which when combined with OCP use increases the risk of thrombotic events. All the other options are incorrect as none of these factors are known to increase the risk of carciovascular and thrombotic events when combined with OCP use.

Task Area: Health Maintenance
Organ System: Cardiovascular

67. c. *Helicobacter pylori* (choice **c**) is the Gram-negative, spiral-shaped bacillus that is responsible for most gastric ulcers and chronic gastritis. This type of bacterium can inhabit many areas of the stomach, but it is primarily found in the antrum. Choice **a**, *Lactobacillus rhamnosus*, is incorrect as this is a friendly bacterium found in healthy human intestines. Choice **b**, *Lactobacillus acidophilus*, is also a friendly bacteria found in the intestines of healthy animals and humans. Choice **d**, *Streptococcus agalactiae*, is incorrect as this bacterium is native to the female urogenital tract and rectum. Choice **e**, *Legionella pneumophila*, is incorrect as this bacterium is the causative agent of Legionnaire's disease.

Task Area: Applying Basic Science Concepts
Organ System: Gastrointestinal/Nutrition

68. e. Abdominal aortic aneurysm (choice **e**) is a very serious condition that is associated with a very poor prognosis in the event of rupture; however, if the aneurysm is detected prior to rupture, it can be corrected with surgery. The pain is generally mild, but it can be characterized by its pulsating nature and central location. A pulsating central abdominal mass on physical examination is a fairly specific sign. Umbilical hernia (choice **a**) is another possible cause of a central abdominal mass, but this mass is unlikely to be pulsating. Rhabdomyolysis (choice **b**) is a rare complication of atorvastatin therapy, but again, it is unlikely to produce a pulsating mass. Gastric carcinoma (choice **c**) is not usually palpable on physical examination and usually presents with a very different set of symptoms, the exact nature of which will depend on the location of the tumor within the stomach. Ischemic bowel disease (choice **d**) usually presents with a severe pain without any significant physical examination findings.
Task Area: Formulating Most Likely Diagnosis
Organ System: Cardiovascular

69. d. The correct answer is choice **d**, hordeolum. Hordeolum, commonly known as a stye, is characterized by acute onset of pain and swelling in the affected eye. In addition, there is a palpable, indurate area with a central area of purulence and surrounding redness. Choice **a**, orbital cellulitis, should not be a consideration because this condition is accompanied by a fever and decreased vision, which this patient does not report experiencing. Choice **b**, dacryostostenosis, is common in newborn children and usually resolves around nine months of age, so this is not a proper diagnosis for a 40-year-old man. Choice **c**, chalazion, is the closest possibility. However, this disorder is of insidious onset and minimal irritation. Choice **e**, blepharitis, is incorrect because this disorder is characterized by redness around the rims of the eyelid and possible scaly, dandrufflike deposits.
Task Area: History Taking and Performing Physical Examinations
Organ System: EENT (Eye, Ear, Nose, and Throat)

70. d. The correct answer is choice **d**, fibromyalgia. Lyrica is the only FDA-approved drug for the treatment of fibromyalgia pain. Fibromyalgia symptoms can include pain, muscle stiffness, muscle tenderness, fatigue, difficulty falling asleep, and difficulty staying asleep. Choice **a**, Huntington's disease, is treated with medications such as Haldol, clozapine, and Xenazine. Choice **b**, scleroderma, is treated with a variety of medications such as calcium channel blockers, antacids, and proton pump inhibitors. Choice **c**, multiple sclerosis, is also treated with a variety of medications such as Klonopin, Neurontin, and Prozac. Choice **e**, systemic lupus erythematosus, is commonly treated with NSAIDs, corticosteroids, and hydroxychloroquine.

Task Area: Pharmaceutical Therapeutics
Organ System: Musculoskeletal

71. c. The correct answer is choice **c**, Dressler's syndrome. Dressler's syndrome, also referred to as post-MI syndrome, usually occurs one to two weeks after a myocardial infarction. Patients with Dressler's syndrome can experience pericarditis, fever, leukocytosis, pericardial effusions, and pleural effusions. Choice **a**, pulmonary embolism, should not be considered because of the presence of fever, pericarditis, and pleural effusions. Choice **b**, cardiogenic shock, is associated with anxiety, altered mental state, hypotension, and a weak pulse, which the patient is not experiencing. Choice **d**, cardiac tamponade, is associated with hypertension, jugular venous distention, and muffled heart sounds. Choice **e**, congestive heart failure, is associated with shortness of breath, fatigue, and fluid collection in the lungs, the liver, the gastrointestinal tract, and the arms and legs. As a result, there is a lack of oxygen and nutrition to organs, which damages them and reduces their ability to work properly.

Task Area: History Taking and Performing Physical Examinations
Organ System: Cardiovascular

72. c. The correct answer is choice **c**, start regular physical exercise, which is an important component of health maintenance. Normal body weight is defined as a body mass index (BMI) of <25 kg/m^2. This patient is obese. Choice **a**, keep a BMI between 25 and 29, is incorrect because this range of BMI is overweight. Choice **b**, maintain a diet with no carbohydrates but high in fat, is incorrect because it is not a balanced diet. Choice **d**, this patient is still young, so no health maintenance discussions are necessary, is incorrect because health maintenance applies to all ages. Choice **e**, none of the above, is incorrect given that choice **c** is correct.

Task Area: Health Maintenance
Organ System: Gastrointestinal/Nutritional

73. c. Hypoplastic left heart syndrome (choice **c**) is a congenital heart defect in which the left side of the heart, including the aorta, aortic valve, left ventricle, and mitral valve, fails to develop properly. The patient will present with cyanosis, shock, heart failure, and respiratory distress. Auscultation of the chest reveals a single S2 sound. Choice **a**, pulmonary atresia, is a form of congenital heart disease in which the pulmonary valve does not form properly. This might be a viable option; however, auscultation of the chest should reveal a hyperdyanamic apical impulse and a single S1 and S2 sound. Choice **b**, Tetralogy of Fallot, may also be a consideration; however, this condition is often associated with shortness of breath, agitation, dizziness, and fainting. Choice **d**, transposition of the great vessels, might also be a consideration; however, this condition is associated with blue skin, clubbing of fingers and toes, poor feeding, and shortness of breath. Auscultation of the chest will reveal a single loud S2 and a systolic murmur. Choice **e**, patent ductus arteriosus, should be excluded as this condition is associated with bounding pulse, fast breathing, poor growth, tiring easily, and sweating while eating.

Task Area: History Taking and Performing Physical Examinations
Organ System: Cardiovascular

74. d. While different antibiotics can cause a wide range of gastrointestinal adverse effects, the most common is a nonspecific GI upset due to their effect on the normal flora of the gut (choice **d**). Almost all antibiotics cause this effect, so it is important to ensure that patients are aware that it is likely a temporary situation that will usually resolve spontaneously after the antibiotic treatment regimen is completed. Pseudomembranous colitis (choice **a**) is a much more significant form of antibiotic-induced diarrhea that is caused by proliferation of *Clostridium difficile* after the competing gut bacteria are killed by the antibiotics; however, this is far less likely. Viral gastroenteritis (choice **b**) is no more likely in this patient than in the general population, while bacterial gastroenteritis (choice **c**) is even less likely because of the recent course of antibiotics. Irritable bowel syndrome (choice **e**) is a diagnosis that is generally reserved for situations in which the etiology of a patient's bowel symptoms is unclear.

Task Area: Pharmaceutical Therapeutics
Organ System: Gastrointestinal/Nutritional

75. b. Blue crystals on parallel light indicate the presence of calcium pyrophosphate seen in pseudogout (choice **b**). On parallel light, urate crystals seen in gout (choice **a**) are yellow. Osteoarthritis (choice **c**), psoriactic arthritis (choice **d**), and septic arthritis (choice **e**) do not produce crystals.

Task Area: Formulating Most Likely Diagnosis
Organ System: Musculoskeletal

76. a. The correct answer is choice **a**, decreased breath sound in left lower lobe of lung field, which is consistent with left lower lobe fluid infiltration happening during an infectious process. Choice **b**, pericardial friction rub, is incorrect because it is a physical finding in pericarditis. Choice **c**, diastolic decrescendo murmur at left upper sternal border, is incorrect because it is most consistent with aortic regurgitation. Choice **d**, hyperresonance in left lower lung field, is incorrect because hyperrsonance is more consistent with pneumothorax when air replaces normal lung tissue. Choice **e**, all of the above, is therefore incorrect.

Task Area: History Taking and Performing Physical Examinations
Organ System: Pulmonary

77. a. Aortic dissection (choice **a**) is caused by an intimal tear, which causes ripping or tearing chest pain and unequal distal pulses. Patients typically have history of uncontrolled hypertension. Choice **b**, acute myocardial infarction, is incorrect because the chest pain is typically more pressurelike without unequal distal pulses. Choice **c**, anxiety attack, is incorrect because the normal heart rate and the unequal distal pulses are not typical in anxiety attacks. Choices **d**, gastroesophageal reflux disease (GERD), and **e**, pulmonary embolism, are also incorrect given that the physical findings are not typically present in these conditions.

Task Area: Formulating Most Likely Diagnosis
Organ System: Cardiovascular

78. b. This is a case of fetal distress, as signified by the fetal tachycardia and the elevated fetal levels of lactic acid. While the cause of fetal distress is unclear in this situation, the safest course of action is to immediately conduct an emergency caesarean delivery (choice **b**) in order to relieve the distress. Choices **a**, **c**, **d**, and **e** are incorrect because fetal distress must be discontinued immediately in order to avoid fetal death.

Task Area: Clinical Intervention
Organ System: Reproductive

79. b. A positive Dix-Hallpike manuever is a specific test for benign paroxysmal positional vertigo (choice **b**). Meniere's disease (choice **a**) usually presents with tinnitus and hearing loss. An acoustic neuroma (choice **c**) and schwannoma (choice **d**) describe the same condition that causes unilateral hearing loss. A foreign body within the ear canal (choice **e**) would cause obstructive hearing loss.

Task Area: Formulating Most Likely Diagnosis
Organ System: EENT (Eye, Ear, Nose, and Throat)

80. a. Schizophrenia is a condition that is caused by overproduction of dopamine and/or overstimulation of dopamine receptors in the brain (choice **a**). Dopaminergic neurons are present in various parts of the brain and serve a variety of different functions; over-stimulation of these receptors usually manifests as psychosis. Typical antipsychotic drugs such as haloperidol usually function as antidopaminergics, thereby attempting to normalize the patient's dopamine activity. Understimulation of dopamine receptors (choice **b**) is found in Parkinson's disease, a condition that affects dopamine-producing neurons in the substantia nigra. Serotonin receptors (choices **c** and **d**) are affected in several psychiatric conditions, the most prominent of which is major depressive syndrome; schizophrenia, however, is not one of these conditions. Epinephrine may be over-produced (choice **e**) in schizophrenia because of its relationship with dopamine, but it is not affected by haloperidol or other antipsychotic drugs.

Task Area: Applying Basic Science Concepts
Organ System: Psychiatry/Behavioral Science

81. a. Testicular ultrasound (choice **a**) is now the gold standard for evaluating testicular torsion. A nuclear medicine testicular scan (choice **b**) would be an alternative to a testicular ultrasound if a testicular ultrasound were unavailable; however, testicular ultrasound is the study of choice for this disorder. Choices **c**, **d**, and **e** are all incorrect as they would have no benefit in the diagnosis of testicular torsion.

Task Area: Using Laboratory and Diagnostic Studies
Organ System: Genitourinary

82. d. While various fungal infections can often cause similar and nonspecific symptoms, it is often possible to make the distinction based on a patient's recent travel history. Coccidioidomycosis (choice **d**), in particular, is caused by *Coccidioides immitis*, a fungal species that is usually found in the southwestern United States; the condition is often known as California disease or San Joaquin Valley Fever. The disease is characterized by fever, arthralgia, pulmonary edema, and erythema nodosum in the lower legs. Bacterial pneumonia (choice **a**) is usually characterized by considerable malaise and a productive cough. Candidiasis (choice **b**) can cause systemic disease and sepsis, but does not usually cause isolated respiratory symptoms. Histoplasmosis (choice **c**) is caused by *Histoplasma spp.*, a type of fungus that is native to the Ohio and Mississippi River Valleys. Blastomycosis (choice **e**) is caused by *Blastomyces spp.*, which is usually found in the midwestern and northern United States.

Task Area: Formulating Most Likely Diagnosis
Organ System: Infectious Diseases

83. a. Down syndrome, or trisomy 21, is the most common chromosomal abnormality in the general population. While it is fairly rare in most patients, its incidence has increased in recent years as women choose to delay pregnancy. The general frequency of Down syndrome is approximately 1 in 800 live births, but this frequency increases significantly with maternal age (choice **a**); the frequency is lower than 1 in 1000 in mothers age 25 and as high as 1 in 35 in mothers age 45. Most patients will undergo a nuchal translucency scan between 11 and 14 weeks gestation in order to better establish the risk of chromosomal abnormalities. Nulliparity (choice **b**) may be associated with a decreased risk of chromosomal abnormalities, while obesity (choice **c**) and a history of polycystic ovarian syndrome (choice **e**) have not been shown to be associated with chromosomal abnormalities. A family history of Down syndrome (choice **d**) has been correlated with a slightly higher risk (possibly due to the nature of the patient's genetic processing systems), but this risk is far less significant than that for maternal age.

Task Area: History Taking and Performing Physical Examinations
Organ System: Reproductive

84. b. Polymyalgia rheumatica (choice **b**) is characterized by bilateral pain and stiffness in the neck, shoulder, and pelvic girdles. Patients with this disorder often experience fever, fatigue, weight loss, and depression. The pain and stiffness most often occurs, and is most severe, after rest and in the morning. Choice **a**, polymyositis, should be ruled out because this disorder causes muscle weakness along with other symptoms such as difficulty eating, swallowing, and speaking. Choice **c**, polyarteritis nodosa, should be ruled out because this disorder causes mild joint pain and muscle aches; however, this disorder also causes other symptoms such as abdominal pain and weakness, and mostly affects individuals suffering from hepatitis B and C. Choice **d**, systemic sclerosis, or scleroderma, should be excluded immediately because this condition is characterized by symmetric thickening of the skin. Choice **e**, fibromyalgia, might be a consideration, but in order to be diagnosed with this disorder, the patient must have pain in at least 11 of 18 areas including buttocks, chests, thighs, and rib cage for a duration of at least three months.

Task Area: Formulating Most Likely Diagnosis
Organ System: Musculoskeletal

85. b. Individuals suffering from anorexia nervosa (choice **b**) have a distorted body image and an intense fear of becoming overweight even though they are underweight. Physical signs of this disorder include emaciation, orthostatic hypotension, bradycardia, hypothermia, and dry skin. Lab work can reveal leukopenia, hypochloremia, hypokalemia, elevated blood urea nitrogen, and metabolic acidosis. Choice **a**, binge eating disorder, is incorrect as this disorder is characterized by routinely overeating, Individuals with this disorder are often obese, not underweight and emaciated as stated in the patient's presentation. Choice **c**, bulimia nervosa, might be a consideration; however, this disorder is characterized by binge eating followed by forced purging. Choice **d**, narcissistic personality disorder, is incorrect as this disorder is characterized by increased self-importance, need for admiration, and self-absorption. Choice **e**, body dysmorphic disorder, might be a consideration; however, this disorder typically does not revolve around weight loss as much as minor imperfections over the whole body. Individuals with this disorder tend to have many plastic surgeries to correct these minor physical flaws.

Task Area: History Taking and Performing Physical Examinations

Organ System: Psychiatry/Behavioral Science

86. d. Choice **d**, The Safe Medical Devices Act, requires users of medical devices to report any incidents that could in any way suggest that the device caused death, serious injury, or illness to a patient. This act is a medical device amendment to the Federal Food, Drug, and Cosmetic act that was signed into law by President Bush in 1990 and is administered by the Food and Drug Administration. A death that occurs as a result of improper function of a medical device is reportable to the FDA and to the device manufacturer. An injury that occurs as a result of improper function of a medical device is reportable to the device manufacturer, and to the FDA only if the manufacturer is unknown. Choice **a**, HIPAA, is incorrect as this legislation is designed to insure the privacy and security of personal health information. Choice **b**, MIPPA, is incorrect as this legislation is designed to adjust Medicare reimbursement to certain facilities. Choice **c**, EMTALA, is incorrect as this legislation legally obligates health care facilities to provide emergent care regardless of citizenship, legal status, or ability to pay. Choice **e**, Patient's Bill of Rights, is incorrect as this legislation requires health care providers to inform all patients of their rights as patients receiving medical treatment.

Task Area: Using Laboratory and Diagnostic Studies

Organ System: Genitourinary

87. b. This patient appears to have a basal cell carcinoma, the world's most common form of skin cancer. Basal cell carcinoma generally carries a very low malignancy potential, but is still usually treated with surgical excision. However, for patients who are uncomfortable with the idea of excision, topical imiquimod therapy (choice **b**) is also safe and effective. Imiquimod is a topical immunomodulatory treatment that has been shown to be beneficial for treatment of basal cell carcinoma, squamous cell carcinoma, actinic keratosis, and several other types of skin lesions. Prednisone (choice **a**) is often useful for allergic skin reactions, but is of little benefit in the case of a cancer. Erythromycin (choice **c**) and tetracycline (choice **d**) are antibiotics that may be used as topical formulations, but again, are of no use for a cancerous lesion. Lidocaine (choice **e**) is often used as a topical local anesthetic and is not necessary because the nodule is painless.

Task Area: Pharmaceutical Therapeutics
Organ System: Dermatologic

88. d. Thrombotic thrombocytopenic purpura (TTP) is a condition in which von Willebrand factor (vWF) (choice **d**) is able to grow into abnormally large multimers. This is caused by autoimmune destruction of the protein that normally cleaves vWF polymers. The extra-long vWF molecules attract platelets and coagulation factors, leading to excessive thrombosis throughout the circulation. Due to the thrombotic events, the patient's platelet count is depleted, thereby also causing bleeding and purpura. It is usually treated with plasmapheresis and, in some cases, immunosuppression. Tyrosine kinase (choice **a**) is affected in chronic myelogenous leukemia. Abnormalities of vitamin K (choice **b**) may cause symptoms similar to those seen in warfarin therapy. Abnormality or deficiency of factor VIII (choice **c**) causes hemophilia A, a condition that is characterized by excessive bleeding. Tissue factor (choice **e**) is not generally affected in any well-characterized pathological process.

Task Area: Applying Basic Science Concepts
Organ System: Hematologic

89. **e.** Placenta previa (choice **e**) is a disorder of pregnancy in which the placenta partially or completely covers the cervical os. This disorder will prevent a vaginal delivery; therefore, a Cesarean section is required. This disorder routinely occurs in women who have had several pregnancies, are of advanced age, and who smoke cigarettes. Choice **a**, spontaneous abortion, should be ruled out because of the lack of open cervix upon physical examination. Choice **b**, ectopic pregnancy, might be a consideration; however, this condition is associated with abdominal or pelvis pain, dizziness, and fatigue, which this patient does not present. Choice **c**, gestational trophoblastic disease, might also be a consideration; however, this condition is associated with increased uterine size, nausea, vomiting, and hypertension, which this patient does not present. Choice **d**, abruptio placentae is associated with a rigid, hard uterus upon physical examination, regular contractions, and abdominal or back pain, which this patient does not present.

Task Area: Formulating Most Likely Diagnosis
Organ System: Reproductive

90. **e.** Osteoporosis is not affected by metformin (choice **e**). The most concerning side effect of metformin is lactic acidosis. Liver failure (choice **a**), heart failure (choice **b**), alcoholism (choice **c**), and renal failure (choice **d**) would worsen this side effect.

Task Area: Pharmaceutical Therapeutics
Organ System: Endocrine

91. **a.** Neurofibrillary tangles (choice **a**) are aggregated hyperphosphorylated tau proteins within the neurons that are known primary markers for Alzheimer's disease. Lewis bodies (choice **b**) are more commonly seen in Parkinson's disease and in Lewis body dementia. Basal ganglion degeneration (choice **c**) can be seen in Huntington's disease. Atherosclerosis (choice **d**) is more indicative of vascular dementia. Subdural hematomas (choice **e**) can occur in many degenerative CNS conditions and would not indicate Alzheimer' disease alone.

Task Area: Applying Basic Science Concepts
Organ System: Neurologic

92. **c.** The correct answer is (choice **c**), subtype 13. Gardisil covers subtypes 6 (choice **a**) and 11 (choice **b**), which cause 50% of genital warts. It also covers subtypes 16 (choice **d**) and 18 (choice **e**), which cause 70% of cervical cancers.

Task Area: Health Maintenance
Organ System: Genitourinary

93. **d.** Burn victims are at risk of developing bacterial infections specifically with *P. aureginosa*. Silver sulfadiazin (choice **d**) is the best choice to prevent this infection. Penicillin (choice **a**) does not cover *P. aureginosa*. Corticosteroids (choice **b**) may promote infection. Fluconazole (choice **c**) is effective only against fungal agents. Doxycycline (choice **e**) is known to cause skin irritation.

Task Area: Clinical Intervention
Organ System: Dermatologic

94. d. Reed-Sternberg cells are pathognomonic for Hodgkin's lymphoma (choice **d**). Non-Hodgkin's lymphoma (choice **e**) would have a very similar clinical presentation. The only way to truly distinguish them is through analysis of a fine needle biopsy, looking for Reed-Sternberg cells. Patients with chronic lymphocytic leukemia (choice **c**) have smudge cells, which are artifacts due to damaged lymphocytes during the slide preparation. Acute myeloid leukemia cells (choice **b**) have Auer rods, which are abnormal, needle-shaped or round, pink-staining inclusions in the cytoplasm of myeloblasts and promyelocytes in acute myelogenous, promyelocytic, or myelomonocytic leukemia. Chronic myeloid leukemia (choice **a**) is associated with a 9/22 translocation.

Task Area: Formulating Most Likely Diagnosis
Organ System: Hematologic

95. b. This patient's presentation is typical of hyperthyroidism, which can be due to a variety of causes; often, these causes can be classified based on TSH levels. In Graves' disease and other primary hyperthyroid conditions of the thyroid gland itself, TSH is low due to negative feedback. In more rare cases, TSH is high; this suggests either feedback compensation of underproduction of thyroid hormone or overproduction of TSH in the pituitary. In this case, because the patient is clinically hyperthyroid and has high thyroxine levels, overproduction in the pituitary is much more likely; this is probably due to a TSH-secreting pituitary tumor. Overgrowth of a pituitary tumor often causes it to press on the optic chiasm, which leads to a bitemporal hemianopia (choice **b**). Homonymous hemianopia and binasal hemianopia, (choices **a** and **c**), can also happen as a result of a mass effect, but they are not common consequences of a pituitary tumor. Exophthalmos (choice **d**) is a feature that is highly specific for Graves' disease, but this patient's high TSH levels exclude Graves' Disease. Endophthalmos (choice **e**) can be related to a variety of rare causes, but none of these is common.

Task Area: History Taking and Performing Physical Examinations
Organ System: Endocrine

96. a. This patient most likely suffers from Wernicke's encephalopathy, a neurological condition characterized by ataxia, anterograde amnesia, ophthalmoplegia, and expressive dysphasia. Wernicke's encephalopathy is usually caused by thiamine (Vitamin B1) deficiency in chronic alcohol abusers, and if left untreated, it can progress to Korsakoff's psychosis. While much of the damage is irreversible, an IV thiamine infusion (choice **a**) can provide some benefit. This patient's symptoms are somewhat similar to what would be expected for a cerebrovascular attack, but this specific combination of symptoms is much more consistent with Wernicke's; consequently, thrombolytic therapy (choice **b**) and anticoagulation (choice **c**) are unlikely to provide any benefit. Craniotomy and drainage (choice **d**) may be useful in the event of a subdural hemorrhage, but they are of no use for this patient. Certain types of antibiotic therapy (choice **e**) are indicated for meningitis, but a patient with meningitis would be expected to have a fever, headache, and/or neck stiffness.

Task Area: Clinical Intervention
Organ System: Neurologic

97. e. A sore throat, headache, and fever are generally suggestive of an upper respiratory tract infection (URTI). While most URTIs are viral, the presence of a tonsillar exudate is strongly suggestive of a bacterial pharyngitis, which is most commonly caused by *Streptococcus pneumoniae*. Streptococcal pharyngitis is usually treated with a penicillin group antibiotic, but because of this patient's history of an allergy to penicillin, it is advisable to consider an alternate option if possible. Drugs from within the penicillin group (choice **a**) carry a very high risk of cross-reactivity in patients who are allergic to penicillin. Cephalosporins (choices **b** and **c**) are somewhat less likely to provoke an allergic response, but are still associated with approximately 10% cross-reactivity; consequently, macrolides are usually used as for Gram-positive coverage in patients with a penicillin allergy. Erythromycin (choice **d**), however, is contraindicated in liver failure because it is hepatically eliminated. Azithromycin (choice **e**) is renally eliminated, which makes it safe for this patient.

Task Area: Pharmaceutical Therapeutics
Organ System: Infectious Diseases

98. d. The correct answer is choice **d**, Bell's palsy, given the unilateral peripheral facial palsy. Choice **a**, status epilepticus, is incorrect because it is inconsistent with the physical findings. Choice **b**, stroke, is incorrect because the neurologic deficit is peripheral in this case, not central as in stroke. Choice **c**, Guillain-Barré syndrome, is incorrect because paralysis in this disorder usually involves distal extremities. Choice **e**, migraine headache, is incorrect because there is no mention of headaches in the case.

Task Area: History Taking and Performing Physical Examinations
Organ System: Neurologic

99. d. A persisting fever with a cough, decreased air entry, and dullness to percussion are highly suggestive of a pneumonia. Different forms of pneumonia may exhibit different symptoms; *Mycoplasma* pneumonia (choice **d**), also known as walking pneumonia because patients are well enough to walk around, is a form of atypical pneumonia that is not associated with significant sputum production. While *Mycoplasma pneumoniae* is considered an atypical bacterium because it lacks a cell wall, it is the most common form of community-acquired pneumonia in young adults (18 to 40 years). *Mycoplasma* is generally resistant to cephalosporins and is notorious for being difficult to grow in culture, so it is fairly common for the diagnosis to be made on clinical features without microbiological confirmation. The treatment regimen will often depend heavily on the severity of the patient's symptoms, but generally comprises broad-spectrum bacteriostatic antibiotics. Respiratory syncytial virus (choice **a**) is a common cause of pneumonia and bronchiolitis in children, but it is far less common than *Mycoplasma* in adults. Influenza pneumonia (choice **b**) is rare in all populations. *Candida* (choice **c**) can cause a systemic (or pulmonary) infection called candidiasis, but it is very different from pneumonia. Tuberculosis (choice **e**) usually presents with a highly productive cough, noticeable weight loss, and gradual onset; additionally, while tuberculosis is very common worldwide, it is less common than *Mycoplasma* in the United States.
Task Area: Formulating Most Likely Diagnosis
Organ System: Pulmonary

100. b. The correct answer is choice **b**, sertraline, which is an SSRI (selective serotonin receptor inhibitor). Therefore choice **e**, none of the above, is incorrect. Choice **a**, lithium, is incorrect because it is indicated for treatment of bipolar disorder. Choice **c**, risperidone, is incorrect because it is indicated for treatment of bipolar disorder and psychosis. Choice **d**, haloperidol, is incorrect because it is an antipsychotic.
Task Area: Pharmaceutical Therapeutics
Organ System: Psychiatry/Behavioral Science

101. d. The correct answer is choice **d**, varicella zoster virus infection (also known as herpes zoster, or shingles). This condition often affects patients with impaired immunity. The rash is painful and generally has a dermatomal distribution. Choice **a**, tinea corporis, is incorrect because this rash is usually annular and itchy. Choice **b**, psoriasis, is incorrect because this rash typically affects patients at a younger age and does not have a dermatomal distribution. Choice **c**, acanthosis nigricans, is incorrect because it is typically not painful and is not consistent with the appearance of this patient's rash. Choice **e**, rosacea, is incorrect because it typically affects the face and is nonpainful.
Task Area: Formulating Most Likely Diagnosis
Organ System: Dermatologic

102. c. The correct answer is choice **c**, magnesium sulfate. Magnesium sulfate is administered to pregnant women who are experiencing premature labor in order to slow down or stop uterine contractions. Signs of magnesium sulfate overdose, or toxicity, include respiratory depression and loss of deep tendon reflexes. If an individual exhibits these signs of overdose, calcium gluconate can be administered to counteract the effects of the overdose. Choice **a**, ACE inhibitor overdose, is rare and is commonly treated with activated charcoal and intravenous fluids. Choice **b**, overdose of ritodrine, is commonly treated with the administration of beta blockers. Choice **d**, overdose of calcium channel blockers, is treated by calcium and atropine. With respect to choice **e**, data is lacking on acute overdose of clomiphene citrate; however, supportive measures and gastric lavage would be the course of action.
Task Area: Pharmaceutical Therapeutics
Organ System: Reproductive

103. e. The correct answer is choice **e**, MRI (magnetic resonance imaging), with gadolinium enhancement; this is the most effective diagnostic tool for the visualization of white matter lesions in the central nervous system associated with multiple sclerosis. Choice **a**, PET scanning, is primarily used to assess the brain for dementia. Choice **b**, angiography, is used to assess blood flow to the brain. Choice **c**, CT scanning, can be used in an attempt to visualize white matter lesions associated with multiple sclerosis; however, an MRI can visualize lesions that may be invisible on CT, which makes an MRI far more sensitive for this application. Choice **d**, nuclear medicine, is used for dementia, infarcts, or brain death but are of no use for visualizing white matter lesions.
Task Area: Using Laboratory and Diagnostic Studies
Organ System: Neurologic

104. d. The correct answer is choice **d**, pneumococcal vaccine and annual influenza vaccinations, which will prevent superinfections. Given the history, this patient has mild persistent asthma symptoms and needs to be treated with a combination of an anti-inflammatory agent and a short-acting bronchodilator. Choice **a**, none at this time other than using bronchodilators as needed, is incorrect because this patient needs preventive vaccinations. Choice **b**, moderate tobacco use, is incorrect because complete smoking cessation should be advised to prevent asthma flare. Choice **c**, influenza vaccination during worsening of symptoms, is incorrect because influenza vaccination should be given annually. Choice **e**, avoid physical activity, is incorrect because moderate physical activity should be encouraged to maintain lung function.
Task Area: Health Maintenance
Organ System: Pulmonary

105. **a.** The nature of this patient's pain is characteristic of gallstones, which are particularly common in middle-aged overweight females (a common mnemonic for the risk factors is *fat, female, fertile, forty*). While her jaundice and the persisting nature of her pain suggest a higher likelihood of choledocholithiasis, it is difficult to distinguish cholelithiasis from choledocholithiasis based solely on history and physical examination. An ultrasound provides additional information to demonstrate the presence of a gallstone, but endoscopic retrograde cholangiopancreatography (ERCP) (choice **a**) is generally used to confirm the diagnosis and, if possible, to mechanically clear the blockage by removing the stone or inserting a stent. Magnetic resonance cholangiopancreatography (MRCP) (choice **b**) is also a reasonable choice for diagnostic purposes, but it does not provide any therapeutic benefit and is generally reserved for situations in which ERCP is contraindicated. Cholecystectomy (choice **c**) may prove to be necessary based on the results of the ERCP/MRCP, but it is not indicated at this stage. Pancreaticoduodenectomy (choice **d**) is a major procedure with many risks and is usually used only in the case of a pancreatic cancer. Antibiotic therapy (choice **e**) may be useful in the case of ascending cholangitis, but this is unlikely in the absence of a fever.

Task Area: Clinical Intervention
Organ System: Gastrointestinal/Nutritional

106. **d.** Glaucoma is an optic neuropathy that is usually caused by an increased intraocular pressure; however, it is important to recognize that the changes in intraocular pressure are merely a risk factor for glaucoma rather than a diagnostic factor. The optic neuropathy is generally diagnosed and monitored based on the change in size of the optic cup (choice **d**). While the elevated cup-to-disc ratio is not adequate to make a diagnosis by itself, the increasing ratio (due to increased optic cup size) is more specific for glaucoma than any other diagnostic factors. Peripheral vision loss (choice **a**) is the key sign that is evident in glaucoma patients, and while it is a critical feature, it is not specific for glaucoma. High intraocular pressure (choice **b**) is merely a risk factor for glaucoma, and it is possible not only for the disease to occur in a patient with a normal pressure, but also for a patient to be completely free of pathology despite a severely elevated pressure. Variation in intraocular pressures (choice **c**) is irrelevant. Decreased optic disc size (choice **e**) would be concerning, but the increased cup-to-disc ratio in this patient is caused by a large cup rather than a small disc.

Task Area: History Taking and Performing Physical Examinations
Organ System: EENT (Eye, Ear, Nose, and Throat)

107. **e.** Dobutamine (choice **e**) is an inotrope and can increase heart contractility. Flecainide and verapamil (choices **a** and **b**) are antiarrhythmics. Nifedipine (choice **c**) is an antihypertensive. Dapsone (choice **d**) is an antibiotic.

Task Area: Pharmaceutical Therapeutics
Organ System: Cardiovascular

108. **c.** The patient has a history, examination, and reversible obstructive pattern consistent with asthma (choice **c**). She is too young to have chronic obstructive pulmonary disease (COPD) (choice **a**). Acute viral bronchitis (choice **b**), cystic fibrosis (choice **d**), and upper respiratory tract infection (choice **e**) would present differently and give a different spirometry pattern.

Task Area: Formulating Most Likely Diagnosis
Organ System: Pulmonary

109. **a.** This question tests your knowledge of physical exam findings in ACL injury. Given the positive anterior drawer sign, the correct answer is choice **a**, anterior cruciate ligament (ACL) tear. Choice **b**, posterior cruciate ligament (ACL) tear, is incorrect because the posterior drawer sign is negative. Choice **c**, Baker's cyst, is incorrect because there is no palpable lesion in the popliteal area. Choice **d**, cellulitis, is incorrect because there are no superficial signs suggestive of cellulitis. Choice **e**, genu varum, is incorrect because the knee is well aligned.

Task Area: History Taking and Performing Physical Examinations
Organ System: Musculoskeletal

110. **a.** Lidocaine (choice **a**) is a commonly used antiarrhythmic medication as well as a local anesthetic. Choice **b**, adenosine, is incorrect as this is the drug of choice for the treatment of supraventricular tachycardia. Choice **c**, diltiazem, is incorrect as this is a calcium channel blocker that is effective in treating atrial fibrillation. Choice **d**, nitroglycerin, is incorrect as this medication is the first-line treatment for chest pain. Choice **e**, furosemide, is incorrect as this medication is a diuretic that is used to rid the body of excess fluids associated with congestive heart failure.

Task Area: Pharmaceutical Therapeutics
Organ System: Cardiovascular

111. **b.** The correct answer is choice **b**, greenstick fracture, which is a very common injury among children. This type of fracture is classically defined as a fracture in which one side of the bone is broken while the other side is bent. Choice **a**, transverse fracture, is incorrect as this type of fracture occurs at a right angle to the bone's axis. Choice **c**, Colles' fracture, is incorrect as this fracture only occurs at the distal radius that causes posterior displacement of the wrist. Choice **d**, open fracture, is incorrect as this type of fracture is a compound fracture in which the bone is protruding through the skin. Choice **e**, comminuted fracture, is incorrect as this type of fracture is characterized by the bone splintering into several pieces.

Task Area: Using Laboratory and Diagnostic Studies
Organ System: Musculoskeletal

112. b. Macular degeneration (choice **b**) is a disorder that is characterized by permanent central vision loss. Macular degeneration may simply be caused by old age, or by the toxic effects from phenothiazine medications such as Compazine. Choices **a**, **c**, **d**, and **e** are all incorrect as none of these disorders can be caused by overuse and toxic effects from phenothiazine medications such as Compazine.

Task Area: Pharmaceutical Therapeutics
Organ System: EENT (Eye, Ear, Nose, and Throat)

113. a. Cystic fibrosis is a debilitating multisystem disease that affects chloride channels in the lungs, pancreas, and various other parts of the body. Usually, the pulmonary complications are the most significant, and despite advances in medical therapy, most patients do not live past the age of 40. One of the key poor prognostic factors is early pulmonary bacterial colonization with *Pseudomonas aeruginosa* (choice **a**) or *Staphylococcus aureus*; in order to avoid this, patients are often treated with aggressive antibiotic therapy. Frequent upper respiratory tract infections (choice **b**) may increase the risk of pulmonary colonization, but they are not a life-limiting concern in themselves. Continuous airway clearance (choice **c**) and bronchodilator therapy (choice **d**) are both beneficial forms of cystic fibrosis management. Intussusception (choice **e**) is more common in patients with cystic fibrosis, but it can be corrected with surgical intervention.

Task Area: Health Maintenance
Organ System: Pulmonary

114. a. Because a wide range of antihypertensive drugs is available on the market, it is possible to craft a very specific regimen that is optimal for each patient. While hydrochlorothiazide (choice **a**) is not contraindicated in patients with hypercholesterolemia, it should be avoided due to its tendency to elevate cholesterol levels further. Hydrochlorothiazide can also cause hypercalcemia, hypokalemia, hyponatremia, hyperuricemia, and hyperglycemia, and should consequently be avoided in patients at risk for ion abnormalities, gout, or diabetes. Furosemide (choice **b**) can cause hypokalemia and hyponatremia, but it does not generally affect lipid levels. Spironolactone (choice **c**) is more likely to cause hyperkalemia and androgenic effects. Ramipril (choice **d**) has been associated with a severe cough, hypoglycemia, and a range of other nonspecific consequences. Metoprolol (choice **e**) is associated with antiadrenergic side effects such as bronchospasm, drowsiness, and other systemic consequences.

Task Area: Pharmaceutical Therapeutics
Organ System: Cardiovascular

115. e. A scaphoid fracture is a common consequence of a fall onto an outstretched hand in a young patient. Although the nature of the pain is often nonspecific, the presence of tenderness in the anatomical snuffbox (choice **e**) is highly suggestive of a scaphoid injury. Though an X-ray will often confirm this provisional diagnosis, many scaphoid fractures are not clearly evident on initial radiographs; a follow-up X-ray may be needed in about ten days to verify the diagnosis. A scaphoid fracture may also affect range of motion (choices **a** and **b**), but it is unusual for these effects to be dramatic. Swelling (choices **c** and **d**) is also often present, but this is a nonspecific sign that may be caused by a variety of other types of fractures.

Task Area: History Taking and Performing Physical Examinations
Organ System: Musculoskeletal

116. b. Postural hypotension (choice **b**), otherwise known as orthostatic hypotension, is characterized by a drop in blood pressure greater than 20 mmHg when transferring from a supine to a sitting position or from a sitting to standing position. Postural hypotension is a major cause of syncope and a leading cause of falls among the elderly. Choices **a** and **c**, primary hypertension and malignant hypertension, are clearly incorrect as this is a hypotensive condition and not a hypertensive condition. Choice **d**, hypoglycemia, is incorrect; although it may cause lightheadedness, the fact that blood pressure falls when transferring positions makes this a clear case of postural hypotension. Choice **e**, cardiac arrhythmia, may also be a consideration and should be evaluated; however, the fact that blood pressure falls when transferring positions makes this a clear case of postural hypotension.

Task Area: Formulating Most Likely Diagnosis
Organ System: Cardiovascular

117. **b.** *Pneumocystis* pneumonia (choice **b**) is the most common infection occurring in HIV-positive patients. CD4 counts of less than 200 cells/μL are typical with this disorder. Patients may present with fever, tachypnea, dyspnea, and a nonproductive cough. Chest X-ray will typically show diffuse or perihilar infiltrates but no pleural effusions. Blood work will show lymphopenia and low CD4 count. Choice **a**, nosocomial pneumonia, is incorrect as this is a hospital-acquired pneumonia that is characterized by symptoms of productive cough, nausea, vomiting, and chest pain. Choice **c**, community-acquired pneumonia, is incorrect as this condition is associated with productive cough and has no association with CD4 counts. Choice **d**, tuberculosis, is incorrect as this condition is characterized by symptoms such as weight loss, night sweats, fatigue, and loss of appetite. Choice **e**, cystic fibrosis, is incorrect as this condition is associated with cough, foul-smelling stools, and distended abdomen.
Task Area: Formulating Most Likely Diagnosis
Organ System: Pulmonary

118. **b.** Choice **b**, lap band procedure, is a form of bariatric surgery in which a restrictive, circular band is implanted around the upper part of the patient's stomach. A lap band is normally implanted using a laparoscopic approach. The band can be tightened or loosened easily by either adding or removing the quantity of saline filling the band. Choice **a**, gastric bypass, is incorrect as it involves a surgical division of the stomach. This procedure involves connecting the upper pouch of the stomach to the jejunum while closing off the distal part of the stomach. Choice **c**, liposuction, is incorrect as this involves surgical removal of fat by using suction. Choice **d**, stomach stapling, is incorrect as this is a restrictive technique using both band and staples to make the stomach smaller to slow the passage of food. Choice **e**, partial gastrectomy, is incorrect as this is a surgical procedure used to remove part of the stomach entirely and is usually done if a tumor is present.
Task Area: History Taking and Performing Physical Examinations
Organ System: Gastrointestinal/Nutritional

119. **a.** This question tests your knowledge of hearing tests. The correct answer is choice **a**, conductive hearing loss of the right ear, which is consistent with a positive Weber test lateralized to the right ear (the impaired ear), and with a Rinne test showing sound is heard through bone longer than it is through air in the right ear. Choices **b**, **d**, and **e** are incorrect because the question states the Weber test is positive for lateralization to the right ear, not the left ear or bilateral. Choice **c** is incorrect because the Rinne test shows conductive hearing loss, not sensorineural.
Task Area: Using Laboratory and Diagnostic Studies
Organ System: EENT (Eye, Ear, Nose, and Throat)

120. b. Antihistamines (choice **b**) are the most appropriate medications for this condition because symptoms associated with allergic rhinitis such as sneezing, itching, and runny nose occur when mast cells degranulate and release histamine. Choice **a**, antibiotics, is incorrect as there is no evidence of infection, so antibiotics are not warranted. Choice **c**, corticosteroids, may be used to alleviate inflammation in the nasal cavity and reduce symptoms; however, these medications can cause side effects if used longer than a few days, so antihistamines are the better option. Choice **d**, NSAIDs, is incorrect as these medications might relieve the headache but will not address the allergies. Relieving the allergies should also relieve the headache. Choice **e**, anti-inflammatories, is incorrect as these medications may alleviate inflammation in the nasal cavity and reduce symptoms, but they will have no effect for treatment of the allergy.

Task Area: Pharmaceutical Therapeutics
Organ System: Pulmonary

Section 3

121. d. This clinical scenario suggests bone marrow aplasia; in a 15-year-old boy, this would most likely be caused by either aplastic anemia or acute lymphoblastic leukemia (ALL). These two conditions can be fairly difficult to distinguish based on clinical features or a complete blood count. However, before jumping to a bone marrow biopsy, it is often possible to use a peripheral blood smear (choice **d**) to help gain some clinical direction. Both smears will show hypocellularity and pancytopenia; however, aplastic anemia will feature cells that are morphologically normal, while ALL will reveal immature leukocytes with condensed genetic material, absent nucleoli, and very little agranular cytoplasm. Choices **a**, **b**, **c**, and **e** are incorrect because aplastic anemia and ALL will both present with pancytopenia, so levels of all types of blood cells will be low.

Task Area: Using Laboratory and Diagnostic Studies
Organ System: Hematologic

122. d. Heberden's and Bouchard's nodes present as nodules on the DIP and PIP joints (choice **d**) and are commonly seen in osteoarthritis. Early morning joint pain (choice **a**) that is relieved by movement (choice **b**) is indicative of an inflammatory arthritis. Ulnar deviation (choice **c**) and nodules underneath the elbow (choice **e**) can be found in rheumatoid arthritis.

Task Area: History Taking and Performing Physical Examinations
Organ System: Musculoskeletal

123. d. Choice **d**, quantitative measurement of fecal fat, is correct. Stool is collected for three days, and a quantitative measure of fecal fat is performed in order to diagnose the condition of malabsorption. This is performed by weighing the stool sample, extracting the lipids, and then performing a simple mathematical equation to determine the amount of fat present in the sample. Normal fecal fat is equal to or less than 7.0 grams per day. Choice **a**, D-xylose absorption test, is incorrect as this exam is performed to assess how the intestines absorb a simple sugar if the quantitative fecal fat is abnormal. Choice **b**, bile acid breath test, is used for steatorrhea caused by suspected bacterial overgrowth. Choice **c**, microscopic study of the stool, is incorrect because although this, technically, would be a useful method, it is limited by the accuracy of the microscope and the individual performing the exam. Choice **e**, urea breath test, is incorrect as this exam is used to evaluate for the presence of *Helicobacter pylori* bacteria in the stomach.
Task Area: Using Laboratory and Diagnostic Studies
Organ System: Gastrointestinal/Nutritional

124. c. Choice **c**, excision biopsy, is correct as this procedure requires the entire lesion be removed in order to test for clean tissue margins after the surgical procedure. Choice **a**, fine-needle aspiration, is incorrect as this procedure involves the collection of cells from a mass that is just under the skin, and most of the mass is left in place. Choice **b**, incision biopsy, is incorrect as this procedure involves cutting into the lesion or tissue to be examined and removing a portion of the lesion or tissue to be sent for further evaluation. Choice **d**, sentinel node biopsy, is incorrect as this procedure is used to identify the sentinel node, which is the first lymph node from which a cancerous tumor will spread. Choice **e**, endoscopic biopsy, is incorrect as this is generally used to assess tumors of a bronchus, and most of the lesion remains in place.
Task Area: Applying Basic Science Concepts
Organ System: Pulmonary

125. **c.** Cardiogenic shock (choice **c**) is a type of shock that can arise from myocardial infarctions, arrhythmias, heart failure, valvular abnormalities, myocarditis, cardiac contusions, and myocardiopathies. Shock can cause low blood pressure, tachycardia, orthostatic changes, and altered mental status. Choice **a**, congestive heart failure, is incorrect as there is no evidence of fluid retention, and this condition does not cause alteration of mental status. Choice **b**, orthostatic hypotension, is incorrect as this patient's hypotension is not due to change in physical location, such as transferring from sitting to standing position. Choice **d**, cardiac arrest, is incorrect as this patient is experiencing tachycardia, whereas in cardiac arrest the patient would have a cardiac rhythm of asystole or ventricular fibrillation. Choice **e**, septic shock, is incorrect as this patient has no history of severe infection.

Task Area: Formulating Most Likely Diagnosis
Organ System: Cardiovascular

126. **b.** Mesalamine (choice **b**) belongs to the drug family of anti-inflammatory agents, which means they inhibit the body from producing substances that cause pain or inflammation. Mesalamine is effective for the treatment of Crohn's disease because it inhibits inflammation in part of or the entire colon. Choice **a**, antacids, is incorrect as these medications are effective in treating symptoms associated with Crohn's disease but do not promote healing. Choice **c**, aminosalicylates, might be a consideration; however, these medications do not stop symptoms from returning during remission. Choice **d**, immunodilators, is incorrect as these medications would be a consideration only if other medications such as prednisone or mesalamine failed. Choice **e**, prednisone, is incorrect as this medication is only indicated for acute attacks of Crohn's disease.

Task Area: Health Maintenance
Organ System: Gastrointestinal/Nutritional

127. **c.** When using laboratory tests, it is important to understand the relative sensitivities and specificities of various options. A sensitive test may help to raise the suspicion of certain diseases, while a specific test is more likely to suggest one specific diagnosis. Systemic lupus erythematosus (SLE) is a complex disease for which there is no test that is both sensitive and specific; consequently, a range of tests must be used when the diagnosis is suspected. The anti-dsDNA antibody (choice **c**), if detected, is highly specific for SLE; in other words, its presence is highly suggestive of a diagnosis of SLE. However, because anti-dsDNA is only 70% sensitive, some patients with SLE will not have the antibody. Antineutrophil cytoplasmic antibody (choice **a**) is a fairly sensitive test for autoimmune vasculitides but is not specific for other diseases such as SLE. Antinuclear antibody (choice **b**) is highly sensitive for SLE, but it is not highly specific; it can also be elevated in the presence of several other autoimmune diseases. Rheumatoid factor (choice **d**) is specific for rheumatoid arthritis and Sjögren's syndrome. C-reactive protein (choice **e**) is very nonspecific and is elevated in almost all inflammatory conditions.

Task Area: Using Laboratory and Diagnostic Studies

Organ System: Musculoskeletal

128. **d.** Abdominal pain is a common nonspecific symptom that may be associated with a wide range of possible diagnoses. The presence of boardlike rigidity (choice **d**), however, is a fairly specific sign that should raise the suspicion of an intestinal perforation or a perforated peptic ulcer. In most cases, surgical intervention is necessary to correct the perforation. Diffuse abdominal tenderness (choice **a**) may be caused by a wide range of gastrointestinal conditions. Hypotension (choice **b**) is often found in gastrointestinal perforations associated with bleeding, but it may also be caused by any other sort of internal bleeding. Guarding (choice **c**) is caused by tensing of the abdominal muscles, which may be associated with any abruptly painful abdominal condition. High-pitched bowel sounds (choice **e**) are likely to be found in a bowel obstruction.

Task Area: History Taking and Performing Physical Examinations

Organ System: Gastrointestinal/Nutritional

129. **b.** Labyrinthitis (choice **b**) is a disorder that involves irritation and inflammation of the inner ear. Patients may present with difficulty focusing due to involuntary eye movements, dizziness, vertigo, one-sided hearing loss, nausea, and vomiting. Choice **a**, central vertigo, is often associated with nausea, vomiting, and loss of balance, which are not exhibited by this patient. Choice **c**, barotrauma, would not be a consideration because there is no history of airplane travel or scuba diving. Lack of drainage from the ear and tinnitus should rule out choice **d**, tympanic membrane rupture. The symptoms of difficulty focusing and involuntary eye movements should rule out choice **e**, otitis media.

Task Area: Formulating Most Likely Diagnosis

Organ System: EENT (Eye, Ear, Nose, and Throat)

130. d. The correct answer is choice **d**, daily anti-inflammatory agent (either inhaled corticosteroid or cromolyn) plus a daily short-acting bronchodilator. Given the history, this patient has mild persistent asthma symptoms and needs to be treated with a combination of an anti-inflammatory agent and a short-acting bronchodilator. Therefore choice **e**, none of the above, is incorrect. Choice **a**, a short-acting bronchodilator as needed, is incorrect because it is appropriate treatment for patients with mild intermittent symptoms. Choice **b**, a daily short-acting bronchodilator, is incorrect because this patient's symptom severity will benefit from the addition of an anti-inflammatory agent. Choice **c**, daily anti-inflammatory agent (either inhaled corticosteroid or cromolyn), is incorrect because the patient will always need a short-acting bronchodilator for acute attacks.
Task Area: Pharmaceutical Therapeutics
Organ System: Pulmonary

131. d. The correct answer is **d**, pericarditis, given the pericardial friction rub and diffuse ST elevations on the electrocardiogram (EKG). Choices **a**, gastroesophageal reflux disease (GERD), and **b**, mitral valve stenosis, are incorrect because neither of them will induce ST elevations on the EKG. Choice **c**, acute myocardial infarction, is incorrect because in an acute myocardial infarction, it is not typical to find pericardial friction rub, which indicates pericardium involvement. Choice **e**, anxiety attack, is incorrect because an anxiety attack will not create a pericardial friction rub or diffuse ST elevation.
Task Area: Formulating Most Likely Diagnosis
Organ System: Cardiovascular

132. d. The correct answer is choice **d**, metabolic disorder. Osteoporosis is the most common metabolic bone disease that produces diffusely decreased bone density and strength. All the other options are incorrect.
Task Area: Applying Basic Scientific Concepts
Organ System: Musculoskeletal

133. d. Dialysis (choice **d**) is the proper course of treatment when the plasma sodium level is in excess of 200 mEq/L. Rapid correction of this disorder via dialysis is required in order to avoid complications that may arise from excessively high plasma sodium. Choices **a**, **b**, and **c** are all viable options for minor increases in serum sodium levels; however, sodium elevations at this level require dialysis to resolve. Choice **e**, intravenous potassium, would be contraindicated as this will compound the condition.
Task Area: Clinical Intervention
Organ System: Genitourinary

134. e. Obstructive sleep apnea (choice **e**) is a common condition caused by nighttime airway obstruction leading to awakening and snoring. The condition is characterized by excessive daytime somnolence, often in inappropriate situations; additionally, most patients also have a long history of snoring. Obese patients are at particularly high risk, although a low BMI does not preclude the diagnosis. The most appropriate next step is to conduct a monitored sleep study, and if the diagnosis is confirmed, the condition can be relieved with a device that provides continuous positive airway pressure (CPAP). Narcolepsy (choice **a**) is another possible cause of daytime somnolence, but it is far less common than obstructive sleep apnea and is not usually associated with snoring. Because a medical diagnosis is present, there is no reason to suspect idiopathic hypersomnolence (choice **b**) or chronic insufficient sleep (choice **c**). Central sleep apnea (choice **d**) is a similar condition, but it is less common and is less likely to be associated with snoring.

Task Area: Formulating Most Likely Diagnosis
Organ System: Pulmonary

135. c. A somatization disorder is a condition in which physical symptoms are caused by a psychiatric condition; irritable bowel syndrome, by contrast, is a condition in which no physical or psychological cause can be identified for a patient's bowel symptoms. While the distinction is subtle, it is important to recognize because of the significant difference in therapeutic strategies. One key feature of somatization disorders is that the symptoms often resemble symptoms that the patient has witnessed in a close family member. A recent diagnosis of colorectal cancer in the patient's mother (choice **c**), for example, is a possible stressor that can cause a patient to experience similar nonspecific symptoms. The family history of colorectal cancer may also be suggestive of a bowel malignancy, but this is unlikely in a young patient. It may be advisable to refer this patient for mental health counseling in order to identify and treat the source of the patient's symptoms. Normal findings on laboratory investigation (choice **a**) and physical examination (choice **b**) are characteristic of both somatization disorder and irritable bowel syndrome. Exacerbation of symptoms with stress choice and physical examination (choice **d**) and a past history of major depressive disorder choice and physical examination (choice **e**) have been strongly linked to irritable bowel syndrome, but may also be present in somatization disorder.

Task Area: History Taking and Performing Physical Examinations
Organ System: Psychiatry/Behavioral Science

136. d. Acute lymphocytic leukemia (choice **d**) is primarily diagnosed in children three to seven years of age. Children with this disorder may present with fatigue, fever, lethargy, headache, and bone pain in the sternum, tibia, and femur. Blood work will reveal pancytopenia with circulating blasts. Terminal deoxynucleotidyl transferase is present in 95% of acute lymphocytic leukemia cases. A chest X-ray may reveal a mediastinal mass. Choice **a**, cystic fibrosis, should be excluded immediately because of the lack of mucus buildup, coughing, nasal congestion, and repeated bouts of pneumonia. You should exclude choice **b**, polycythemia vera, based on the blood work, since polycythemia vera is characterized by overproduction of red blood cells. Other factors that exclude polycythemia vera are dizziness, headache, shortness of breath, and redness of the face. The blood work also excludes choice **c**, thrombocytopenia, since thrombocytopenia is characterized by low platelet count. Other factors that exclude thrombocytopenia are the lack of bruising and abnormal bleeding of the mouth and gums. Choice **e**, acute myelogenous leukemia, should be excluded simply based on the patient's age, as acute myelogenous leukemia normally affects individuals over the age of 65.
Task Area: Formulating Most Likely Diagnosis
Organ System: Hematologic

137. a. Avascular necrosis (choice **a**) of the hip is a result of inadequate blood supply to the trabecular bone, which will ultimately cause collapse of the femoral head. A crescent sign on a lateral hip radiograph is a classic finding for avascular necrosis. Choice **b**, septic arthritis, is incorrect as this disorder is not classically diagnosed with X-ray but rather by evaluation of synovial fluid from the joint space. Choice **c**, Osgood-Schlatter disease, is incorrect as this disorder affects the anterior tibial tubercle, which is located just below the knee. Choice **d**, slipped capital femoral epiphysis, is incorrect as this condition is associated with a Klein's line or metaphyseal blanch sign on hip radiographs. Choice **e**, acute hip fracture, is incorrect as this condition is diagnosed by a clear fractured hip bone on an X-ray.
Task Area: Using Laboratory and Diagnostic Studies
Organ System: Musculoskeletal

138. **e.** Informed consent (choice **e**) is classically defined as the consent of a patient to undergo a medical procedure or to participate in a clinical trial after achieving an understanding of the medical facts and risks involved. Choice **a**, HIPAA, is incorrect as this legislation is designed to insure the privacy and security of personal health information. Choice **b**, time out, is incorrect as this is the universal protocol to verify the correct patient, procedure, site, and implants. Choice **c**, Safe Medical Devices Act, is incorrect as this piece of legislation requires users of medical devices to report any incidents that could in any way suggest that the device caused death, serious injury, or illness to a patient. Choice **d**, Patient's Bill of Rights, is incorrect as this legislation requires health care providers to inform all patients of their rights as patients receiving medical treatment.

Task Area: Clinical Intervention
Organ System: Genitourinary

139. **c.** This patient's clinical presentation and lab results are consistent with cholecystitis (choice **c**). All the other choices are incorrect because the patient should not be jaundiced, and liver enzymes and bilirubin should not be elevated in these conditions.

Task Area: Formulating Most Likely Diagnosis
Organ System: Reproductive

140. **e.** The correct answer is choice **e**, tinea corporis, which is also called dermatophytosis, a fungal infection of the skin. This question tests your knowledge of using a KOH (potassium hydroxide) preparation to diagnose fungal infections. A KOH preparation will show hyphae. All the other choices are incorrect because they are inconsistent with the itchiness or the positive KOH test result.

Task Area: Using Laboratory and Diagnostic Studies
Organ System: Dermatologic

141. **d.** Congestive heart failure (choice **d**) is characterized by dyspnea and the abnormal retention of water and sodium. Patients may experience exertional dyspnea, nonproductive cough, leg and ankle edema, and fatigue. They may also experience orthopnea, paroxysmal nocturnal dyspnea, and exercise intolerance. Chest X-ray should reveal cardiomegaly, bilateral pleural effusions, and perivascular or interstitial edema. Auscultation of the chest should reveal basilar rales and cardiac gallops. Symptoms and patient presentation may vary according to the side of the heart that is failing. Choices **a** and **b** are incorrect because pneumothoraces do not present with cardiomegaly or perivascular edema. Choice **c**, cystic fibrosis, should be excluded based on the age of the patient and on the lack of symptoms such as wheezing and distended abdomen. Choice **e**, pulmonary embolism, should be excluded because this condition does not present with nonproductive cough, cardiomegaly, or perivascular edema.

Task Area: Formulating Most Likely Diagnosis
Organ System: Cardiovascular

142. b. The correct answer is choice **b**, lumbar puncture to evaluate CSF. When meningitis is suspected, a prompt lumbar puncture must be performed in order to evaluate the cerebrospinal fluid. With meningitis, CSF may appear cloudy to purulent, CSF pressure will be elevated, white blood cells will be increased, protein concentrations will be increased, and glucose levels will be decreased. A Gram stain and culture is diagnostic in 80% of the cases. Choice **a**, inserting pledgets, is used to evaluate a CSF leak in the case of rhinorrhea. Choices **c**, **d**, and **e** are incorrect because, while imaging modalities are useful for recognizing complications associated with meningitis such as hydrocephalus and cerebral abscess, a lumbar puncture with CSF evaluation is the only true method to confirm a meningitis diagnosis.

Task Area: Clinical Intervention
Organ System: Neurologic

143. e. The correct answer is choice **e**, decrease the influx of intracelluar calcium ions. Calcium channel blockers effectively stop premature uterine contractions because these medications inhibit smooth muscle contractility and relax the uterine muscles by decreasing the influx of intracellular calcium ions. Choices **a**, **b**, **c**, and **d** are all incorrect because calcium channel blockers do not treat pre-term uterine contractions in these ways.

Task Area: Pharmaceutical Therapeutics
Organ System: Reproductive

144. a. Wegener's granulomatosis is ANCA associated vasculitis (choice **a**). Therefore, ANCA negative (choice **b**) is incorrect. Anti-dsDNA (choices **c** and **d**) is associated with lupus. Anti-basement membrane (BM) antibody (choice **e**) is associated with Goodpasture syndrome.

Task Area: Using Laboratory and Diagnostic Studies
Organ System: EENT (Eye, Ear, Nose, and Throat)

145. c. The correct answer is choice **c**, hyperparathyroidism. Hyperparathyroidism is characterized by generalized weakness, body aches, nausea, loss of appetite, and increased thirst along with an elevated serum calcium level. The parathyroid glands produce PTH, or parathyroid hormone, which regulates calcium levels in the body. Overfunctioning parathyroid glands lead to elevated serum calcium levels. You might also consider choice **a**, hypothyroidism, because of weakness, body aches, and loss of appetite, but the calcium level is the key component with this patient that should exclude hypothyroidism. Choice **b**, hyperthyroidism, is incorrect because of the elevated serum calcium level. Choice **d**, hypoparathyroidism, is incorrect because this condition can be associated with low serum magnesium levels as well as with symptoms such as abdominal pain, dry skin, brittle nails, and dry hair. You might consider choice **e**, diabetes mellitus, based on increased thirst, but the elevated calcium level indicates a different disorder.

Task Area: Formulating Most Likely Diagnosis
Organ System: Endocrine

146. a. The correct answer is choice **a**, extensor carpi radialis brevis (ECRB). Tennis elbow, scientifically known as lateral epicondylitis, is a disorder that involves the tendinous insertion of the extensor carpi radialis brevis muscle. This disorder is the most common overuse injury associated with the elbow. Patients with tennis elbow experience pain when lifting objects or when the arm is pronated. Choices **b**, **c**, **d**, and **e** are all incorrect as tennis elbow is defined as a disorder that involves the tendinous insertion of the extensor carpi radialis brevis muscle.

Task Area: Applying Basic Science Concepts
Organ System: Musculoskeletal

147. d. The correct answer is choice **d**, felbamate. Felbamate, marketed under the name of Felbatol, is an anticonvulsant medication used in children and adults with epilepsy whose seizures have not improved with other treatments. This medication is also used when serious side effects, such as aplastic anemia and hepatic failure, occur with other combinations of treatments. Choice **a**, tegretol, is used to treat and prevent partial seizures and to treat trigeminal neuralgia, which causes facial nerve pain. Choice **b**, valproic acid, is a common treatment for epilepsy that has more than likely already been attempted with this patient. Choice **c**, phenytoin, is also a first-line medication for treatment of epilepsy and has probably already been attempted for treatment of this patient. Choice **e**, gabapentin, is a first-line medication for treatment of some forms of epilepsy and has more than likely already been attempted with this patient.

Task Area: Pharmaceutical Therapeutics
Organ System: Neurologic

148. b. The correct answer is choice **b**, acute bronchitis. Acute bronchitis presents with cough (with or without sputum), shortness of breath, fever, sore throat, headache, and body aches. Auscultation of the chest will reveal expiratory rhonchi and wheezes. A chest X-ray will be negative. Choice **a**, chronic obstructive pulmonary disease (COPD), might be a possibility, but the presence of other symptoms such as sore throat, headache, and body aches should suggest other disorders. The lack of a sudden fever, sore throat, and muffled voice should eliminate choice **c**, acute epiglottitis, from consideration. The absence of anorexia, weight loss, and hemoptysis should rule out choice **d**, tuberculosis. Choice **e**, pneumonia, should be ruled out because of the negative chest X-ray. Pneumonia will show on a chest X-ray.

Task Area: History Taking and Performing Physical Examinations
Organ System: Infectious Diseases

149. a. Cats are the primary host for *Toxoplasma gondii*, which causes toxoplasmosis (choice **a**) in immunocompromised populations such as pregnant women. Herpes (choice **b**) can cross the placenta, but it is not transmissible to humans by cats. The influenza virus (choice **c**) is not usually carried by cats. Sarcoidosis (choice **d**) is not an infection. Syphilis (choice **e**) is sexually transmitted.

Task Area: Health Maintenance
Organ System: Reproductive

150. b. The patient most likely has a prolactin-producing tumor that is large enough to compress the optic chiasm (choice **b**). A microscopic adenoma (choice **c**) is less than 10 mm wide and is therefore too small to compress surrounding structures. A craniopharyngioma (choice **d**) usually presents at a younger age and has a more insidious onset. A berry aneurysm (choice **e**) can produce bitemporal hemianopia (also called hemianopsia) but cannot cause endocrine derangement. McCune-Albright syndrome (choice **a**) causes early puberty in young girls.

Task Area: Formulating Most Likely Diagnosis
Organ System: Endocrine

151. c. Lichen simplex chronicus (LSC) (choice **c**) is a thickening of the skin with variable scaling that arises as a result of repetitive scratching or rubbing. LSC can be due to a number of factors, the most common being an itch-scratch cycle that has gotten out of control. When diagnosing the disorder of lichen simplex chronicus, a potassium hydroxide preparation is commonly used to rule out fungal infection associated with this disorder. Choice **a**, contact dermatitis, is incorrect as this disorder is diagnosed primarily by physical examination of the affected area. Patch testing may be used to determine the allergen causing the condition. Choice **b**, seborrheic dermatitis, is incorrect as this condition is primarily diagnosed by physical examination of the affected area. Choice **d**, pityriasis rosea, is incorrect as this disorder is primarily diagnosed by physical exam of the lesion, or a biopsy of the lesion, may be performed to confirm the diagnosis. Choice **e**, psoriasis, is incorrect as this condition is diagnosed by microscopic evaluation of a sample of the affected skin patch.

Task Area: Using Laboratory and Diagnostic Studies
Organ System: Dermatologic

152. c. Oxybutynin (choice **c**) is an antimuscarinic agent used to treat urinary incontinence. It can trigger dementia by centrally blocking ACh receptors. Acetaminophen (choice **a**) is an analgesic agent. Atorvastatin (choice **b**) is a HMG-coA reductase inhibitor used for hypercholesterolemia. Ramipril (choice **d**) is an ACE inhibitor used for hypertension. Metformin (choice **e**) is generally used for type 2 diabetes.

Task Area: Pharmaceutical Therapeutics
Organ System: Neurologic

153. e. The correct answer is choice **e**, all of the above. Increased social interaction (choice **a**), antioxidant supplements (choice **b**), physical exercise (choice **c**), and memory training (choice **d**) are all considered to be potentially helpful against the progression of cognitive decline and predementia.

Task Area: Health Maintenance
Organ System: Psychiatry/Behavioral Science

154. e. Benign prostatic hyperplasia (choice **e**) is the most common cause of lower urinary tract symptoms in elderly men. A normal urinalysis would make the diagnosis of urinary tract infection (choice **a**), nephrolithiasis (choice **b**), and prostatitis (choice **c**) less likely. A normal PSA and prostate biopsy would rule out prostate cancer (choice **d**).

Task Area: Formulating Most Likely Diagnosis
Organ System: Genitourinary

155. b. Quinidine (choice **b**) is a Class I antiarrhythmic agent that is effective because it binds to open sodium channels and prevents sodium influx, which is necessary for treatment of supraventricular tachycardia. Choices **a** and **c** are incorrect as lidocaine and mexiletine are also sodium channel blockers but have a greater use in the management of ventricular arrhythmias. Choice **d**, verapamil, is incorrect as this medication is most effective when used to slow ventricular rate in patients with atrial fibrillation or atrial flutter. This medication is also a calcium channel blocker, not a sodium channel blocker. Choice **e**, adenosine, is incorrect because even though this medication is very useful for treatment of supraventricular tachycardia, it is a purine nucleoside that acts to relax smooth muscles that line the artery walls.

Task Area: Pharmaceutical Therapeutics
Organ System: Cardiovascular

156. e. HHV-8 has been found to be associated with Kaposi's sarcoma in immunosuppressed patients. This presents as a brown macular lesion (choice **e**) on the lower extremities, face (especially the nose), oral mucosa, and genitalia. Diarrhea (choice **a**) can occur with a *Cryptosporidium* infection. Leukoplakia (choice **b**) can be caused by *Candida* or EBV infection. Scleral icterus (choice **c**) and jaundice (choice **d**) can occur in hepatic failure.

Task Area: History Taking and Performing Physical Examinations
Organ System: Dermatologic

157. e. The correct answer is choice **e**, omeprazole, because proton pump inhibitors reduce gastric acid production and allow mucosal healing. Choice **a**, aspirin, is incorrect because aspirin can cause gastric ulcers with prolonged use at high doses. Choice **b**, clopidogrel, is incorrect because this antiplatelet medication is not indicated in gastric ulcers. Choice **c**, ciprofloxacin, is incorrect because this antibiotic is not indicated in this condition. Choice **d**, acetaminophen, is incorrect because it is does not address mucosal healing.

Task Area: Pharmaceutical Therapeutics
Organ System: Gastrointestinal/Nutritional

158. d. Echocardiograms (choice **d**) are essential to the work-up of anatomical heart problems. Electrocardiograms and chest X-rays (choices **a** and **b**) may give qualitative indications of structural abnormality but not quantitative ones. A CT angiogram (choice **c**) is the investigation of choice for an acute coronary syndrome. An MRI (choice **e**) will not give any dynamic information about the heart.

Task Area: Using Laboratory and Diagnostic Studies
Organ System: Cardiovascular

159. **b.** In some cultures, there is a fear that early menopause is a predictor of early death. This may be related to the fact that early menopause is more common in cigarette smokers, who have a shorter life expectancy for a variety of other reasons. To the contrary, early menopause actually decreases the chances of developing certain diseases, including breast cancer and ovarian cancer, because of the decreased circulating levels of estrogen. These decreased estrogen levels do, however, lead to an increased risk of osteoporosis (choice **b**); this increased risk can be attenuated with hormone replacement therapy and the standard regimen of lifestyle changes, including resistance weight training to strengthen the bones by the mobilization of osteclasts. Risk of osteoarthritis (choice **a**) and osteomalacia (choice **c**) are unrelated to estrogen levels and age at menopause. Breast cancer (choice **d**) and ovarian cancer (choice **e**) are less common in women who experience early menopause.

Task Area: Health Maintenance
Organ System: Reproductive

160. **a.** In the presence of a growing neck nodule, it is important to consider the possibility of thyroid cancer. If the nodule moves with swallowing, it is probably associated with the thyroid. Most thyroid malignancies lead to a clinically euthyroid presentation, and the patient generally complains of neck enlargement or tightness. Investigations may show an increase in carcinoembryonic antigen and increased uptake of Tc-99m into the thyroid. A fine-needle aspiration biopsy should generally be used in order to confirm the diagnosis, and the most effective therapy is surgical excision (choice **a**). The amount of tissue excised will usually depend on the extent of the malignancy. Antithyroid therapy (choice **b**) is useful for hyperthyroid conditions, and thyroid hormone supplementation (choice **c**) is useful for hypothyroid conditions, but neither is likely to help in the case of a euthyroid condition. Radioiodine therapy (choice **d**) improves prognosis when used as an adjuvant to surgery but is not the first-line option. Observation (choice **e**) may be a reasonable option if the nodule is benign.

Task area: Clinical Intervention
Organ System: Endocrine

161. **b.** The correct answer is choice **b**, obstruction of the meibomian gland. Choice **a**, bacterial infection of the meibomian gland, is incorrect because it is more consistent with hordeolum. Choice **c**, basal cell carcinoma of the eyelid, is incorrect because chalazion is a benign nodule. Choice **d**, increased intraocular pressure, is incorrect because it is more consistent with glaucoma. Choice **e**, vascular occlusion, is incorrect because chalazion is not a vascular disorder.

Task Area: Applying Basic Science Concepts
Organ System: EENT (Eye, Ear, Nose, and Throat)

162. c. If you suspect a patient is suffering from schizophrenia, a CT scan of the brain (choice **c**) should be obtained in order to confirm the diagnosis. Individuals who suffer from schizophrenia will show enlarged ventricles and cortical atrophy on a CT scan, both of which are indicative of chronic schizophrenic disease. Choice **a**, electroencephalogram, is incorrect as this diagnostic tool is used to assess electrical activity of the brain. Choice **b**, MRI of the brain, might be an option; however, recent studies have shown that MRI is more effective in detecting changes in gray matter, which may predispose individuals to developing schizophrenia. CT scanning is still the primary imaging tool of choice for the diagnosis of schizophrenia. Choice **d**, SPECT scan of the brain, is incorrect as this imaging modality is typically used for diagnosis of dementia. Choice **e**, cerebral angiogram, is incorrect as this imaging modality is used to assess vascular flow to the brain.

Task Area: Using Laboratory and Diagnostic Studies

Organ System: Psychiatry/Behavioral Science

163. b. Cryptococcosis (choice **b**) is a potentially fatal fungal disease that is particularly damaging to individuals with weakened immune systems, such as HIV patients. Intravenous amphotericin B combined with oral flucytosin has been proven to be an effective treatment for this disorder, and this medical intervention does not further weaken the immune system. Choice **a**, malaria, is incorrect as this disorder is most effectively treated with medications such as doxycycline or chloroquine. Choice **c**, shigellosis, is incorrect as this disorder is most effectively treated with antibiotics and fluid replacement. Choice **d**, salmonellosis, is incorrect as this condition is most effectively treated with antibiotics and fluid replacement. Amphotericin and flucytosin are antifungal agents and are not to be confused with antibiotics used to treat bacterial infections such as shigellosis and salmonellosis. Choice **e**, botulism, is incorrect as this condition is most effectively treated with an antitoxin that blocks the action of neurotoxins circulating in the blood.

Task Area: Clinical Intervention

Organ System: Infectious Diseases

164. d. Placenta previa is a condition that occurs when the placenta blocks the path between the fetus and the uterine canal. It typically presents as painless (choice **d**) vaginal bleeding and should be investigated with an ultrasound in order to localize the placenta. If the diagnosis is confirmed, the fetus must be delivered by cesarean section. Uterine contractions (choice **a**) may be present in placenta previa, but they are unlikely to be painful. Any abdominal or pelvic pain (choices **b** and **c**) should raise the suspicion of a placental abruption. A digital vaginal examination (choice **e**) should never be attempted due to the risk of provoking a life-threatening hemorrhage.

Task Area: History Taking and Performing Physical Examinations
Organ System: Reproductive

165. b. This question tests your knowledge of medical treatment options in type 2 diabetes and their side effects. The correct answer is choice **b**, metformin (biguanide), which may have the potential risk of lactose acidosis. All the other choices are incorrect because they are not known to cause lactose acidosis. Therefore, choice **e**, all of the above, is incorrect.

Task Area: Clinical Intervention
Organ System: Endocrine

166. b. The correct answer is choice **b**, supraventricular tachycardia. Supraventricular tachycardia appears as rapid sinus rhythm without the presence of p-waves. Supraventricular tachycardia can cause symptoms such as shortness of breath, dizziness, and chest pressure. Choice **a**, atrial flutter, would not be considered because of the absence of the characteristic "sawtooth" pattern of the p-waves. Choice **c**, ventricular tachycardia, is incorrect because the heart beats on the EKG shown are normal and rapid, while QRS complexes in ventricular tachycardia are wide, abnormal, and rapid. Choice **d**, atrial fibrillation, is incorrect because atrial fibrillation contains no p-waves and is an irregular rhythm, whereas supraventricular tachycardia is a regular rhythm. Choice **e**, sinus tachycardia, can often be mistaken for supraventricular tachycardia; however, the rhythms differ in that sinus tachycardia contains QRS complexes with associated p-waves, whereas p-waves are absent with supraventricular tachycardia.

Task Area: Using Laboratory and Diagnostic Studies
Organ System: Cardiovascular

167. **d.** The correct answer is choice **d**, labyrinthitis. Meclizine is a common medication prescribed for the treatment of dizziness caused by disorders of the inner ear. Meclizine is available in regular and chewable tablets and in suppository form. The underlying cause of labyrinthitis is unknown, but it is believed to be caused by an otitis or viremia. Choice **a**, barotrauma, is commonly treated medically with antihistamines, steroids, or decongestants. Choice **b**, acute vertigo, is often treated with diazepam. Choice **c**, motion sickness, is most commonly treated with scopolamine. Choice **e**, presbycusis, is not treatable, but hearing loss is often ameliorated with hearing aids.

Task Area: Pharmaceutical Therapeutics
Organ System: EENT (Eye, Ear, Nose, and Throat)

168. **e.** While acute episodes of dyspnea, dizziness, and palpitations can have a fairly wide range of differential diagnoses, the slurred upstroke in the QRS complex (also known as a delta wave) is very specific for Wolff-Parkinson-White (WPW) syndrome, also known as pre-excitation syndrome. This is a syndrome caused by the presence of a second conduction pathway between the atrial and ventricular systems; this accessory pathway is distinct from the AV node. Catheter ablation (choice **e**) is curative for 90 to 95% of patients and is generally considered to be the most effective therapeutic option. Amiodarone (choice **a**) is an option for therapy in acute arrhythmic episodes but is not used regularly because of its tendency to cause interstitial lung disease and thyroid dysfunction. Cardioversion (choice **d**) may also be useful in an acute episode, but it is not useful for preventing future episodes. Adenosine (choice **b**) and beta blockers (choice **c**) are not useful in WPW syndrome because they act at the AV node and are ineffective at accessory conduction pathways.

Task Area: Clinical Intervention
Organ System: Cardiovascular

169. a. In a patient with a long history of smoking, an FEV_1/FVC ratio below 70% is almost always indicative of chronic obstructive pulmonary disease (COPD). Continued smoking generally leads to further deterioration in lung function, which manifests as a progressive increase in the patient's dyspnea and cough. If the patient quits smoking, however, the deterioration in her lung function will revert to that of the general population; while the current damage to her lungs is mostly irreversible, smoking cessation (choice **a**) may still provide her with a reasonable chance of avoiding long-term respiratory failure. While an aerobic exercise program (choice **b**) is nearly always a good recommendation, it is unlikely to be sustainable in a patient with irreversible exertional dyspnea. Bronchodilator therapy (choice **c**) and inhaled corticosteroid therapy (choice **d**) have been shown to be mildly beneficial to COPD patients, but their effect is relatively mild, and they will not prevent long-term deterioration if the patient is still smoking. Chemotherapy (choice **e**) may be effective if the patient develops a lung cancer, but this patient's presentation is much more likely to be associated with COPD. For this patient, it is still valuable to recommend inhaled therapy as well as aerobic exercise. If these actions are combined with smoking cessation, they are likely to provide considerable long-term benefits. However, smoking cessation is most powerful as a single independent recommendation to maximize prognosis.
Task Area: Health Maintenance
Organ System: Pulmonary

170. a. In the presence of a chronic gnawing stomach pain associated with fatigue, weight loss, and early satiety, a diagnosis of peptic ulcer disease is highly likely. However, gastric adenocarcinoma (choice **a**) can also present in a similar way; often, the diagnosis is missed until the patient presents with symptoms of metastatic disease. In this case, the presence of painful defecation and sexual intercourse (signs of metastasis via peritoneal spread to the Pouch of Douglas) is suggestive of malignancy. Chronic gastritis (choice **b**) and *H. pylori* infection (choice **c**) can cause the initial symptoms and would be resistant to initial therapy, but they are unlikely to cause obstructive vaginal or rectal symptoms. Pelvic inflammatory disease (choice **d**) and cervical cancer (choice **e**) are less likely to initially present with gastrointestinal symptoms.
Task Area: Formulating Most Likely Diagnosis
Organ System: Gastrointestinal/Nutritional

171. b. A sudden-onset severe tearing chest pain should always raise the suspicion of an aortic dissection. This is a medical emergency that will often lead to death without immediate surgical intervention (choice **b**). The presentation usually features a unilateral diminished pulse, systemic hypertension, and mediastinal widening on a chest X-ray. Often, there is a long history of poorly-controlled hypertension. Thrombolytic therapy (choice **a**) may be useful in the case of a thromboembolic event such as a myocardial infarction or a pulmonary embolism, both of which usually present with dyspnea and less severe pain. Angiogram and stenting (choice **c**) is more likely to be beneficial for relief of coronary artery disease. Thoracentesis (choice **d**) may be used for a pneumothorax, which will usually present with tracheal deviation and mediastinal shift, but it is characterized by acute onset of dyspnea. Pain relief (choice **e**) should probably be used, but it is far less important than immediate surgery.

Task area: Clinical Intervention
Organ System: Cardiovascular

172. e. Pulse oximetry (choice **e**) will give the percentage of saturated haemoglobin in a non-invasive manner. Venous blood gas (choice **a**) can be used to measure bicarbonate, carbon dioxide, and pH. Arterial blood gas (choice **b**) is an invasive test that gives accurate blood concentrations of oxygen. A full blood count (choice **c**) is useful for working up anemia. Spirometry (choice **d**) differentiates obstructive versus restrictive disease.

Task Area: Using Laboratory and Diagnostic Studies
Organ System: Pulmonary

173. a. Antibody blockage and destruction of acetylcholine receptors (choice **a**) at the neuromuscular junction causes the symptoms of myasthenia gravis. Antibody blockage of calcium channels (choice **b**) causes Lambert-Eaton syndrome. Demyelination of Schwan cells (choice **c**) can be seen in Guillain-Barré syndrome. Demyelination of astrocytes (choice **d**) can describe multiple sclerosis. T-cell inflammation of myocytes (choice **e**) can be seen in inclusion body myositis.

Task Area: Applying Basic Science Concepts
Organ System: Musculoskeletal

174. b. The most appropriate initial treatment for congestive heart failure is treatment with diuretics (choice **b**). Diuretics are effective in reducing the fluid volume in the lungs, which will relieve the symptoms associated with congestive heart failure. Choice **a**, ACE inhibitors, are used to control blood pressure, which is a common risk factor for congestive heart failure. However, diuretics are most effective in ridding the body of fluid collection associated with congestive heart failure. Choices **c**, β-adrenergic antagonists, and **d**, calcium channel blockers, are incorrect as they have the potential to worsen the condition of congestive heart failure. Choice **e**, corticosteroids, is incorrect as the use of corticosteroids can also cause the body to retain fluid, so these medications are definitely contraindicated for patients with congestive heart failure.

Task Area: Pharmaceutical Therapeutics
Organ System: Cardiovascular

175. c. The presence of normal ventilation and multiple perfusion defects on lung V/Q scan are the classic indicators for pulmonary embolism (choice **c**). Because of the evidence of renal impairment, further work-up for kidney function would be indicated. Choices **a**, **b**, **d**, and **e** are all incorrect.

Task Area: Using Laboratory and Diagnostic Studies

Organ System: Pulmonary

176. a. This patient is suffering from a thromboembolism in his femoral artery, a condition that often causes severe pain followed by necrosis of peripheral muscle. Risk factors are similar to those for coronary artery disease; this patient's history of a myocardial infarction puts him at particularly high risk. The diagnosis is highly likely based on the deficiency of peripheral pulses. Femoral embolectomy (choice **a**) is the most definitive treatment option. Medical thrombolytic (choice **b**) or anticoagulant (choice **c**) therapy can also be used, but these are less likely to be effective, especially in a patient who has already suffered muscle damage due to infarction. Pain relief (choice **d**) is helpful, but will not provide any long-term benefit. Amputation (choice **e**) only becomes necessary in the case of severe necrosis.

Task Area: Clinical Intervention

Organ System: Cardiovascular

177. c. Cholangitis (choice **c**) is a condition characterized by infection or inflammation due to obstruction of the hepatic duct or the bile duct by a gallstone. It typically presents with fever, right upper quadrant pain, and bile-tinged urine. Bile duct dilation on an ultrasound is also suggestive of the presence of an obstruction in the biliary tree. In addition to initiating antibiotic therapy, it may be necessary to clear the obstruction via endoscopic retrograde cholangiopancreatography or surgical intervention. Cholecystitis (choice **a**) and cholelithiasis (choice **b**) also present in a similar way but are unlikely to cause bile duct dilation. Cholangiocarcinoma (choice **d**) is unlikely to cause an acute presentation and is far less common than cholangitis. Appendicitis (choice **e**) typically presents with right lower quadrant pain and does not affect the bile duct.

Task Area: Formulating Most Likely Diagnosis

Organ System: Gastrointestinal/Nutritional

178. e. Anorexia nervosa is an eating disorder that involves complex psychological issues. The correct answer is choice **e**, all of the above, because this disorder requires a multidisciplinary approach to address the multiple dimensions of this illness.

Task Area: Clinical Intervention

Organ System: Psychiatry/Behavioral Science

179. d. The physical presentation of this child should prompt high suspicion for epiglottitis (choice **d**). The "thumb sign" on X-ray is indicative of an enlarged epiglottis. Choice **e**, none of the above, is therefore incorrect. Choice **a**, tonsillitis, is incorrect because the oral exam does not show signs of tonsillitis. Choice **b**, foreign body obstruction of the oral pharynx, is incorrect because the X-ray finding is more consistent with epiglottitis, although a foreign body remains part of the differential diagnosis. Choice **c**, scarlet fever, is incorrect because the normal oral exam is inconsistent with this diagnosis.

Task Area: Using Laboratory and Diagnostic Studies

Organ System: EENT (Eye, Ear, Nose, and Throat)

180. c. For individuals who are diagnosed with pulmonary embolism, anticoagulation therapy (choice **c**), preferably with heparin, should be initiated immediately. For individuals at risk of recurrence of pulmonary embolism or intolerant of anticoagulants, vena cava filter is the indicated intervention. Choice **a**, surgical clot removal, might be a consideration; however, this option is usually only indicated if anticoagulation fails or if the patient's health is in such serious jeopardy that it requires immediate clot removal. Choice **b**, vena cava interruption, is incorrect as this option is used to prevent blood clots from traveling to the lungs. Vena cava interruption is most commonly referred to as placement of a Greenfield filter. Once the blood clots have reached the lungs, anticoagulation therapy must be initiated. Choice **d**, hyperbaric treatment, is incorrect as this option is useful to minimize damage to the brain, which occurs if a blood clot reaches the brain and causes a stroke. Choice **e**, lithotripsy, is incorrect as this option is used to eliminate stones from the kidneys, bladder, or urethra, and will have no therapeutic benefit for blood clots.

Task Area: Clinical Intervention

Organ System: Pulmonary

Section 4

181. e. This question tests your knowledge of the physical manifestations of cirrhosis. The correct answer is choice **e**, liver cirrhosis. These physical findings are consistent with portal hypertension as a result of worsening cirrhosis of the liver. All the other choices are incorrect because they are inconsistent with the physical findings.

Task Area: History Taking and Performing Physical Examinations

Organ System: Gastrointestinal/Nutritional

182. e. Like most allergic conditions, asthma is characterized by inappropriate activation of mast cells (choice **e**) and eosinophils. When a mast cell degranulates, it releases several molecules that are partly responsible for the airway hyperresponsiveness that characterizes an asthma exacerbation. This process is utilized for several diagnostic tests and is inhibited by several drugs that are often used for asthma. Neutrophils (choice **a**) are generally produced in response to bacterial infection. Basophils (choice **b**) are involved in several inflammatory processes but make up an insignificant portion of white blood cells. B-lymphocytes (choice **c**) act to produce antibodies in response to different types of antigens. Giant cells (choice **d**) are usually involved in granulomatous processes.

Task Area: Applying Basic Science Concepts

Organ System: Pulmonary

183. d. Propafenone (choice **d**) contains some beta adrenergic receptor blocking properties and may further exacerbate the condition of heart failure. Choice **a**, amiodarone, is incorrect as this medication has been proven effective to increase functional capacity in patients with heart failure. Choice **b**, dofetilide, is incorrect as this medication has little to no effect on heart failure in the presence of atrial fibrillation. Choice **c**, digoxin, is incorrect as this medication has been the drug of choice for many years for the treatment of heart failure and is not contraindicated in a person with both heart failure and atrial fibrillation. Choice **e**, adenosine, is incorrect as this medication is used to convert the rhythm of supraventricular tachycardia and has no therapeutic value for atrial fibrillation.

Task Area: Pharmaceutical Therapeutics

Organ System: Cardiovascular

184. b. The correct answer is choice **b**, control blood glucose. The main cause of retinopathy among adults in the United States is diabetes. Controlling blood glucose levels is critical to preventing the progression of retinopathy. Patients with this disorder should have yearly dilated opthalmoscopic examinations. Choices **a**, **c**, **d**, and **e** are all incorrect as they will have no benefit for the prevention of retinopathy.

Task Area: Health Maintenance

Organ System: EENT (Eye, Ear, Nose, and Throat)

185. a. Zollinger-Ellison syndrome (choice **a**) is characterized by a gastrin-secreting tumor called a gastrinoma that causes hypergastrinemia, which results in a resistant form of peptic ulcer disease. A patient may present with exactly the same symptoms as for peptic ulcer disease, such as abdominal pain that feels like a burning or gnawing, belching, bloating, heartburn, nausea, and black tarry stools. A fasting gastrin level greater than 150 pg/mL indicates hypergastrinemia. Endoscopy is useful in localizing the tumor. Choice **b**, gastric adenocarcinoma, might be a consideration; however, the elevated gastric level should rule this out in favor of Zollinger-Ellison syndrome. Choice **c**, carcinoid stomach tumor, is incorrect as these tumors can cause carcinoid syndrome, which provokes symptoms such as flushing, wheezing, and diarrhea. Choice **d**, gastric lymphoma, is incorrect because of the patient's age (most gastric lymphomas occur over the age of 60) and the lack of symptoms such as feeling full, fatigue, and weight loss. Choice **e**, gastroparesis, is incorrect as this condition is characterized by vomiting and feeling full after a few bites of food.
Task Area: Using Laboratory and Diagnostic Studies
Organ System: Gastrointestinal/Nutritional

186. c. Metformin (choice **c**) is effective because it reduces hepatic glucose production. It effectively lowers blood glucose levels without risk of hypoglycemia. This medication is also effective in promoting weight loss and lowering triglycerides. Choice **a**, glimepiride, is incorrect as this medication causes the pancreas to increase insulin production, which does have a risk for hypoglycemia. Choice **b**, glyburide, is incorrect as this medication causes the pancreas to increase insulin production and causes the liver to decrease sugar production, which could potentially cause hypoglycemia. Choice **d**, exenatide, is effective for glucose control and promoting weight loss; however, it requires caution to avoid hypoglycemia and pancreatitis. Choice **e**, glipizide, is incorrect as it stimulates the pancreas to increase production of insulin, which could cause hypoglycemia.
Task Area: Pharmaceutical Therapeutics
Organ System: Endocrine

187. c. Bronchiolitis with the presence of respiratory syncytial virus (RSV) is an indication for treatment with ribavirin (choice **c**). A three- to seven-day regimen of ribavirin has been proven to reduce mortality, length of hospitalization, and duration of mechanical ventilation for patients with RSV-induced bronchiolitis. Choice **a**, sulfamethoxazole/trimethoprim, is incorrect as this is an antibiotic medication that is used to treat bacterial infections and is not indicated for a viral infection. Choice **b**, erythromycin, is incorrect as this is an antibiotic medication that is used to treat bacterial infections and is not indicated for a viral infection. Choice **d**, cyclosporine, is incorrect as this medication is commonly used to prevent transplant rejection and offers no benefit against a viral infection. Choice **e**, ciprofloxacin, is incorrect as this is an antibiotic medication that is used to treat bacterial infections and is not indicated for a viral infection.

Task Area: Clinical Intervention
Organ System: Pulmonary

188. d. Weight-bearing exercise (choice **d**) will cause further degenerative damage to the joint. Weight loss (choice **a**), physical therapy (choice **b**), and occupational therapy (choice **c**) can reduce degenerative damage to the knee joint. Heat pads (choice **e**) can offer symptomatic relief.

Task Area: Health Maintenance
Organ System: Musculoskeletal

189. a. Dilation of arteries results in a reduced cardiac output, which is compensated through homeostatic mechanisms by raising the heart rate (choice **a**). The heart rate would not be expected to decrease (choice **b**), remain constant (choice **c**), or fluctuate (choices **d** and **e**).

Task Area: Applying Basic Science Concepts
Organ System: Cardiovascular

190. c. The correct answer is choice **c**, fibromyalgia. Pregabalin was the first FDA-approved drug for the treatment of fibromyalgia pain. In 2007, duloxetine hydrochloride was also approved for the treatment of fibromyalgia. Fibromyalgia symptoms can include pain, muscle stiffness, muscle tenderness, fatigue, difficulty falling asleep, and difficulty staying asleep. Choices **a**, **b**, **d**, and **e** are all incorrect because, at this time, pregabalin, milnacipran, and duloxetine hydrochloride are the only FDA-approved medications for the treatment of fibromyalgia.

Task Area: Pharmaceutical Therapeutics
Organ System: Musculoskeletal

191. a. The correct answer is choice **a**, broad-spectrum fluoroquinolones, because of their activity against *S. pneumoniae*. Therefore choice **e**, none of the above, is incorrect. Choice **b**, acetaminophen, is incorrect because it does not address the underlying bacterial infection. Choice **c**, isonizide, is incorrect because it is part of the treatment regimen for pulmonary tuberculosis. Choice **d**, metronidazole, is incorrect because it is generally used for parasitic or anaerobic organisms, which are not common in community-acquired pneumonia.

Task Area: Clinical Intervention
Organ System: Pulmonary

192. a. The correct answer is choice **a**, acute anteroseptal infarct, given what is shown on the electrocardiogram (EKG). This makes choice **e**, none of the above, incorrect. Choice **b**, acute lateral wall infarct, is incorrect because it is more consistent with ST elevation in leads I and aVL. Choice **c**, acute inferior myocardial infarction, is incorrect because it is more consistent with ST segment elevation in leads II, III, and aVF. Choice **d**, pericarditis, is incorrect because an EKG usually shows diffuse ST elevation or more generalized ST and T wave changes.

Task Area: Using Laboratory and Diagnostic Studies

Organ System: Cardiovascular

193. b. Sciatica is a condition in which mechanical pressure on the sciatic nerve or the L5/S1 nerve roots causes back pain that shoots into the posterior aspect of a patient's leg. This is often caused by a disc herniation or other injury to the vertebral column. The L5/S1 nerve root is also responsible for the ankle jerk reflex, which is often diminished (choice **b**) in a sciatic nerve compression. Exaggerated ankle jerk reflex (choice **a**) would be expected in an upper motor neuron lesion. The knee jerk reflex (choices **c** and **d**) is mediated by the L4/L5 nerve roots, which may offer some contribution to the sciatic nerve but is less specific for sciatica than the L5/S1 root. Uniformly exaggerated lower limb reflexes (choice **e**) may be found in an upper motor neuron lesion above the level of L5.

Task Area: History Taking and Performing Physical Examination

Organ System: Musculoskeletal

194. c. The correct answer is choice **c**, calcium channel blockers. Calcium channel blocker medications prevent calcium from entering cells of the heart and blood vessel walls. These medications relax and therefore allow the blood vessels to dilate by affecting the muscle cells of arterial walls. These medications are the best choice for peripheral vasodilatation. Calcium channel blockers are also the best choice among the African-American and the elderly populations. Choice **a**, diuretics, is incorrect as these medications are useful for ridding the body of excess fluids and do not achieve peripheral vasodilatation to the extent that is achieved by calcium channel blockers. β-adrenergic antagonists (choice **b**) are effective because they work by blocking signals from the sympathetic nervous system, but they do not achieve peripheral vasodilatation to the extent that is achieved by calcium channel blockers. Choice **d**, ACE inhibitors, is incorrect as these medications work by regulating the renin-angiotensin system but do not achieve peripheral vasodilatation to the extent that is achieved by calcium channel blockers, corticosteroids (choice **e**), is incorrect as these are not a class of antihypertensive medications.

Task Area: Pharmaceutical Therapeutics

Organ System: Cardiovascular

195. **b.** Gonorrhea (choice **b**) is a sexually transmitted disease that occurs in men and women primarily between the ages of 15 and 29. This disorder is caused by the *Neisseria gonorrhoeae* bacterium. Men afflicted with gonorrhea complain of painful, burning urination and a serous or milky white discharge. One to three days after symptoms begin, the pain and burning becomes more pronounced, and the discharge becomes yellow, creamy, profuse, and tinged with blood. Choice **a**, epididymitis, is associated with fever, chills, and a heavy sensation in the scrotum that gets worse with pressure. Choice **c**, syphilis, should be excluded because of the lack of skin lesions and lymph node enlargement. The lack of testicular tenderness and rectal pain or discharge should rule out choice **d**, chlamydia. Choice **e**, HIV, should be ruled out because of the lack of fever, sore throat, enlarged lymph nodes, and muscle pains. Any person who comes in with any type of STD should be tested for *N. gonorrhoeae*, *Chlamydia trachomatis*, HIV, and syphilis. Oral, anal, penile, and vaginal swabs should be taken.

Task Area: Formulating Most Likely Diagnosis
Organ System: Infectious Diseases

196. **d.** This patient's presentation is typical of rheumatoid arthritis, an inflammatory condition that most commonly affects the peripheral joints. However, the presence of a rash with a silvery scale (choice **d**) is fairly specific for psoriasis, which commonly presents with symptoms similar to those for rheumatoid arthritis. Approximately one-third of patients with psoriasis will develop a psoriatic arthritis, but the presence of a rash with silvery scale is a good way to clinically differentiate the two conditions. Asymmetry (choice **a**), redness (choice **b**), tenderness (choice **c**), and raised areas (choice **e**) are fairly nonspecific signs that may be present in psoriasis but are not strongly suggestive of a diagnosis.

Task Area: History Taking and Performing Physical Examinations
Organ System: Dermatologic

197. **e.** The correct answer is choice **e**, warfarin, which is never indicated for immediate anticoagulation in acute coronary syndrome. Morphine (choice **a**), oxygen (choice **b**), metoprolol (choice **c**), and aspirin (choice **d**) are considered standard treatment for acute coronary syndrome.

Task Area: Clinical Intervention
Organ System: Cardiovascular

198. c. Scabies (choice **c**) is a common condition that is caused by the arthropod *Sarcoptes scabiei*, which is often transferred among children who have close contact with one another. It typically presents with a rash that features multiple papules, burrows, and pustules. Unlike most viral and bacterial infectious conditions, scabies does not cause a fever because there is generally no systemic infection. Dermatitis (choice **a**) and eczema (choice **b**) may present with a diffuse rash, but they are unlikely to cause multiple localized nodular lesions; additionally, the recent history involving other children in the patient's class is suggestive of a contagious condition. Chickenpox (choice **d**) and measles (choice **e**) typically present with considerable fever and malaise and have been drastically reduced in incidence since the institution of widespread vaccination programs.

Task Area: Formulating Most Likely Diagnosis
Organ System: Dermatologic

199. a. This question tests your knowledge of common anemia conditions during pregnancy. Folate deficiency anemia (choice **a**) is common especially in multiple gestations because of increased maternal and fetal demands, and is indicated in this patient by the megaloblastic anemia and low serum folate. Folate supplementation is crucial. All the other choices are incorrect because they are inconsistent with the laboratory panel in this case.

Task Area: Using Laboratory and Diagnostic Studies
Organ System: Reproductive

200. b. The correct answer is choice **b**, antisocial personality disorder. Adults with this type of disorder often have behavior problems starting in childhood. Choice **a**, delusional disorder, is incorrect because this patient does not have false beliefs that affect his daily activities. Choice **c**, borderline personality disorder, is incorrect because there is no mention of difficulties with interpersonal relations. Choice **d**, narcissistic personality disorder, is incorrect because this patient's clinical history makes antisocial personality disorder a more likely diagnosis. Choice **e**, schizoid personality disorder, is incorrect because this type of patient typically has odd or eccentric thoughts or behavior.

Task Area: Formulating Most Likely Diagnosis
Organ System: Psychiatry/Behavioral Science

201. e. Bradycardia is a common phenomenon that is often not considered to be an abnormality, especially in the case of a young athlete. However, in a middle-aged patient, it may warrant further investigation in order to rule out the possibility of heart block. While first-degree heart block is usually inconsequential, second-degree heart block may manifest as a regularly irregular heart rate (choice **e**). If this is the case, it is likely due to a Wenckebach rhythm, in which the interval between two beats progressively increases until the heart effectively skips a beat. Usually, the rhythm repeats after every three to five beats. A change in the patient's pulse pressure (choices **a** and **b**) may be caused by a problem that affects the patient's blood pressure. A regularly regular heart rate (choice **c**) is a normal finding that is present in most patients. An irregularly irregular heart rate (choice **d**) is usually found in atrial fibrillation and other forms of arrhythmia.

Task Area: History Taking and Performing Physical Examinations
Organ System: Cardiovascular

202. **c.** A nosebleed that occurs from the Wood-ruff's plexus (choice **c**) is often arterial, which explains the presence of bright red blood. This disorder is a result of trauma. Blood will often be appreciated in the posterior pharynx. Choice **a**, fractured sinus, should be excluded because of the lack of forehead swelling and forehead paresthesia. Choice **b**, epistaxis from Kiesselbach's plexus, should be excluded almost immediately because of the posterior location of the bleeding; Kiesselbach's plexus is in the anterior aspect of the nose. Choice **d**, epiglottitis, should be excluded because of the lack of high fever, sore throat, difficulty swallowing, and cyanosis. Choice **e**, sinusitis, should be excluded because of the lack of headache, bad breath, stuffy nose, and fever.

Task Area: Formulating Most Likely Diagnosis
Organ System: EENT (Eye, Ear, Nose, and Throat)

203. **b.** The correct answer is choice **b**, secondary hypothyroidism. Choice **a**, primary hypothyroidism, is incorrect because TSH is usually elevated. Given the low free T4, choices **c**, euthyroid goiter; **d**, primary hyperthyroidism; and **e**, secondary hyperthyroidism, are incorrect.

Task Area: Using Laboratory and Diagnostic Studies
Organ System: Endocrine

204. **e.** This patient's painful lesion has a dermatomal distribution, which is typical for herpes zoster. It is caused by reactivation of varicella-zoster virus. The correct answer is choice **e**, famciclovir. Choices **a**, topical antibiotic cream, and **b**, topical antifungal cream, are incorrect because this patient has a viral infection. Choice **c**, surgical excision, is incorrect because the condition is not malignant and therefore excision is not necessary. Choice **d**, fluconazole, is incorrect because this medication is indicated for the treatment of candidiasis infection.

Task Area: Pharmaceutical Therapeutics
Organ System: Infectious Diseases

205. **b.** Nasal polyps (choice **b**) in children are indicative of cystic fibrosis. Asthmatics have many atopic symptoms (choice **c**). They also have shortness of breath (choice **a**), wheeze (choice **d**), and cough (choice **e**).

Task Area: History Taking and Performing Physical Examinations
Organ System: Pulmonary

206. a. Herpes simplex virus (HSV) is generally divided into two subtypes: HSV1 and HSV2. HSV1 (choice **a**) is usually responsible for oropharyngeal, eye, and central nervous system infections, while HSV2 is more likely to cause anogenital infections. Although many patients are distressed by the stigma of a herpes infection, HSV1 is highly prevalent, is not generally associated with sexual transmission, and does not usually cause significant symptoms beyond the simple oral ulcers that are often described as cold sores. HSV2 (choice **b**) is also a common cause of cold sores, but is significantly less common than HSV1 in oral infections. Epstein-Barr virus (choice **c**) usually causes infectious mononucleosis (also known as glandular fever) and is not usually implicated in oral ulcers. Rhinovirus (choice **d**) is the cause of the common cold, but it does not usually cause cold sores. *Streptococcus pneumoniae* (choice **e**) often causes pharyngitis, tonsillitis, pneumonia, and a wide range of other respiratory tract infections.
Task Area: Applying Basic Science Concepts
Organ System: EENT (Eye, Ear, Nose, and Throat)

207. b. The correct answer is choice **b**, frontotemporal dementia. Frontotemporal dementia presents similarly to Alzheimer's dementia except that this disorder is characterized by degeneration of the frontal lobe of the brain and may include the temporal lobe. Patients with this disorder may present with memory loss, abrupt mood swings, inability to function in social situations, lack of personal hygiene, and obsessive-compulsive behavior. A physical examination will reveal increased rigidity in the muscles and loss of coordination. An MRI will reveal atrophy in the frontal lobe and/or the anterior temporal lobe. Choice **a**, pseudodementia, is incorrect because patients with this disorder have a psychiatric illness that causes them only to *appear* to be demented. Patients will present with the appearance of being distressed or upset and will complain of memory problems. Choice **c**, vascular dementia, is incorrect because this disorder is caused by prolonged decrease of blood flow to the brain, normally as a result of multiple strokes. Choice **d**, Alzheimer's disease, is incorrect because, although Alzheimer's presents much like frontotemporal dementia with memory loss and mood swings, this disorder is also associated with diminished vocabulary and word fluency. Choice **e**, Huntington's disease, is associated with hallucinations, paranoia, psychoses, and abnormal involuntary muscle movements.
Task Area: History Taking and Performing Physical Examinations
Organ System: Neurologic

208. b. The correct answer is choice **b**, ritodrine, which is no longer available for use in the United States for treatment of pre-term labor. Choices **a**, **c**, **d**, and **e** are all incorrect because all of these medications are available for use in the United States for treatment of pre-term labor.

Task Area: Pharmaceutical Therapeutics
Organ System: Reproductive

209. b. The correct answer is choice **b**, appendectomy, which is the standard treatment to prevent complications such as perforation. Choice **a**, give antibiotic treatment and observe, is incorrect because although antibiotic is indicated, surgical removal of the inflamed appendix is indicated to prevent complications such as perforation. Choice **c**, give acetaminophen for pain, is incorrect because it does not address the inflammatory process of acute appendicitis. Choices **d**, observe and repeat abdominal CAT scan in one week to confirm, and **e**, perform a colonoscopy, are incorrect because they are not the standard of treatment.

Task Area: Clinical Intervention
Organ System: Gastrointestinal/Nutritional

210. a. The correct answer is choice **a**, clear. If cerebrospinal fluid obtained from a lumbar puncture is negative for subarachnoid hemorrhage, the cerebrospinal fluid will be crystal clear in color. If the color of the cerebrospinal fluid is found to be any color other than clear, then the result of the cerebrospinal fluid evaluation is not negative. Cloudy (choice **c**) cerebrospinal fluid is an indicator of infection and buildup of white blood cells. Milky (choice **d**) cerebrospinal fluid is an indicator of bacterial meningitis. Yellow (choice **b**) or bloody (choice **e**) cerebrospinal fluid may be indicative of subarachnoid hemorrhage.

Task Area: Using Laboratory and Diagnostic Studies
Organ System: Neurologic

211. c. Turner syndrome (choice **c**) is the most common cause of primary amenorrhea. It is a chromsomal abnormality resulting in ovarian failure. Noonan syndrome (choice **d**) presents in a similar way to Turner syndrome, but it has a normal karyotype. Down syndrome (choice **a**) usually has a trisomy 21 karyotype. Klinefelter syndrome (choice **b**) has a karyotype of 47XXY. Marfan sydrome (choice **e**) is caused by a mutation in the fibrilin gene.

Task Area: Formulating Most Likely Diagnosis
Organ System: Reproductive

212. **b.** β-andrenergic antagonists (choice **b**) have been proven effective to decrease heart rate and cardiac output. This class of medication has been proven most effective in younger white males. Choice **a**, a higher dose of diuretics, is incorrect because his hypertensive condition has been proven to be resistant to diuretic therapy. Choices **c**, ACE inhibitors, and **d**, calcium channel blockers, could be considered; however, β-andrenergic antagonists have been proven most effective in treating hypertension in young Caucasian males. Choice **e**, nitrates, should not be a consideration because this type of medication is commonly used for treatment of chest pain.

Task Area: Pharmaceutical Therapeutics
Organ System: Cardiovascular

213. **d.** The symptoms of acromegaly are caused by abnormal production of growth hormone (choice **d**) from a benign tumor in the pituitary gland. Somatostatin (choice **a**) and dopamine (choice **c**) can be used to treat this condition. Thyroxine (choice **e**) elevation causes thyrotoxicosis. Erythropoietin (choice **b**) elevation causes polycythemia.

Task Area: Applying Basic Science Concepts
Organ System: Endocrine

214. **b.** The correct answer is choice **b**, colchicine, which is indicated for acute gouty attacks. Choice **a**, allopurinol, is incorrect because it is a urate-lowering agent that is indicated after an acute attack subsides. Choices **c**, acetaminophen, and **d**, oxycodone, are incorrect because they do not address the underlying inflammatory process. Choice **e**, omeprazole (proton pump inhibitor), is incorrect because it is indicated for acid reflux disease.

Task Area: Pharmaceutical Therapeutics
Organ System: Musculoskeletal

215. **b.** A hepatitis B vaccination (choice **b**) will prevent another cause of hepatic damage. Hepatitis C vaccinations (choice **c**) do not exist. Increasing salt (choice **a**) does not improve the patient's health. Although protein intake should be monitored, an increased protein intake (choice **d**) can cause hepatic decompensation, and a decreased protein intake (choice **e**) can cause muscle wasting.

Task Area: Health Maintenance
Organ System: Gastrointestinal/Nutritional

216. **d.** Multiple sclerosis demyelinates axons throughout the central nervous system (CNS). This produces intermittent neurological symptoms that occur at different sites within the CNS and at different times. This produces multiple CNS lesions, which are best detected using MRI (choice **d**) rather than CT (choice **c**). Choices **a** and **b** are incorrect because multiple sclerosis produces multiple CNS lesions. Multiple sclerosis produces oligoclonal bands within the CNS rather than monoclonal bands (choice **e**).

Task Area: Using Laboratory and Diagnostic Studies
Organ System: Neurologic

217. **a.** This patient's presentation is typical of Horner's syndrome, a set of features caused by a unilateral defect in the sympathetic nervous supply of the face. One possible cause of Horner's syndrome is a Pancoast tumor, an apical lung tumor that often causes a sympathetic nerve palsy via a mass effect. A Pancoast tumor also often presents with ipsilateral shoulder pain (choice **a**), and in any patient with this constellation of signs and symptoms, it is important to rule out the possibility of lung cancer. Chest and back pain (choices **b**, **d**, and **e**) may be associated with a bronchocarcinoma or other form of lung cancer, but this would not cause Horner's syndrome. Right shoulder pain (choice **c**) may cause similar symptoms on the right side.

Task Area: History Taking and Performing Physical Examinations
Organ System: Pulmonary

218. **e.** The patient has bipolar disorder and is currently having a manic episode. The symptoms she describes are consistent with diabetes insipidus, which can be caused by lithium (choice **e**). Haloperidol (choice **a**) may cause diabetes mellitus, which would have raised her serum and urine glucose levels. Valproate (choice **b**) and carbamazepine (choice **c**) are sodium channel blockers. Clozapine (choice **d**) may cause agranulositosis.

Task Area: Clinical Intervention
Organ System: Psychiatry/Behavioral Science

219. **d.** Loss of protein in the urine results in hypoalbuminemia. The decrease in serum oncotic pressure causes edema (choice **d**). Kausmaul breathing (choice **a**) occurs more in diabetic ketoacidosis, which is far more common in type 1 diabetes. Hematuria (choice **b**) and dysuria (choice **c**) are not typical in a nephrotic picture. Melena (choice **e**) is a gastrointestinal symptom.

Task Area: History Taking and Performing Physical Examinations
Organ System: Genitourinary

220. **d.** Patients with the sickle cell trait can present with hematuria and an inability to concentrate urine (choice **d**). Full-blown sickle cell anemia (choice **a**) and bone marrow expansion (choice **b**), or accelerated hematopoiesis which damages surrounding bones, only occur in sickle cell disease, where two copies of the gene are present. Peripheral neuropathy (choice **c**) and obesity (choice **e**) are not associated with the sickle cell trait.

Task Area: Health Maintenance
Organ System: Hematologic

221. **d.** When evaluating causes of infertility among couples, a hysterosalpingogram is useful to evaluate tubal patency (choice **d**) as a cause of infertility. This exam can also evaluate any uterine abnormalities that may contribute to infertility. Choice **a**, ovulation, is incorrect as a hysterosalpingogram will have no diagnostic value to evaluate a female's ovulation. Choices **b**, sperm survival; **c**, sperm penetration; and **e**, sperm count, are all incorrect as these can be evaluated by a simple semen analysis performed in a laboratory.

Task Area: Using Laboratory and Diagnostic Studies
Organ System: Reproductive

222. e. Otitis externa (OE) is also called swimmer's ear. Swimming is a common cause of OE because the excess moisture leads to a breakdown of the cerumen barrier. The correct answer is choice **e**, all of the above. Choices **a** to **d** are all appropriate steps to prevent infection of the external ear canal.

Task Area: Health Maintenance

Organ System: EENT (Eye, Ear, Nose, and Throat)

223. c. Pityriasis rosea (choice **c**) is characterized by a herald patch, which precedes symmetrical papular eruption. A herald patch is a solitary round or oval pink plaque with a raised border and fine scales in the margin. The associated rash will appear as round or oval salmon-colored lesions approximately 1 cm in diameter. Choice **a**, seborrheic keratosis, should be excluded because this condition is associated with wartlike growths on the face, chest, and back, which are usually painless and without redness. Choice **b**, dermatophytosis (such as tinea or ringworm) might be considered; however, this condition may also affect the finger and/or toenails, causing them to thicken and discolor, which should exclude this diagnosis. Choice **d**, scabies, should be excluded because of the lack of night itching and thin pencil marks on the skin. Choice **e**, vitiligo, should be excluded immediately because this disorder is associated with loss of skin pigmentation.

Task Area: Formulating Most Likely Diagnosis
Organ System: Dermatologic

224. b. Hyperparathyroidism (choice **b**) is classically diagnosed by elevated levels of serum calcium, or hypercalcemia. Hyperparathyroidism is primarily caused by a parathyroid adenoma, a malignant tumor of the parathyroid gland. Parathyroid cancer is an extremely rare type of cancer. Choice **a**, hypoparathyroidism, is characterized by low blood calcium levels and low blood magnesium levels. Choice **c**, hypothyroidism, is characterized by elevated thyroid stimulating hormone levels and low T3 and T4 levels. Choice **d**, hyperthyroidism, is characterized by decreased levels of thyroid stimulating hormone and elevated T3 and T4 levels. Choice **e**, euthyroidism, is the condition of normal thyroid function, and all levels of thyroid hormones should be within normal limits.

Task Area: Using Laboratory and Diagnostic Studies
Organ System: Endocrine

225. c. In patients with stress-related symptoms, it is often difficult to establish whether the etiology is mostly psychological or physical. However, in this case, the patient's presentation is very typical of vasovagal syncope (choice **c**), an inappropriate parasympathetic response that is often triggered by stressful situations. In many cases, a particular trigger will continue to cause syncopal episodes, even after the stress associated with the trigger is no longer present. Somatization disorders (choice **a**) and malingering (choice **b**) might be considered if there is no physiological explanation for the patient's symptoms, but in this case, vasovagal syncope is more likely. Epilepsy (choice **d**) may present with episodes that appear similar to syncope, but it is not associated with stress-related triggers. A normal response to stress (choice **e**) may include focal neurological symptoms, but cardiovascular involvement suggests that it may be advisable to initiate clinical intervention.
Task Area: Formulating Most Likely Diagnosis
Organ System: Psychiatry/Behavioral Science

226. a. In the presence of a growing scrotal mass, it is important to consider the possibilities of hydrocele, hematocele, and tumors. The lack of transillumination eliminates the possibility of a hydrocele, but in order to make a further distinction, it is important to examine the mass via ultrasound (choice **a**). History and physical examination may help to narrow down the diagnoses to some extent, but only an ultrasound can be used to distinguish between a testicular lesion and an extratesticular lesion. If the lesion is testicular, malignancy is the most likely diagnosis. X-ray (choice **b**) and MRI (choice **c**) are not particularly useful for examination of scrotal masses, but they may help in the search for metastases if the mass is found to be malignant. A fine-needle aspiration biopsy (choice **d**) should never be performed on a testicular mass; the procedure significantly increases the likelihood of tumor metastasis into the scrotal wall. Inguinal orchiectomy and biopsy (choice **e**) may be performed by a urologist after extratesticular masses are excluded with the help of ultrasound.
Task Area: Using Laboratory and Diagnostic Studies
Organ System: Genitourinary

227. b. Hypovolemic shock (choice **b**) is the result of conditions that result in a life-threatening loss of blood volume. This type of shock is commonly caused by hemorrhage, loss of plasma, or loss of fluid and electrolytes. This condition is an emergency condition in which severe blood and fluid loss makes the heart unable to pump enough blood to the body. This type of shock can also be the result of third space sequestration. Choice **a**, cardiogenic shock, is incorrect as this condition is caused when the heart has been damaged to the point where it cannot adequately supply the bodily organs with blood. Choice **c**, obstructive shock, is incorrect because this condition is caused by obstruction of the great vessels, such as pulmonary embolism. This condition is very similar to cardiogenic shock. Choice **d**, septic shock, is incorrect as this condition is caused by severe infection that leads to vasodilatation. Choice **e**, neurogenic shock, is incorrect as this condition is caused by trauma to the spinal cord.

Task Area: Applying Basic Science Concepts
Organ System: Cardiovascular

228. c. HELLP syndrome (choice **c**) is defined as severe preeclampsia with the addition of hemolysis, elevated liver enzymes, and low platelets. HELLP syndrome is a life-threatening complication associated with pregnancy, and it can even occur after childbirth. Patients may present with headache, nausea, vomiting, bandlike pressure around the abdomen, blurred vision, and tingling in the extremities. Choice **a**, chronic hypertension, is incorrect as this condition is only associated with uncontrolled high blood pressure during pregnancy. Choice **b**, eclampsia, might be an option; however, the presence of hemolysis, elevated liver enzymes, and low platelets should rule this out. Choice **d**, pre-term labor, is incorrect as this condition is associated with discharge from the vagina, leaking from the vagina, and vaginal bleeding. Choice **e**, leiomyomata, is incorrect as this condition is characterized by benign masses (fibroids) within the uterus.

Task Area: History Taking and Performing Physical Examinations
Organ System: Reproductive

229. c. Bulimia nervosa (choice **c**) involves binge eating followed by inducing vomiting or using laxatives and diuretics. Individuals with bulimia nervosa present with dental erosion, esophagitis, calluses on the knuckles, and atrophy of the salivary glands. Blood work reveals hypochloremic hypokalemic alkalosis and hypomagnesemia. Choice **a**, binge eating disorder, is incorrect as this disorder is characterized by obesity, not by being underweight and emaciated. Choice **b**, anorexia nervosa, is incorrect as this condition is not characterized by dental erosion, esophagitis, and calluses on the knuckles. Choice **d**, narcissistic personality disorder, is incorrect as this is a psychological condition of increased sense of one's self and is not associated with any physical symptoms. Choice **e**, body dysmorphic disorder, is incorrect as this is a psychological condition in which an individual is excessively obsessed with flaws in his or her appearance and is not associated with any physical symptoms.

Task Area: Using Laboratory and Diagnostic Studies
Organ System: Psychiatry/Behavioral Science

230. d. The correct answer is choice **d**, ciproflaxin. Ciproflaxin, a member of the fluoroquinolone family of medications, is a powerful antibiotic. In older men, epididymitis is generally caused by a bacterium rather than by a sexually transmitted disease. Ciproflaxin will effectively eliminate the bacterium causing the epididymitis. Choice **a**, ACE inhibitors, is incorrect as this class of medications will have no therapeutic effects for epididymitis and should not be considered as a treatment option for this condition. Choice **b**, ceftriaxone, might be a consideration; however, this medication has more use if the epididymitis is caused by a sexually transmitted disease rather than a bacterium. Choice **c**, tolterodine, is incorrect as this medication is used to treat urinary incontinence. Choice **e**, warfarin, is incorrect as this medication is an anticoagulant and will have no therapeutic benefit for this condition.

Task Area: Pharmaceutical Therapeutics
Organ System: Genitourinary

231. **a.** The correct answer is choice **a**, echocardiogram to assess the function of the heart valves. A "swishing" sound upon auscultation of the heart is a classic signal of mitral valve prolapse. An echocardiogram is the easiest, noninvasive method to evaluate the function of the heart valves. Choice **b**, cardiac catheterization, would not be appropriate because the test is invasive and the patient is asymptomatic, with a normal electrocardiogram (EKG) and normal blood pressure. Choice **c**, a 24-hour Holter monitor, would not be appropriate because the patient is not experiencing palpitations or any other symptoms, and the baseline electrocardiogram was normal. Choice **d**, cardiac stress testing, would not be appropriate because the patient is asymptomatic, with a normal EKG and normal blood pressure. Choice **e**, cardiac PET scan, would be inappropriate because there is no previous cardiac history such as ischemia or myocardial infarction.

Task Area: Using Laboratory and Diagnostic Studies
Organ System: Cardiovascular

232. **e.** The correct answer is choice **e**, pneumothorax. A pneumothorax is characterized by acute onset of chest pain and shortness of breath. A physical exam may show one-sided chest expansion, hyperresonance, and decreased breath sounds. A chest X-ray may show presence of pleural air, but often a visceral pleural line is the only radiographic evidence of a small pleural effusion. Choice **a**, bronchiectasis, should not be considered because of the lack of cough, sputum, and wheezing. Choice **b**, pulmonary embolism, might be a viable choice; however, a pulmonary embolism does not cause one-sided chest expansion. Choice **c**, pleural effusion, should be ruled out after examination of the chest X-ray, in which a pleural effusion was not recognized. Choice **d**, pulmonary hypertension, is often associated with dizziness, fainting, swelling in the extremities, and bluish skin and lips, which this patient is not experiencing.

Task Area: History Taking and Performing Physical Examinations
Organ System: Pulmonary

233. c. The correct answer is choice **c**, motion sickness. For individuals who suffer from severe motion sickness associated with severe vertigo, scopolamine is the most effective treatment. Scopolamine is most often administered via transdermal patch, which releases a dose of 330 micrograms per day. Choice **a**, barotrauma, is commonly treated medically with antihistamines, steroids, or decongestants. Choice **b**, acute vertigo, is often treated with diazepam. Choice **d**, labyrinthitis, will commonly resolve on its own after a few days; however, meclizine is often prescribed for treatment of this disorder. Choice **e**, presbycusis, is not treatable, but hearing loss is often ameliorated with hearing aids.

Task Area: Pharmaceutical Therapeutics
Organ System: EENT (Eye, Ear, Nose, and Throat)

234. a. This patient most likely has giant cell arteritis (GCA), an autoimmune vasculitis that usually affects the temporal arteries (which is why it is often called *temporal arteritis*). GCA typically presents with intermittent visual acuity loss, which leads to permanent visual impairment in as many as 60% of patients, along with irreversible blindness in advanced cases. Visual symptoms are often associated with jaw claudication, tenderness in the region of the temporal artery, fever, or new-onset headache. Autoimmune diseases often present in clusters; in particular, GCA is known to be strongly associated with polymyalgia rheumatica (choice **a**). Rheumatoid arthritis (choice **b**), Wegener's granulomatosis (choice **c**), sarcoidosis (choice **d**), and systemic lupus erythematosus (choice **e**) are all associated with a variety of different autoimmune conditions, but none has been linked to GCA.

Task Area: Formulating Most Likely Diagnosis
Organ System: Cardiovascular

235. e. In a patient with severe pain with mild physical examination findings, ischemic bowel disease should always be considered as a likely diagnosis; this notion is strengthened by this patient's past history of hypercholesterolemia and smoking along with a lack of a past history of bowel disease. She most likely has ischemia in the area supplied by the superior mesenteric artery, which includes part of the head of the pancreas and the region of bowel between the lower duodenum and the splenic flexure of the colon (often known as the midgut). Ischemic bowel disease may also occur in the foregut (including the esophagus, the stomach, and the upper duoenum) or the hindgut (including the descending colon and the rectum). The presence of ischemia puts her at higher risk for other forms of ischemic disease, the most common of which is ischemic heart disease (choice **e**). This presentation does appear to be similar to acute pancreatitis, consequences of which may include chronic pancreatitis (choice **a**) and pancreatic cancer (choice **b**); however, this is less likely because the patient does not have a fever, her abdominal tenderness is mild, and she has none of the major risk factors for pancreatitis (which include gallstones, alcohol abuse, trauma, and a few others). Colorectal carcinoma (choice **c**) may be a possible consequence of adenoma, but this is generally asymptomatic until the development of the cancer itself. Ruptured abdominal aortic aneurysm (choice **d**) is an important differential diagnosis to consider when an abdominal aortic aneurysm is suspected, but this is can be excluded here because of the lack of a pulsatile mass along the midline of the abdomen.

Task Area: Health Maintenance
Organ System: Gastrointestinal/Nutritional

236. **a.** This patient's symptoms appear to be consistent with systemic sclerosis, often known by the name *scleroderma* or the acronym CREST (calcinosis, Raynaud's phenomenon, esophageal dysmotility, sclerodactyly, and telangiectasia) syndrome. This is an autoimmune condition that is particularly common in females and leads to a characteristic tightening and thickening of the skin, which in turn leads to pain and stiffness in the joints, particularly in the hands and face. The antibody anti-Scl-70 (choice **a**), an antinuclear antibody that targets DNA topoisomerase I, is highly specific for systemic sclerosis. Anti-dsDNA (choice **b**) and antihistone (choice **c**) are also antinuclear antibodies, but these two are more specific for systemic lupus erythematosus (SLE). Antineutrophil cytoplasmic antibodies (choice **d**) are more likely to cause Wegener's granulomatosis and several autoimmune vasculitides. Anti-IgG (choice **e**) antibodies, also known as *rheumatoid factor* (Rf), usually cause rheumatoid arthritis.

Task Area: Using Laboratory and Diagnostic Studies

Organ System: Musculoskeletal

237. **c.** Treatment with calcium channel blockers (choice **c**) is indicated for patients diagnosed with primary pulmonary hypertension. Calcium channel blockers act to reduce systemic arterial pressure; the decrease in calcium results in less contraction of vascular smooth muscle, thereby increasing arterial diameter. Other medical treatments may include oral anticoagulant therapy and a potent pulmonary vasodilator called prostacyclin, which inhibits the formation of myosin light-chain kinase. This inhibition leads to smooth muscle relaxation and therefore vasodilation. Choice **a**, beta blockers, incorrect as these medications are used to reduce systemic venous pressure. Choices **b**, bronchodilators, and **d**, corticosteroids, are incorrect as these medications may open airways and make breathing easier, but they will do little to decrease systemic arterial pressure. Choice **e**, diuretics, is incorrect as these medications are used to rid the body of excess fluids. Diuretics are not effective in lowering systemic arterial pressure.

Task Area: Pharmaceutical Therapeutics

Organ System: Pulmonary

238. b. A high percentage of volvulus cases can be resolved with endoscopic decompression (choice **b**); therefore, this procedure should be attempted initially. Choice **a**, surgical correction, is incorrect as surgical correction for volvulus is indicated only if endoscopic decompression fails. Choice **c**, colon cleansing, is incorrect as this disorder is not characterized by excessive bowel contents. Choice **d**, abdominal angiogram, is incorrect as this procedure will have no therapeutic value for this condition. Choice **e**, partial colectomy, is incorrect as this procedure is not necessary, since the twisted area of the bowel can generally be corrected using endoscopic decompression.

Task Area: Clinical Intervention
Organ System: Gastrointestinal/Nutritional

239. c. If puncture wounds are present as a result of the patient's fist coming in contact with another person's mouth, antibiotics (choice **c**) should be prescribed to avoid infection in the puncture wounds. *Eikenella corrodens* is an organism specific to the human mouth that can promote infection if it comes into contact with an open wound. Treatment with antibiotics will prevent any infection *Eikenella corrodens* may cause. Choices **a**, anti-inflammatories, and **b**, corticosteroids, are incorrect. Although these medications may reduce the swelling associated with the injury, they have no benefit for reducing the risk of infection from the puncture wounds. Choice **d**, opiate pain medication, is incorrect; though these may be useful to alleviate some of the pain associated with the injury, they offer no benefit for reducing the risk of infection. Choice **e**, sutures, is incorrect and should not be considered if there is a risk of infection.

Task Area: Clinical Intervention
Organ System: Musculoskeletal

240. d. This question tests your knowledge of diagnosing a urologic condition involving the foreskin. Given the history and physical exam, the correct answer is choice **d**, paraphimosis, which is a urologic emergency because of the potential for tissue ischemia of the glans. Choice **a**, phimosis, is incorrect because phimosis describes the inability to retract the foreskin. Choice **b**, testicular torsion, is incorrect because it is inconsistent with the physical exam. Choice **c**, cryptorchidism, is incorrect because it describes undescended testicles. Choice **e**, varicocele, is incorrect because it describes dilation of spermatic veins, which is inconsistent with the presentation.

Task Area: History Taking and Performing Physical Examinations
Organ System: Genitourinary

Section 5

241. a. The correct answer is choice **a**, diuretics and salt restriction. Most individuals who are diagnosed with Meniere's disease can easily manage this disorder by restricting their salt consumption combined with a daily regimen of diuretic medication. If this treatment option is unsuccessful, surgical intervention is required to treat this disorder. Choices **b**, **c**, **d**, and **e** are all incorrect as none of these medications provide any therapeutic benefit for Meniere's disease. Some medicinal options may include anti-vertigo medications such as meclizine, and antinausea medications such as promethazine.

Task Area: Pharmaceutical Therapeutics
Organ System: EENT (Eye, Ear, Nose, and Throat)

242. b. In inpatients with pneumonia or exacerbations of COPD, it is important to monitor their respiratory status periodically. The best assessment can be obtained by measuring the patient's arterial blood gases after allowing the patient to breathe room air for several minutes (choice **b**). Arterial blood gases provide the most accurate and precise picture of a patient's oxygenation; a few minutes of room air exposure is necessary in order to ensure that the patient's natural respiratory capacity is being measured. A patient's current oxygen requirement (choice **a**) is also often used as a way to estimate current lung function, but this is inaccurate because a large current dose of oxygen does not necessarily indicate that the patient is unable to function on room air. Because of its noninvasive nature, pulse oximetry (choices **c** and **e**) may be used for regular monitoring, but it provides a less precise measurement than arterial blood gases. Any levels taken while the patient's nasal prongs are inserted (choice **d**) will provide meaningless results because the supplemental oxygen will correct most abnormalities.

Task Area: Using Laboratory and Diagnostic Studies
Organ System: Pulmonary

243. c. Mitral stenosis (choice **c**) is a disorder that impedes the flow of blood between the left atrium and ventricle. Patients will present with dyspnea, fatigue, cough, nocturnal dyspnea, hemoptysis, or hoarseness. Auscultation of the chest reveals a mid-diastolic murmur at the apex with little radiation. Auscultation also reveals S1 accentuated opening snap following S2. Choice **a**, aortic stenosis, is incorrect as this condition is associated with a mid-systolic murmur at the second right intercostal space radiating to the neck and left sternal border. Choice **b**, aortic regurgitation, is incorrect as this condition is associated with a soft systolic and diastolic decrescendo from the second to the fourth left intercostal space radiating to the apex and right sternal border. Choice **d**, pulmonic stenosis, is incorrect as this condition is associated with a systolic murmur between the second and third left intercostal space radiating to the left shoulder and neck. Auscultation will also reveal an early pulmonic ejection sound. Choice **e**, tricuspid regurgitation, is incorrect as this condition is associated with a soft holosystolic murmur that increases in intensity with inspiration or with pressure on the liver.

Task Area: Formulating Most Likely Diagnosis
Organ System: Cardiovascular

244. **c.** A Colles' fracture (choice **c**) is a distal radius fracture with dorsal angulation. This type of fracture is the most common injury of the wrist, and it results from a fall onto the dorsiflexed hand. Silver fork deformity on X-ray is characteristic of this type of fracture. Choice **a**, buckle (torus) fracture, is incorrect as this is an incomplete fracture in which one side of the bone is fractured without the other side being disrupted. Choice **b**, greenstick fracture, is incorrect as this is very similar to a torus fracture in which one side of the bone is fractured without the other side being disrupted. The difference between a greenstick fracture and a torus fracture is that a greenstick fracture occurs in the diaphysis of the bone, whereas a torus fracture occurs in the distal epiphysis of the bone. Choice **d**, open fracture, is incorrect as this condition is characterized by the broken bone protruding through the skin. Choice **e**, compound fracture, is also incorrect as this is identical to an open fracture in which the broken bone is protruding through the skin.

Task Area: Applying Basic Science Concepts
Organ System: Musculoskeletal

245. **c.** Celiac disease is characterized by inflammation of the small bowel. A small bowel biopsy (choice **c**) is needed in order to confirm the diagnosis of celiac disease. Choices **a**, CT scan of the abdomen, and **e**, endoscopy, can detect small bowel inflammation; however, these exams cannot confirm a diagnosis of celiac disease. Choice **b**, barium enema, is incorrect as this exam is used to detect tumors, ulcers, and diverticulum in the large intestine. Choice **d**, gastrointestinal bleeding study, should not be considered as this exam is used to determine the site of gastrointestinal bleeding.

Task Area: Clinical Intervention
Organ System: Gastrointestinal/Nutritional

246. **b.** For patients with chronic obstructive pulmonary disease, such as emphysema or chronic bronchitis, anticholinergic medications (choice **b**), such as ipratropium or tiotropium, are superior to β-adrenergic agonists in achieving bronchodilation. Short-acting bronchodilators should be on hand to treat acute exacerbations of dyspnea. Choice **a**, antibiotics, is incorrect as these medications are used to treat infections. Choice **c**, inhaled corticosteroids, is incorrect as these medications are commonly used to treat chronic asthma. Choice **d**, β-adrenergic agonists, is incorrect as this type of medication is commonly used to treat acute attacks of asthma. Choice **e**, diuretics, is incorrect as these medications are used to rid the body of excess fluids and have no bronchodilatory effects.

Task Area: Health Maintenance
Organ System: Pulmonary

247. c. Shock (choice **c**) is defined as severe cardio-vascular failure caused by poor blood flow, inadequate distribution of blood flow, and inadequate oxygen delivery to the tissues. Shock can lead to multisystem organ failure or death. Choice **a**, cardiac arrest, is incorrect because this condition results from the lack or cessation of blood flow due to failure of the heart to contract normally. Choice **b**, hypovolemia, is incorrect as this condition is characterized by a decrease in blood volume. Choice **d**, congestive heart failure, is incorrect as this condition involves the heart not being able to adequately pump blood to the rest of the body. Choice **e**, myocardial infarction, is incorrect as this condition is characterized by blockage of coronary blood vessels, which prevents the heart from receiving adequate oxygen.

Task Area: Applying Basic Science Concepts
Organ System: Cardiovascular

248. b. Unike the acute version of thrombocytopenia, chronic thrombocytopenia will rarely resolve spontaneously. Chronic thrombocytopenia is classically treated with high doses of prednisone (choice **b**). Choice **a**, erythropoietin, is incorrect because administration of this medication may make the condition of chronic thrombocytopenia more severe. Choice **c**, folic acid, is incorrect: although this might be a consideration if the thrombocytopenia was secondary due to folic acid deficiency anemia, folic acid will not assist in this disorder secondary to SLE. Choice **d**, vitamin B12, is incorrect because although this may be a consideration if the thrombocytopenia was secondary due to vitamin B12 deficiency anemia, vitamin B12 will not assist in this disorder secondary to SLE. Choice **e**, vitamin K, may also be used if the cause of thrombocytopenia is a vitamin K deficiency; however, vitamin K will have little effect when SLE is the cause.

Task Area: Pharmaceutical Therapeutics
Organ System: Hematologic

249. d. Ulcerative colitis (choice **d**) rarely has inflammation past the first two layers of the intestinal wall. Bowel cancer (choice **a**) tends to occur in older populations and is associated with the presence of polyps on colonoscopy. Irritable bowel syndrome (IBS) (choice **b**) is a diagnosis of exclusion. Granulomatous inflammation is seen in Crohn's disease (choice **c**). Celiac disease (choice **e**) is usually associated with foul-smelling stools caused by malabsorption in the small intestine.

Task Area: Formulating Most Likely Diagnosis
Organ System: Gastrointestinal/Nutritional

250. e. The correct answer is choice **e**, chronic obstructive pulmonary disease (COPD). COPD includes emphysema and chronic bronchitis. Patients will present with shortness of breath getting progressively worse, excessive cough, and sputum production. Auscultation of the lungs will reveal decreased breath sounds and early inspiratory crackles. Percussion yields increased resonance. A chest X-ray will reveal hyperinflation of the lungs and a flattened diaphragm. Choice **a**, alveolitis, is associated with fever, chills, and chest tightness, which this patient is not experiencing. Choice **b**, bronchiectasis, might be a viable option, but this disorder is associated with chest pain and clubbing of the hands. Bronchiectasis is often caused by recurrent inflammation or infection of the airways. It most often begins in childhood as a complication from infection or from inhaling a foreign object. Choice **c**, pulmonary hypertension, is often associated with dizziness, fainting, swelling in the extremities, and bluish skin and lips, which this patient is not experiencing. Choice **d**, pulmonary embolism, is incorrect because of the progressive shortness of breath and excessive cough and sputum production; individuals with pulmonary embolism experience rapid onset of shortness of breath and chest pain.
Task Area: History Taking and Performing Physical Examinations
Organ System: Pulmonary

251. e. The correct answer is choice **e**, tonsillectomy. Tonsillectomy is indicated in cases of peritonsillar cellulitis when symptoms have progressed to include airway obstruction causing sleep apnea and persistent marked asymmetry of the tonsils. Choice **a**, treatment with penicillin or erythromycin, is appropriate with streptococcal or viral pharyngitis, but this is not sufficient when peritonsillar cellulitis has progressed to the extent described above. The same is true for choice **b**, hospital admission, in order to treat with intravenous antibiotics. This course of treatment is not sufficient for peritonsillar cellulitis that has progressed to the extent described above. Choices **c**, aspiration of the tonsils, and **d**, incision and drainage, are appropriate for this disorder but are precluded by the progression of the disorder to the point of airway obstruction.
Task Area: Clinical Intervention
Organ System: EENT (Eye, Ear, Nose, and Throat)

252. d. Given the X-ray and MRI findings, slipped capital femoral epiphysis (SCFE) is the most likely diagnosis, so the correct answer is choice **d**. Choice **e**, none of the above, is therefore incorrect. Choice **a**, septic hip, is incorrect because there is no mention of fever, elevated white count, or elevated erythrocyte sedimentation rate (ESR), which are typical findings in septic hip. Choice **b**, avascular necrosis of the left hip, is incorrect, although it may be a complication of chronic SCFE; however, the duration of one week makes this option less likely. Choice **c**, malignant tumor of the femur, is incorrect because the MRI finding is inconsistent with evidence of malignancy.
Task Area: Formulating Most Likely Diagnosis
Organ System: Musculoskeletal

253. b. This question tests your knowledge of liver cirrhosis and its complications. The correct answer is choice **b**, esophageal varices, which are dilated submucosal veins that develop in cirrhotic patients due to portal hypertension. Choice **a**, Mallory-Weiss tear, is incorrect because this patient denies vomiting. Choice **c**, lung cancer, is incorrect because the negative chest X-ray makes this diagnosis less likely. Choice **d**, hemothorax, is incorrect because of the benign chest X-ray. Choice **e**, tuberculosis, is incorrect because this patient's history and physical findings are more consistent with cirrhosis.

Task Area: History Taking and Performing Physical Examinations

Organ System: Gastrointestinal/Nutritional

254. e. This question tests your ability to differentiate antifungal agents from antibiotics in treatment of thrush. Thrush is oral candidiasis. The correct answer is choice **e**, fluconazol, which is the only antifungal agent among all the choices. All the other options are incorrect because they are antibiotics, which are not indicated in thrush.

Task Area: Clinical Intervention

Organ System: EENT (Eye, Ear, Nose, and Throat)

255. c. The correct answer is choice **c**, pulmonary tuberculosis, because *M. tuberculosis* is identified on acid-fast smear, which is diagnostic. Choice **a**, acute asthma exacerbation, is incorrect because asthma patients should not test positive for acid-fast bacilli, and presentation is much more acute. Choice **b**, pneumonia, is incorrect because of the positive acid-fast bacilli test, and there is no mention of fever. Choice **e**, chronic obstructive pulmonary disease (COPD), is incorrect because it typically affects people with a history of tobacco use, and they do not test positive for acid-fast bacilli. Choice **d**, cystic fibrosis, is incorrect because it is a hereditary disorder caused by abnormalities in a membrane chloride channel, and a sweat test is the test of choice.

Task Area: Formulating Most Likely Diagnosis

Organ System: Pulmonary

256. e. The correct answer is choice **e**, diastolic rumble along the lower left sternal border. This heart sound is consistent with tricuspid stenosis, which is usually rheumatic in origin. Choice **a**, prominent S1 heart sound with an opening snap, is incorrect because it is associated with mitral stenosis. Choice **b**, S3 heart sound and pansystolic murmur at the apex that radiates into the axilla, is incorrect because it is associated with mitral regurgitation. Choice **c**, soft, absent S2 heart sound, is incorrect because it is associated with aortic stenosis. Choice **d**, systolic murmur along the left sternal border, is incorrect because it is the typical finding in tricuspid regurgitation.

Task Area: History Taking and Performing Physical Examinations

Organ System: Cardiovascular

257. c. The patient has shingles, which is caused by the varicella-zoster virus. This virus lies dormant in the dorsal root ganglion in multiple cranial nerves, dorsal roots, and autonomic ganglia (choice **c**) after the original infection, which causes chickenpox. A misfolded protein (choice **a**) describes prion diseases. Intracellular bacteria that require an external source of ATP (choice **b**) include *Chlamydia* species. An RNA virus with a reverse transcriptase (choice **d**) describes retroviruses such as HIV. A DNA virus with a reverse transcriptase (choice **e**) describes hepatitis B.

Task Area: Applying Basic Science Concepts
Organ System: Infectious Diseases

258. d. It is important to understand how to recognize a cluster headache (choice **d**). Classically, it features periodic episodes of severe headaches that occur regularly for one to two months, followed by long periods of remission. The headaches are usually unilateral and are characterized by a boring eye pain and, in most cases, ipsilateral neurological symptoms such as lacrimation. Often, patients suffer for years before seeking medical attention. Intracerebral aneurysm (choice **a**) may also present with a severe headache upon rupture, but this causes an acute pain with no history. Migraine (choice **b**) is characterized by an aura, in which patients have certain warning signs before the headache appears. Temporal arteritis (choice **c**) is very rare in patients below 60 to 65 years of age. Chronic sinusitis (choice **e**) typically presents with symptoms such as nasal congestion and coughing; additionally, it does not normally feature long remissions.

Task Area: Formulating Most Likely Diagnosis
Organ System: Neurologic

259. b. A positive interferon-γ release assay (choice **b**) indicates previous exposure to tuberculosis. Once the patient is immunosuppressed with infliximab, tuberculosis can be reactivated. Renal failure (choice **a**) is not thought to affect the metabolism of infliximab. Aspirin (choice **c**) and opioid (choice **d**) use have no effect on infliximab. The BCG vaccination (choice **e**) is not a live attenuated vaccine and therefore does not increase the risk of tuberculosis reactivation.

Task Area: Pharmaceutical Therapeutics
Organ System: Musculoskeletal

260. e. The correct answer is choice **e**, none of the above. Choice **a**, vaginal pH >4.5 (normal: 3.8–4.2), is incorrect because the pH of *Candida* vaginitis is usually less than or equal to 4.5. Choice **b**, green-yellow frothy discharge, is incorrect because the discharge with *Candida* vaginitis is typically white and curdy. Choice **c**, fishy odor on the KOH whiff test, is incorrect because there should not be any fishy odor. Choice **d**, positive bacterial culture, is incorrect because *Candida* is fungal.

Task Area: Applying Basic Science Concepts
Organ System: Reproductive

261. d. Given the clinical findings and elevated TSH, the correct answer is choice **d**, hypothyroidism. Choices **a**, premenopausal syndrome, and **b**, fibromyalgia, are incorrect because they are not associated with an abnormal TSH level, although they are possible differentials. Choice **c**, hyperthyroidism, is incorrect because the TSH level should be lower than normal; also, her symptomatology would present differently. Choice **e**, depression, is incorrect because it is also not associated with abnormal TSH.

Task Area: History Taking and Performing Physical Examinations
Organ System: Endocrine

262. d. The correct answer is choice **d**, peripheral motor system. This patient has Bell's palsy, which is an idiopathic facial paresis of peripheral motor neuron. It affects the patient's ability to move upper and lower facial muscles. Nerve groups of the central sensory system (choice **a**), central motor system (choice **b**) and peripheral sensory system (choice **c**) are not involved; therefore they are incorrect. Choice **e** is incorrect because nerve groups of the peripheral motor system are involved.

Task Area: Applying Basic Science Concepts
Organ System: Neurologic

263. c. Based on the arterial pH, this patient has acidosis. The correct answer is choice **c**, respiratory acidosis, because there is an elevation of PCO_2. Choice **a**, metabolic acidosis, is incorrect because there will be a reduction in serum HCO_3, which is normal in this case. Choices **b**, metabolic alkalosis; **d**, respiratory alkalosis; and **e**, mixed alkalosis, are incorrect because based on the arterial pH, the patient has acidosis, not alkalosis.

Task Area: Formulating Most Likely Diagnosis
Organ System: Genitourinary

264. b. The correct answer is choice **b**, myasthenia gravis. Myasthenia gravis is characterized by muscle weakness and fatigue that improves with rest. Patients may present with ptosis, diplopia, difficulty in chewing or swallowing, respiratory difficulties, and limb weakness. A physical examination will reveal normal sensation and reflexes. This disorder can occur at any age, but it is more common in young women and older men. Choice **a**, Guillian-Barré syndrome, is associated with tingling in the extremities. The first symptoms of this disorder include varying degrees of weakness or tingling sensations in the legs. In many instances the weakness and abnormal sensations spread to the arms and upper body. Choice **c**, Bell's palsy, is associated with weakness and paralysis of the facial muscles. This disorder generally affects only one side of the face. Choice **d**, diabetic peripheral neuropathy, is also associated with tingling in the extremities, generally affecting the feet and legs first. Choice **e**, multiple sclerosis, is associated with abnormal sensations in any area and is generally associated with muscle spasms.

Task Area: History Taking and Performing Physical Examinations
Organ System: Neurologic

265. **d.** The patient comes from a region with a high prevalence of endemic hypothyroidism or cretinism. She also has features of hypothyroidism such as a goiter. Cretinism can be caused by iodine deficiency (choice **d**), an anatomic defect in the gland or an inborn error of thyroid metabolism that causes developmental delay in children. Folate (choice **c**) is important in pregnancy, but its deficiency does not cause cretinism. Vitamin C deficiency (choice **a**) causes scurvy. Thiamine (choice **b**) can be deficient in alcoholics. Iron deficiency (choice **e**) causes a microcytic anemia.

Task Area: Health Maintenance
Organ System: Endocrine

266. **e.** Keratoderma is a condition characterized by a thickening of the horny layer of the epidermis. This condition can be treated successfully with liquid nitrogen (choice **e**). Mild acid treatments have also been proven effective for treatment of this condition. Treatment can be very difficult and will be a lifelong effort. Some patients respond to systemic retinoids or topical creams of salicylic, lactic, or glycolic acids. Dermabrasion and CO_2 laser ablation are the preferred treatments for mechanical debridement. Choice **a**, topical corticosteroids, are most commonly used for treatment of rashes, eczema, and dermatitis. Choice **b**, permethrin, is used as an effective treatment for lice. Choice **c**, lindane, is used as an effective treatment for scabies. Choice **d**, fluconazole, is used as an effective treatment for yeast infections.

Task Area: Clinical Intervention
Organ System: Dermatologic

267. **b.** Esophageal varices (choice **b**) are dilations of the veins of the esophagus; varices normally occur at the distal end of the esophagus. Esophageal varices are normally caused by portal hypertension that is caused by cirrhosis from alcoholism or chronic viral hepatitis. Diagnosis is made with the presence of hematemesis, and endoscopy can confirm presence of esophageal varices. Choice **a**, Mallory-Weiss tear, might be a consideration based on symptoms; however, a tear was not appreciated upon endoscopy. Choice **c**, Budd-Chiari syndrome, is incorrect as this condition presents with abdominal pain, ascites, and hepatomegaly. Choice **d**, esophageal neoplasm, is incorrect as this condition is associated with difficulty swallowing, weight loss, and excessive choking. Choice **e**, reflex esophagitis, is incorrect as this condition is characterized by painful swallowing, excessive belching, hoarseness, and chest pain that is worse when lying flat.

Task Area: History Taking and Performing Physical Examinations
Organ System: Gastrointestinal/Nutritional

268. b. Infective endocarditis is an infectious condition that usually affects the endocardial tissue in the mitral valve, but can also affect the other heart valves. The condition is particularly common in injecting drug users because of the tendency of cutaneous *Staphylococcus aureus* colonies to be injected into the patient's veins along with the drugs. According to the Duke criteria for endocarditis, a diagnosis can be confirmed with positive blood cultures and the presence of regurgitant vegetations on an echocardiogram (choice **b**). An electrocardiogram (choice **a**) is unlikely to demonstrate changes in infective endocarditis. An angiogram (choice **c**) may demonstrate valvular lesions and may be used as a vehicle for a biopsy (choice **e**), but this is more invasive and no more beneficial than an echocardiogram. A chest CT (choice **d**) can provide information in severe cases, but it is less useful than an echocardiogram.

Task Area: Using Laboratory and Diagnostic Studies

Organ System: Cardiovascular

269. c. The patient has an ectopic pregnancy, which is most likely ruptured. This requires immediate surgical intervention (choice **c**). If there were no signs of rupture such as tachycardia or hypotension, methotrexate (choice **a**) could have been indicated. Pain management (choice **b**) is important, but it is not a defintive management. A biopsy of the tumor (choice **d**) is not necessary as a diagnosis can be made from the existing information. Clomiphene (choice **e**) has no role in the management of ectopic pregnancies.

Task Area: Clinical Intervention

Organ System: Reproductive

270. e. Anticoagulant therapy (choice **e**) is the gold standard treatment for deep venous thrombosis as this type of therapy will prevent the blood clot from enlarging and inhibit the formation of an embolus that can travel to the lung. Choice **a**, anti-inflammatories, is incorrect as this may be an effective treatment for superficial thrombophlebitis, but it will have no benefit for deep venous thrombosis. Choice **b**, corticosteroids, is incorrect and has no therapeutic benefit for this condition. Choice **c**, antibiotics, is incorrect and has no therapeutic benefit for this condition. Choice **d**, warm compresses, is incorrect as these may be an effective treatment for superficial thrombophlebitis, but will have no benefit for deep venous thrombosis.

Task Area: Health Maintenance

Organ System: Cardiovascular

271. c. An upgoing plantar (Babinski) reflex on the right is abnormal and indicative of a lesion on the right side of the spinal cord (choice **c**). The lesion can therefore not be on the left spinal cord (choices **b** and **d**). Given that the patient has no other neurological symptoms, it is unlikely that the lesion is in the cervical spinal cord (choice **a**). A parietal lobe lesion on the right side would cause left-sided symptoms (choice **e**).

Task Area: Formulating Most Likely Diagnosis

Organ System: Neurologic

272. e. The correct answer is choice **e**, all of the above. Choices **a** to **d** are all part of the health education that health providers should conduct with their patients.

Task Area: Health Maintenance

Organ System: Cardiovascular

273. d. If a patient is in imminent danger, theraputic privilege gives hospital staff the right to detain the patient (choice **d**). A suicidal patient cannot be considered to be competent until after a proper psychatric evaluation (choice **a**). Since this is an emergency, he should not be allowed to leave (choice **b**). Electroconvulsive therapy (choice **c**) is not considered to be a first-line treatment for suicide ideation. Cognitive behavioral therapy (choice **e**) can be helpful in treatment of depression or anxiety, but not in an emergency situation.

Task Area: Clinical Intervention
Organ System: Psychiatry/Behavioral Science

274. c. α-gluucosidase inhibitors, such as acarbose and miglitol, delay absorption of carbohydrates from the intestine (choice **c**) by inhibiting intestinal enzymes that digest carbohydrates, thus lowering blood glucose levels. Gastrointestinal symptoms are often side effects of these medications. Choices **a, b, d,** and **e** are incorrect because α-glucosidase inhibitors delay absorption of carbohydrates from the intestine and do not act via any other mechanism.

Task Area: Pharmaceutical Therapeutics
Organ System: Endocrine

275. b. This patient's symptoms are likely caused by emphysema due to alpha-1-antitrypsin (AAT) deficiency, one of the most common inherited disorders in the Caucasian population. AAT normally inhibits the trypsin-like proteases such as elastin, which normally promote compliance (or stretching) of the alveoli. A deficiency of AAT leads to an excess of elastin, thereby causing excess lung compliance and, consequently, emphysema. Smokers with AAT deficiency often develop emphysema at relatively young ages and will present with the typical features of emphysema, including exertional dyspnea, productive cough, an obstructive pattern on spirometry, and lung hyperinflation on a chest X-ray. AAT deficiency also causes bronchiectasis (choice **b**), which leads to large amounts of sputum production with the regular productive cough. Bronchitis (choice **a**) is an attractive choice because it accompanies emphysema in patients with chronic obstructive pulmonary disease, but this is far less likely than AAT deficiency in a 34-year-old patient. Bronchiolitis (choice **c**) is usually caused by an acute infectious process, most commonly in young patients. Asthma (choice **d**) typically features acute exacerbations that can be easily relieved with bronchodilators. Pneumothorax (choice **e**) is characterized by a very different presentation, the nature of which depends on the type of pneumothorax.

Task Area: Formulating Most Likely Diagnosis
Organ System: Pulmonary

276. e. UV radiation can easily penetrate and cause DNA damage even on overcast days (choice **e**). Decreased exposure to UV radiation (choices **b** and **c**) would have a beneficial effect. Many studies have shown a link between smoking and skin cancers (choice **d**). Regular check-ups (choice **a**) will allow for detection and removal of premalignant lesions.

Task Area: Health Maintenance
Organ System: Dermatologic

277. c. Imatinib mesylate inhibits BCR-ABL, which is a constitutively active tyrosine kinase (choice **c**). TNF blockers (choice **b**) such as etanercept are used in chronic inflammatory conditions. There are no current pharmaceuticals that act as DNase (choice **a**), Cox-4 (choice **d**), or phospholipase A2 (choice **e**) inhibitors.

Task Area: Pharmaceutical Therapeutics
Organ System: Hematologic

278. b. Retinopathy (choice **b**) primarily occurs secondary to systemic disorders such as diabetes, hypertension, and HIV disease. This disorder is the leading cause of blindness in the United States. Examinations can reveal venous dilatation, microaneurysms, retinal hemorrhages, retinal edema, hard exudates, or vitreous hemorrhages. Choice **a**, glaucoma, is not associated with venous dilatation and retinal edema. Choice **c**, orbital cellulitis, should be excluded immediately because orbital cellulitis is associated with fever, eye pain, and swelling of the upper and lower eyelids. Choice **d**, dacryostenosis, should be excluded because of the lack of excessive tear production. Choice **e**, viral conjunctivitis, should be excluded because of the lack of itching, burning eyes, redness in the whites of the eyes, and crusting of the eyelashes.

Task Area: Formulating Most Likely Diagnosis
Organ System: EENT (Eye, Ear, Nose, and Throat)

279. a. Breast cancer is generally treated with the drug tamoxifen, and women who are treated with tamoxifen for breast cancer are at an increased risk of developing endometrial cancer (choice **a**). Women who fall in this group should have an annual breast exam and pelvic exam and should be questioned about any and all vaginal bleeding; however, if the surgeon, oncologist, or gynecologist recommends, these examinations should be conducted more often than annually. Choices **b**, uterine cancer; **c**, cervical cancer; **d**, ovarian cancer; and **e**, bladder cancer, are incorrect because there is no evidence that women who were previously treated for breast cancer are at greater risk of developing any of these cancers.

Task Area: Applying Basic Science Concepts
Organ System: Reproductive

280. d. The correct answer is choice **d**, spinal stenosis. Individuals who experience pain associated with the disorder of spinal stenosis may be able to obtain relief following a lumbar epidural injection with corticosteroids. Approximately 25% of patients with spinal stenosis who undergo lumbar epidural corticosteroid injections experience sustained relief of their symptoms. Spinal bony metastases (choice **a**) are most commonly treated with radiation therapy. Choice **b**, scoliosis, is commonly treated with brace treatment or surgical correction. Choice **c**, kyphosis, is commonly treated with exercises, brace treatment, and/or surgical correction. Choice **e**, ankylosing spondylitis, can be treated with NSAIDs, exercises, and hot/cold therapies. For advanced cases, surgical correction may be warranted.

Task Area: Clinical Intervention
Organ System: Musculoskeletal

281. b. Graves' disease (choice **b**) is an autoimmune disorder in which the thyroid is overactive and produces an excessive amount of thyroid hormones. Individuals with this disorder can present with weight loss, insomnia, exophthalmos, and a visible goiter. Choice **a**, Addison's disease, should be ruled out because of the presence of exophthalmos and visible goiter and the absence of skin darkening and salt cravings. Choice **c**, Wilson's disease, should be ruled out because of the lack of neurologic symptoms and alterations in personality. Choice **d**, pheochromocytoma, should be ruled out because of the presence of exophthalmos and visible goiter and the lack of hypertension and excessive sweating. Choice **e**, Wilms' tumor, should be ruled out because of the presence of exophthalmos and visible goiter and the lack of abdominal swelling, fever, and blood in the urine.

Task Area: Formulating Most Likely Diagnosis
Organ System: Endocrine

282. e. This patient's symptoms fit with a classic presentation of parkinsonism, which often features a resting tremor, rigidity, bradykinesia/akinesia, and postural instability in advanced cases. Parkinsonism is usually caused by inadequate action of dopamine, which may be caused by inadequate production or by insensitivity of peripheral receptors. However, before making a diagnosis of Parkinson's disease (a condition in which parkinsonism is caused by inadequate production of dopamine by the substantia nigra), it is important to consider the possibility of parkinsonism secondary to iatrogenic causes. Haloperidol (choice **e**) is a dopamine receptor antagonist, and while this is effective for treatment of schizophrenia, it can often cause secondary parkinsonism as a side effect of its primary mechanism of action. Parkinson's disease (choice **a**) is a possibility, but it is especially unlikely in a patient with schizophrenia, which is caused by excessive dopamine production. Schizophrenia (choice **b**) is also exceedingly unlikely to cause these sorts of symptoms. Hyperthyroidism (choice **c**) may cause a resting tremor, but is also likely to cause tachycardia and overactivity rather than bradykinesia. Alcohol withdrawal (choice **d**) may cause seizures, but it is unlikely to produce this constellation of signs and symptoms.

Task Area: Pharmaceutical Therapeutics
Organ System: Psychiatry/Behavioral Science

283. e. Urinary tract infection is a fairly common presentation in general practice and emergency medicine, but it is important to recognize other causes of dysuria. This patient, for instance, most likely has pyelonephritis (choice **e**), as evidenced by her flank pain (or CVA tenderness with light percussion) and tenderness. Her recent history of dysuria was probably caused by a lower urinary tract infection (choice **b**), but the severity of these symptoms is generally mild to moderate; the acute presentation to the emergency department is most likely caused by pyelonephritis. Cystitis (choice **a**), by contrast, usually presents with lower pelvic pressure in the region of the bladder. Nephrolithiasis (choice **c**) and urolithiasis (choice **d**) may present with this pattern of symptoms, but the fever is unlikely, and the pain is more likely to be colicky.

Task Area: Formulating Most Likely Diagnosis
Organ System: Genitourinary

284. b. Preeclampsia (choice **b**) is diagnosed with the classic triad of hypertension, edema, and proteinuria. Patients may present with edema in the face and hands, sudden weight gain, headache, visual disturbances, nausea, vomiting, right upper quadrant pain, and decreased urine output. Physical examination will reveal hypertension, proteinuria, and hyperreflexia. Choice **a**, eclampsia, is incorrect as this is a life-threatening condition associated with seizures and even coma in pregnant females with untreated preeclampsia. Choice **c**, chronic hypertension, is a condition that involves uncontrolled high blood pressure during pregnancy and is often a precursor to preeclampsia. Choice **d**, premature labor, is incorrect as this condition is associated with discharge from the vagina, leaking from the vagina, and vaginal bleeding. Choice **e**, leiomyomata, is incorrect as this is characterized by benign masses (fibroids) within the uterus.

Task Area: History Taking and Performing Physical Examinations
Organ System: Reproductive

285. a. Passive-aggressive disorder (choice **a**) is characterized by procrastination, irritability, stubbornness, negative attitude, and passive resistance toward demands for adequate performance. Individuals with this disorder are often sullen, argumentative, and envious or resentful of people who seem to be more fortunate. Choice **b**, depressive disorder, is incorrect as this disorder is characterized by low mood, low self-esteem, and loss of interest. Choice **c**, sadomasochistic disorder, is incorrect as this condition is associated with pain being inflicted on others and on yourself and often occurs during sexual activity. Choice **d**, sadistic disorder, is incorrect as this disorder is associated with afflicting pain on another person, usually during a sexual encounter. Choice **e**, narcissistic personality disorder, is incorrect as this condition is characterized by increased self-importance, need for admiration, and self-absorption.

Task Area: Applying Basic Science Concepts
Organ System: Psychiatry/Behavioral Science

286. b. The correct answer is choice **b**, ceftriaxone. Ceftriaxone is recommended for epididymitis that occurs as a result of sexually transmitted diseases such as gonorrhea and chlamydia. The Centers for Disease Control states that ceftriaxone administered in conjunction with doxycycline twice a day for ten days is an effective regimen for epididymitis that occurs as a result of sexually transmitted diseases. Choice **a**, ACE inhibitors, is incorrect as this class of medications will have no therapeutic effects for epididymitis. Choice **c**, tolterodine, is incorrect as this medication is used to treat urinary incontinence. Choice **d**, ciproflaxin, might be a consideration; however, this medication is more useful if the epididymitis is caused by a bacterium and not by a sexually transmitted disease. There are a number of STDs caused by bacteria, such as *N. gonorrhea*, *C. trachomatis*, *T. pallidum*, etc. Choice **e**, warfarin, is incorrect as this medication is an anticoagulant and will have no therapeutic benefit for this condition.

Task Area: Pharmaceutical Therapeutics
Organ System: Genitourinary

287. c. The best treatment for alcohol-induced cardiomyopathy is total and permanent alcohol abstinence (choice **c**). Aerobic exercise (choice **a**) and smoking cessation (choice **d**) may also be beneficial, but these modifications are not as important as ceasing all alcohol consumption. There is no evidence regarding the benefits of meditation (choice **b**) or positive thinking (choice **e**) on alcohol-induced cardiomyopathy.

Task Area: Health Maintenance
Organ System: Cardiovascular

288. b. A furuncle (choice **b**) is defined as an infection of a single hair follicle, which is most commonly referred to as a boil. The lesions commonly present as red, hard, tender lesions in the hair-bearing regions of the head, neck, and body. Choice **a**, pimple, is incorrect as this condition is a result of excessive oil getting trapped in and clogging the pores of the skin. Choice **c**, carbuncle, is incorrect as this is an infection of more than one hair follicle as a conglomerate mass. Choice **d**, abscess, is incorrect as this is a collection of pus that has accumulated in a particular area. Choice **e**, eczema, is incorrect as this is a condition characterized by redness, swelling, crusting, and flaking of the skin.

Task Area: Applying Basic Science Concepts
Organ System: Dermatologic

289. a. The correct answer is choice **a**, Crohn's disease, because of the small bowel involvement with confirmation of microscopic cryptitis on colonoscopy biopsy. Choice **b**, colon carcinoma, is incorrect because the biopsy does not mention presence of malignant cells. Choice **c**, ulcerative colitis (UC), is incorrect because UC typically only involves the colon and not the small intestine. Choice **d**, diverticulitis, is incorrect because there is no mention of inflammation of a diverticulum, which is typically in the large intestine. Choice **e**, *C. difficile* colitis, is incorrect because the stool test is negative for infectious etiology.

Task Area: Formulating Most Likely Diagnosis
Organ System: Gastrointestinal/Nutritional

290. d. Chest pain is a very common and nonspecific presenting symptom; it is important to know how to differentiate between different causes. While acute-onset chest pain and ST elevation are highly suggestive of a myocardial infarction, this presentation may also be associated with pericarditis. This is particularly likely if the pain is relieved by leaning forward (choice **d**) or if auscultation reveals a friction rub; these signs are fairly specific for pericarditis. Chest pain associated with dyspnea (choice **a**) or exacerbated by activity (choice **e**) is more suggestive of a myocardial infarction, a pulmonary embolism, or a variety of other conditions. Systolic and diastolic murmurs (choices **b** and **c**) may suggest one of various types of valvular defects.
Task area: History Taking and Performing Physical Examinations
Organ System: Cardiovascular

291. d. Sarcoidosis can present with a range of nonspecific symptoms and is generally a diagnosis of exclusion. The most common symptoms include lethargy, dry cough, and dyspnea, which often suggest tuberculosis; however, it can also feature myalgia, arthralgia, rashes, and various other systemic inflammatory symptoms. It is particularly common in young adult females. Bilateral hilar lymphadenopathy (choice **d**), however, is one of the few signs that is relatively specific for sarcoidosis. Calcification in the lung fields (choice **a**) can suggest a few diagnoses, the most common of which are tuberculosis and lung cancer. Cardiomegaly (choice **b**) is a common sign of congestive heart failure, but it is not common in sarcoidosis. Increased vascular markings (choice **c**) may suggest vascular congestion or vasculitis. Basal consolidation (choice **e**) is common in pneumonia.
Task Area: Using Laboratory and Diagnostic Studies
Organ System: Pulmonary

292. c. This patient most likely has Meckel's diverticulum, a common congenital bowel abnormality that is caused by incomplete closure of the vitelline duct, which connects the fetal midgut to the yolk sac. In patients with Meckel's diverticulum, the distal ileum has an outpouching that contains some gastric or pancreatic tissue. While the condition is present from birth, it usually goes unnoticed until it causes an intussusception (choice **c**), leading to a bowel obstruction that often manifests as fecal bleeding and a palpable mass. Occasional vomiting is also present, and this tends to relieve the patient's symptoms. Diverticulitis (choice **a**) is another possible complication of any sort of diverticulum, but it usually presents with a fever and is not as likely as an intussusception in Meckel's diverticulum. Appendicitis (choice **b**) also seems like an attractive choice because of the patient's age and the presence of a right-sided mass, but the detection of Meckel's diverticulum on the nuclear scan make intussusception more likely. Upper GI bleeds (choice **d**) usually present with dark (occasionally black) blood in the stools. Colitis (choice **e**) is not typically associated with radiologic appearance of pathology in the small intestine.

Task Area: Formulating Most Likely Diagnosis
Organ System: Gastrointestinal/Nutritional

293. a. Nasal polyps are a very common cause of anosmia and nasal congestion that generally manifest as translucent masses on intranasal examination. They may be managed with topical or oral corticosteroid therapy, but in some cases surgical excision is the most appropriate therapeutic option. However, surgical excision of the polyps is associated with a 70% recurrence rate (choice **a**). Infection (choice **b**) and bleeding (choice **d**) are possible risks of any surgical procedure, but they are far less likely than recurrence. In rare cases, nasal polyps may be associated with malignancy (choice **c**) or metastasis (choice **e**), but again, this is far less likely than local recurrence.

Task Area: Health Maintenance
Organ System: EENT (Eye, Ear, Nose, and Throat)

294. c. This patient has post-myocardial infarction pericarditis. This pain is usually described as a pleuritic pain that is relieved by leaning forward (choice **c**). A dull central pain radiating to the arm and jaw (choice **a**) is typical for a myocardial infarction. A persistent tearing pain radiating to the back (choice **b**) is seen in an aortic tear. A chest pain associated with dyspnea (choice **d**) is very nonspecific. A pain that spans across a specific dermatome (choice **e**) is present in shingles.

Task Area: History Taking and Performing Physical Examinations
Organ System: Cardiovascular

295. a. Percutaneous vertebroplasty was first described in 1987 and has since become a widely used intervention for patients with severe back pain from osteoporotic or neoplastic compression fractures. It involves the injection of polymethylmetharylate (PMMA), a synthetic cement, directly into the vertebral body. While the use of a hard compound may suggest a structural benefit, the only proven benefit of vertebroplasty is pain relief (choice **a**); in fact, it is contraindicated in patients with asymptomatic compression fractures. The use of vertebroplasty has grown in recent years, but it is somewhat controversial because of its inability to provide any long-term solutions. It is associated with no proven benefit for repair (choice **b**) or prevention (choice **c**) of compression fractures. Joint mobility (choice **d**) is also unlikely to be affected. Referred pain (choice **e**) may actually increase after the procedure.

Task Area: Clinical Intervention
Organ System: Musculoskeletal

296. b. Endophthalmitis, an infection of the inner eye cavities, is one of the most critical diagnoses in ophthalmology. Most cases occur as a complication of ophthalmic surgery, but it is also often caused by sepsis or a penetrating injury. It causes a significant reduction in visual acuity, and, without early treatment, it can cause permanent visual loss. The most specific physical examination finding is a hypopyon, or a purulent collection in the anterior chamber; however, a hypopyon is also seen in autoimmune conditions such as uveitis. The diagnosis can only be confirmed via culture of a vitreal biopsy (choice **b**). This is a fairly invasive and distressing procedure, but it can be performed by an ophthalmologist with only local anesthetic. Retinal photography (choice **a**) is used to monitor the progression of diabetic eye disease. Aqueous humor biopsy (choice **c**) may be beneficial for some forms of uveitis, but it would not be beneficial in this case. Intraocular pressure (choice **d**) is measured in order to determine the risk of further optic neuropathy in patients with glaucoma and to determine the risk of developing glaucoma for the general population. Ophthalmoscopic examination (choice **e**) may provide more information about disease of the macula (such as age-related macular degeneration), the retina (such as diabetic retinopathy), and the optic nerve (such as glaucoma), but has little value for this patient.

Task Area: Using Laboratory and Diagnostic Studies
Organ System: EENT (Eye, Ear, Nose, and Throat)

297. **c.** Corticosteroids (choice **c**) are effective at controlling inflammation associated with sarcoidosis as well as controlling granuloma formation, which may also occur with this disorder. Choice **a**, diuretics, may be used if sarcoidosis precipitates elevated calcium levels in the urine, but it is not indicated for overall treatment of sarcoidosis. Choice **b**, antibiotics, is incorrect. Some studies show that antibiotics can induce remission for sarcoidosis; however, the gold standard treatment for this disorder is corticosteroids. Choice **d**, anti-inflammatories, should be considered in mild cases of sarcoidosis. However, the possibility of gastrointestinal and cardiovascular side effect lessens the effectiveness of anti-inflammatory medications in treating sarcoidosis. Bronchodilators (choice **e**) are used to enhance breathing efforts for patients with obstructive pulmonary sarcoidosis. However, bronchodilators are not indicated for long-term treatment of sarcoidosis.
Task Area: Pharmaceutical Therapeutics
Organ System: Pulmonary

298. **b.** Rheumatoid arthritis (choice **b**) is commonly characterized by morning stiffness lasting for more than one hour, arthritis, and soft tissue swelling in three or more joints and arthritis in the hand joints all lasting for longer than six weeks. Blood work will reveal elevated erythrocyte sedimentation rate and C-reactive protein. In addition, blood work will be positive for rheumatoid factor and anti-CCP antibodies. Choice **a**, septic arthritis, is caused by bacterial infections in other parts of the body that spreads to the joints. In addition, septic arthritis is associated with joint redness and low-grade fever, which are not exhibited in this patient. Choice **c**, psoriatic arthritis, should be excluded because this disorder is associated with psoriasis (red patches on the skin), which is not presented by this patient. Choice **d**, reactive arthritis, should be excluded because this form of arthritis is usually associated with urinary symptoms and conjunctivitis. Choice **e**, scleroderma, should be excluded immediately because this condition is characterized by symmetric thickening of the skin.
Task Area: Formulating Most Likely Diagnosis
Organ System: Musculoskeletal

299. a. Ceftriaxone (choice **a**) is recommended for epididymitis that occurs as a result of sexually transmitted diseases such as gonorrhea and chlamydia. The Centers for Disease Control and Prevention (CDC) states that ceftriaxone administered in conjunction with doxycycline twice a day for ten days is an effective regimen for epididymitis that occurs as a result of sexually transmitted diseases. Choice **b**, ACE inhibitors, is incorrect as these medications are taken to establish protection of the heart muscle, particularly in patients with congestive heart failure. Choice **c**, tolterodine, is incorrect as it is used as treatment for urinary incontinence. Choice **d**, ciprofloxacin, is incorrect as this medication is a powerful antibiotic similar to doxycycline and is used as a substitute for doxycycline, not in conjunction with it. Choice **e**, diuretics, is incorrect as they are used to rid the body of unwanted fluids and have no antibiotic effect.

Task Area: Pharmaceutical Therapeutics
Organ System: Genitourinary

300. c. A hypertensive urgency (choice **c**) refers to a situation in which the systolic blood pressure is greater than 220 mm/Hg and diastolic blood pressure is greater than 125 mmHg. A hypertensive urgency must be treated within hours to avoid further health consequences. Choice **a**, primary hypertension, is incorrect as this condition is associated with serial readings of systolic greater than 140 and diastolic greater than 90. Choice **b**, malignant hypertension, is incorrect as this condition is generally characterized by a sudden, rapid increase in blood pressure. Choice **d**, hypertensive emergency, might be a consideration; however, hypertensive emergency is defined as diastolic in excess of 130 mmHg and the lack of signs of organ damage such as chest pain, arrhythmias, paresthesias, and altered mental status, which should exclude an emergency. Choice **e**, pheochromocytoma, might also be a consideration, but lack of symptoms such as chest pain, weight loss, sweating, rapid heart rate, and palpitations should rule this out.

Task Area: Applying Basic Science Concepts
Organ System: Cardiovascular

ADDITIONAL ONLINE PRACTICE

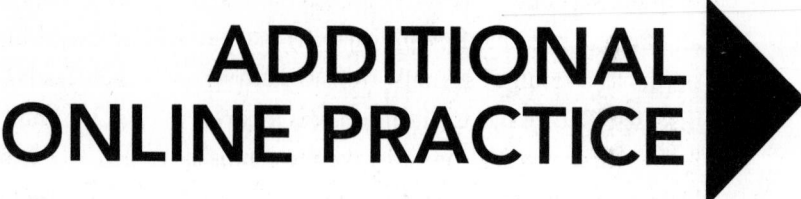

Whether you need help building basic skills or preparing for an exam, visit the LearningExpress Practice Center! On this site, you can access additional practice materials. Using the code below, you'll be able to log in and take an additional one-time use, full-length PANCE practice test. This online practice will also provide you with:

Immediate scoring
Detailed answer explanations
A customized diagnostic report that will assess your skills and focus your study

Log in to the LearningExpress Practice Center by using the URL: **www.learnatest.com/practice**

This is your Access Code: **8974**

Follow the steps online to redeem your access code. After you've used your access code to register with the site, you will be prompted to create a username and password. For easy reference, record them here:

Username: _____   Password: _____

If you have any questions or problems, please contact LearningExpress customer service at 1-800-295-9556 ext. 2, or e-mail us at **customerservice@learningexpressllc.com**